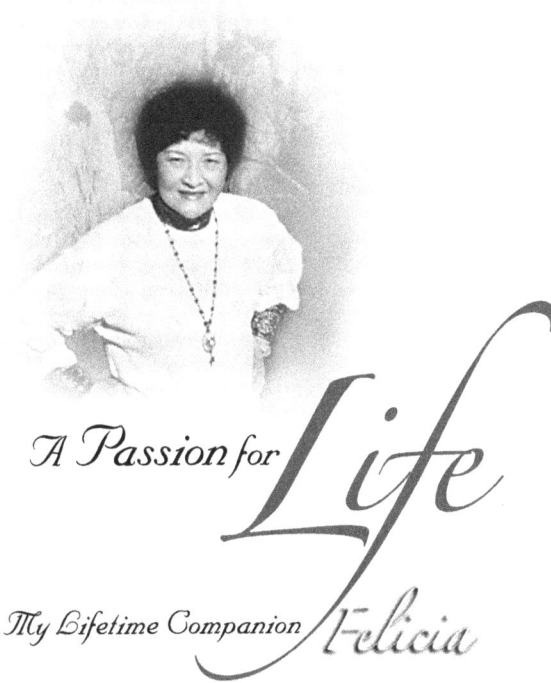

A Passion for Life

My Lifetime Companion Felicia

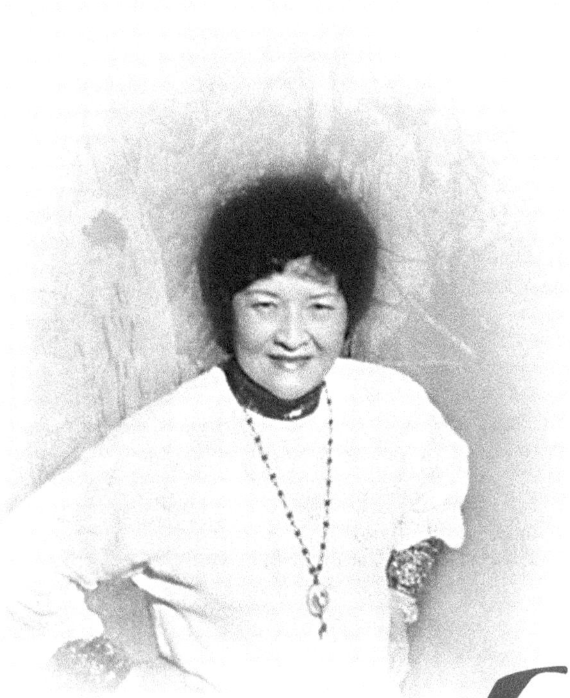

A Passion for Life

My Lifetime Companion Felicia

Cheng-Wen Wu
Founding President, National Health Research Institutes, Taiwan
Chwan-Wen Liu

translated by Cheng-Wen Wu, Annie Chen

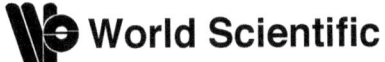

World Scientific
NEW JERSEY • LONDON • SINGAPORE • BEIJING • SHANGHAI • HONG KONG • TAIPEI • CHENNAI

Published by

World Scientific Publishing Co. Pte. Ltd.
5 Toh Tuck Link, Singapore 596224
USA office: 27 Warren Street, Suite 401-402, Hackensack, NJ 07601
UK office: 57 Shelton Street, Covent Garden, London WC2H 9HE

British Library Cataloguing-in-Publication Data
A catalogue record for this book is available from the British Library.

A PASSION FOR LIFE
My Lifetime Companion, Felicia

Copyright © 2010 by World Scientific Publishing Co. Pte. Ltd.

All rights reserved. This book, or parts thereof, may not be reproduced in any form or by any means, electronic or mechanical, including photocopying, recording or any information storage and retrieval system now known or to be invented, without written permission from the Publisher.

For photocopying of material in this volume, please pay a copying fee through the Copyright Clearance Center, Inc., 222 Rosewood Drive, Danvers, MA 01923, USA. In this case permission to photocopy is not required from the publisher.

ISBN-13 978-981-283-839-1
ISBN-10 981-283-839-2
ISBN-13 978-981-283-840-7 (pbk)
ISBN-10 981-283-840-6 (pbk)

Typeset by Stallion Press
Email: enquiries@stallionpress.com

About the Authors

Cheng-Wen Wu, M.D., Ph.D.

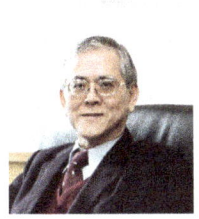

Dr Cheng-Wen Wu is an eminent Taiwanese biomedical scientist who played an instrumental role in the establishment of several important biomedical institutes in Taiwan. He is the founding president of the National Health Research Institutes in Taiwan, and also an academician and distinguished research fellow of Academia Sinica. He obtained his M.D. from the National Taiwan University in 1964, and his Ph.D. in biochemistry from Case Western Reserve University in 1969. Since then, he spent 20 years in the United States devoting himself in biomedical research and teaching in various universities including Cornell University, Yale University and the Albert Einstein College of Medicine. In 1980, he assumed the Catacosinos Chair Professor position at the Department of Pharmacological Sciences at the State University of New York (SUNY), Stony Brook. Best known for his pioneering work on the molecular mechanism of gene transcription, Dr Wu enjoys international repute for his scientific research on cancer, and he once helmed as President of the International Federation for Cell Biology between 2004 and 2008.

This is a touching biography written by Dr Cheng-Wen Wu of his beloved late wife, Dr Felicia Ying-Hsiueh Wu, as a tribute to her extraordinary life as a distinguished scientist with a notable career in cancer research, and to her long, relentless journey fighting against cancer. The words within meld into emotional revelations, strength of human spirit and an undaunted passion for life.

Dr Cheng-Wen Wu is currently the Distinguished Chair Professor at the National Yang-Ming University, Taiwan. Presently, he concentrates his effort on cancer and stem cell research, and is actively steering initiatives to advocate academic and research exchanges in the international scientific community.

Chwan-Wen Liu

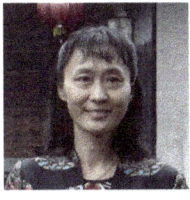

The co-author of this biography — who writes under a pseudonym, Chwan-Wen Liu — is a media practitioner with rich, diverse experience. Liu began her writing and editorial career as newspaper journalist, and subsequently chief editor for magazines. She has published 16 books and took an interest to write this book when she later joined the General Affairs Office of the National Health Research Institutes. Liu currently works with the Health Science Foundation in Taiwan, as she continues her passion in creative writing.

*Dedicated to my lifetime companion,
Felicia,
and our children, David, Faith and Albert*

Contents

ABOUT THE AUTHORS	v
PREFACE I	xiii
The Spirit of Fighting Cancer Remains Eternally Among Mankind	
PREFACE II	xix
Brave, Dedicated and Committed Women are the Most Beautiful	
PREFACE III	xxiii
An Outstanding Researcher of All Time	
PROLOGUE I	xxv
A Book of Life	
PROLOGUE II	xxxi
Touching More Lives	

INTRODUCTION		1
I DAYS OF YOUTH		**3**
Chapter 1	Precocious From the Start	5
Chapter 2	Meeting and Getting to Know Each Other	19
Chapter 3	Lifelong Mutual Commitment	31
Chapter 4	Studying Abroad	45
II LIFE ABROAD		**63**
Chapter 5	Memories of Studying Abroad	65
Chapter 6	Our Research and Life Together	81
Chapter 7	A Sabbatical Year in France	93
Chapter 8	The Long Island Days	107
III TRANSITION PERIOD		**121**
Chapter 9	Discovering Breast Cancer	123
Chapter 10	Imparting Our Knowledge as Our Contribution to Taiwan	137
Chapter 11	Life after Returning to Taiwan	151
Chapter 12	Cancer Recurs	165
IV FIGHTING CANCER		**181**
Chapter 13	Beginning a Long-Term Resistance	183
Chapter 14	Offering Oneself as a Lab Specimen	195
Chapter 15	High Dose Chemotherapy	207
Chapter 16	Autologous Bone Marrow Transplantation	221
Chapter 17	Reborn in Fire, Arisen from the Ashes	235

| V | FIGHTING TO THE END | 247 |

Chapter 18 Cancer Strikes Once Again   249
Chapter 19 Trying Medicine after Medicine   263
Chapter 20 The Last Stage   277
Chapter 21 Death Summons   291

EPILOGUE   315

TIMELINE OF THE MAIN EVENTS IN FELICIA'S LIFE   327

Preface I

The Spirit of Fighting Cancer Remains Eternally Among Mankind
Shu Chien

Felicia and Ken first met at a service counter of the college entrance examination center at Taipei First Girls' High School on July 28, 1957. The simple act of borrowing a water jug was the circumstance that brought about their happy meeting, and their union in marriage to become lifelong partners, accompanying each other through the ups and downs of life for forty-two years. For more than a year, Ken has mustered together a great deal of energy and determination to write *Felicia*, describing her colorful life, their beautiful and blissful union, home and career, in prose overflowing with emotion and affection. This book "casts light on Felicia's unique and amazing life," serving as an inspiration and a source of profound meaning for those of us who survive her.

Though I knew Felicia for twenty years, it was only after reading the first few chapters of this book that I understood the origin of Felicia's serious, tenacious, perfectionist, courageous, determined and warm-hearted personality. Because of her natural talent, upbringing and diligence, Felicia excelled in all things since she was a child. Her diligence enabled her to make it to the "Hall of Fame" throughout her six years at Taipei First Girls' High School. As valedictorian, she was granted admission to National Taiwan University (NTU) without having to take the examination; this sowed the seeds for the lifelong love between Felicia and Ken. Ken was valedictorian of the NTNU Affiliated High School and was also guaranteed admission into National Taiwan University. Because the two of them were exempted from the examination, they had the opportunity to provide support services for other students on the examination day, which brought about their chance meeting. Given that Ken had already heard of Felicia's stellar achievements and seen her picture on the "Hall of Fame," it certainly seemed as if their meeting was destined by fate. After they met, they discovered that they had participated in the Taipei City Model Students' Ceremony in the same year and were pictured in the same photograph when they were in junior high school. That was purely a coincidence, but it could also be said that it was the natural outcome of their superior academic performance.

Ken's flowing prose and emotional sincerity fully expressed the love between him and Felicia. What they achieved together in family life and career is the fruit of their own efforts. After Felicia discovered that she had breast cancer, they both fought the battle together for thirteen years. Their "lifelong interdependence and mutual support" is profoundly moving. After opening the book, I could not put it down. I read it in one breath, felt a multitude of different emotions, and received invaluable inspiration.

Kuang-Cheng and I first met Felicia and Ken at the NTU Medical School reunion at North Sea Fishing Village Restaurant in Queens, New York. They were then faculty members in SUNY Stony Brook's pharmacology department. We just happened to be at the same table and had the opportunity to chat. From the outset, Felicia's spirit, optimism, proactive attitude, warmth and goodwill towards friends, as well as her serious and conscientious attitude towards her work impressed us.

Our chat was quite enjoyable, so we got together again several times. Every time we visited their Long Island home, Felicia always received us with immense kindness and warmth. She was an excellent cook, steadfast and methodical, from that we could imagine how well-organized she was in the laboratory. Her house was dignified and immaculate. Her children,

David, Faith, and Albert were all extremely cute; seeing them filled us with warmth of their household. Felicia and Ken took us for a walk around the neighborhood; we saw the duck pond which was one of Albert's favorite places, and we even walked as far as the Atlantic coast. Today, those happy times still seem as if they had just occurred yesterday.

Since 1984, Ken and I served together on the advisory committee for the Institute of Biomedical Sciences committee at Academia Sinica, so we met on many occasions to do preparatory work for the establishment of the institute. In 1986, Professor Nan-Geng Yu conducted the "Symposium of Recent Advances in Biomedical Sciences" at the Institute of Biomedical Sciences. Felicia was asked to give a lecture; that was the first time I heard her speak. Her research was insightful, in-depth, and at the leading edge of biomedical sciences; her lecture was clear and organized, starting with an introductory opener and then going into the specifics, and elicited the interest of both laymen and medical professionals. Everyone who heard her came away feeling as if they had learned a great deal.

The year 1987 was the thirtieth anniversary of our wedding; our two daughters held a celebration for us in New Jersey. At that time, Felicia had already discovered that she suffered from breast cancer and the chemotherapy that she subsequently underwent had weakened her, but she insisted on attending. Ken and Felicia drove for two hours from Long Island to New Jersey. Since Ken was worried that she would be too tired, they first drove to a motel in New Jersey and spent the night, then attended our dinner the following night. When we saw Felicia, we were certainly excited and touched by the effort she made to attend our celebration. My wife and I danced a tango at the dinner, and Felicia, playful as ever, took a rose and placed it in my mouth. Thinking of it now still brings a smile to our faces. Ken and Felicia gave us a photo frame, photo album, and jewelry box engraved with our names. Even to this day, we still use them, and Felicia is still in our mind.

In 1988, Ken succeeded me as the director of the Institute of Biomedical Sciences, and I returned to the United States, relocating from New York to San Diego, California. Those years when I returned to Taipei, I often visited the Institute of Biomedical Sciences, and had the opportunity to call on Ken and Felicia. During that period, Felicia's medical condition would sometimes hover between good and bad, but she still spent a majority of her time in the laboratory, tirelessly continuing her research. Whether I saw her in the laboratory or at her office, she was always light-hearted and smiling, reflecting the strength, bravery, and enthusiasm with which she committed in her work.

Ken has been in charge of the Institute of Biomedical Sciences and the National Health Research Institutes, the two most important institutions for Taiwanese medical and public health research, for over ten years. They have achieved impressive results, and their success is due in no small part to Felicia's dedication on all fronts. Ken also made the utmost effort in taking care of Felicia's health. Of course, Felicia's success in living with cancer for thirteen years is a credit to her own determination and iron will, but Ken's love and encouragement were also extremely important. "The strength of Felicia's love and her endearing passion for her family enabled her to stand up and overcome her hardship."

In 1995, Felicia's medical condition worsened, requiring her to travel to the United States National Institutes of Health for treatment. At that time, she underwent extremely drastic chemotherapy and had over two hundred bone marrow extractions. Any normal people would not be able to endure what she went through, but Felicia finished the complete sequence of medical treatments by relying on her iron will and love of life.

During that particular treatment, the circumstances became quite dangerous, and Ken remained by Felicia's side throughout. At that time, the National Health Research Institutes' advisory committee and its research grant review committee's yearly meetings were about to convene in Taipei. Although Ken felt that he ought to return to Taipei to preside over the meetings, in the end, he decided to remain in the United States and stay with Felicia until she was completely out of danger.

Felicia loved life and her fellow people, and she was willing to share the experience of her fight against cancer with everyone. She gave many lectures on cancer, speaking from her dual perspective as a cancer researcher and patient; there would be a full house every time she spoke. Felicia's speeches enabled her listeners to understand more about cancer, inspired faith and determination in cancer patients, and created impact on the society for the better.

On July 9, 1999, Kuang-Cheng and I visited Felicia at National Taiwan University Hospital. She was then waiting for a liver transplant; although she passed away just ten days later, she was still full of life. She told us about her latest medical condition and treatment direction, and she became even happier when the topic turned to Ken and the children, demonstrating that she was not yet ready to go. She spoke with great enthusiasm, but we were worried that she might become exhausted, so we said goodbye and left half an hour later. It did not occur to us that not long thereafter, we would receive the sad news of Felicia leaving us. Throughout the forty-two years that Ken and Felicia knew each other, they were together committed to their research, they were of the same heart, and they "were inseparable in everyday life." Undoubtedly, the time they shared together surpasses that of a "diamond" sixtieth anniversary marriage.

Felicia was an exceptional woman who possessed strength beneath the softness, and was overflowing with energy. In action, she was resolute and courageous. Not only was she a natural leader, she was sharp and focused, and also adept at handling interpersonal relations. From beginning to end, she valued her life; she never backed away. Felicia had a great marriage and three capable children who are high achievers and have limitless potential. After receiving a Ph.D. in chemistry from the University of California at Berkeley, David went on to do postgraduate research at the University of Cambridge. He has already made significant contributions to the field of chemistry. Faith worked for the Ministry of Foreign Affairs after graduating from Cornell University; my brother Fu Chien told me that within a few months, she had become indispensable as an English writer in the Ministry. Today she has obtained a J.D. degree in law. Albert is pursuing dual degrees in medicine (M.D. and Ph.D.). He, too, has many great achievements. The fact that Ken and Felicia's children are so accomplished can only be attributed to the parents themselves who were top students too. Without a doubt, Felicia was a virtuous wife and a good mother. Besides caring for her husband and raising the children, she also had great achievements in her career; she served the society incessantly and worked for the common good of people everywhere, thus serving as a role model for modern women.

Ken has succeeded in expressing Felicia's unique and extraordinary life in this biography with earnest warmth and devotion. He said, "I felt closer to her, because her spirit lay within my heart." As her friends, we too, after reading this biography, felt closer to Felicia, and felt that her spirit had a great influence on our hearts.

Today, although Felicia has left us, her personality, her deeds, her achievements, and her influences are still stenciled in our hearts, to be preserved eternally among mankind.

The author of this essay is a member of Academia Sinica.

Preface II

Brave, Dedicated and Committed Women are the Most Beautiful
Jacqueline Peng-Wang

After knowing someone for forty-two years, thirty-seven of which as husband and wife, no matter who leaves first, the burden on the one left behind is virtually impossible to bear. Breast cancer is one of the most common cancers found in Taiwanese women, second only to cervical cancer. There are about five thousand newly diagnosed cases annually. Around a third of these succumb to their illnesses, making breast cancer number four on the cancer mortality list.

Felicia's mother died of breast cancer at the age of seventy, making her a high risk for the illness. Felicia first underwent surgery for breast cancer fifteen years ago. At the time, many of her axillary lymph nodes were positive. This hinted at the malignant nature of her particular cancer and that she was at a high risk for relapse. Thus, she received intense chemotherapy subjecting her to comparatively severe side effects. The intensity of the treatment paid off and the cancer was kept in check for eight years. During intensive chemotherapy and in the subsequent eight disease-free years,

Felicia carried the onus of running her family. She successfully integrated the supervision of her lively children, making sure they grew up healthy, happy and well. She ensured that the household matters were run smoothly, enabling her husband Ken to focus on his vocation of directing and spearheading Taiwan's medical and health research, with the eventual establishment of the National Health Research Institutes.

Though I was not directly responsible for Felicia as a medical oncologist, I was a member of her medical team. I inevitably saw her in the hospital room waiting patiently to hear the results of her latest treatment. When we told her good news, she excitedly thanked each of us in turn for giving her hope for the next treatment. When we gave her bad news, she always quickly asked what the next step would be. She always urged us to look for new treatment methods, and she was always willing to try newly released drugs. I think that was also the reason why, after surgery, when her breast cancer spread, she was able to rely on her own spirit and determination to keep going, cool and composed, for five painful, yet happy and satisfying years.

Seeing her get up after falling down caused us, the medical caregivers, to feel for her time after time. Originally, this book was to be written by Felicia. She wanted to tell every patient she met about her long thirteen years of experience fighting cancer. She wanted to prepare them to face their treatment without fear. Even she herself did not realize that her time was ticking away and that writing her own book was already an impossible task.

I met Ken and Felicia in 1995. Ken and I were elected to become members of Academia Sinica at the same time. After that, we worked together to help establish the Institute of Biomedical Sciences. Felicia's pretty eyes and beautiful voice prompted all who saw her to take a second glance. She was an extremely rare individual who excelled in everything.

Her talent was apparent from early childhood. She not only possessed great intellect, she also had perfect attendance throughout her six years of secondary school and graduated first from the high school. She earned admission to National Taiwan University without having to take the entrance examination.

Felicia also played the piano brilliantly and had held many solo concerts. In athletics, she was not to be beaten either. She once won first place in the China Youth Corps' All-Taiwan High School Bicycle Race. She was praised as an all-rounded person and keen on five Chinese virtues: morals, intellect, physique, team spirit, and aesthetics. After entering society, she married and raised a family, but she continued her research with the same amount of zeal. Vitamin K3 was originally a drug that was used as a coagulant; however, it was discovered that its effectiveness in killing cancer cells far exceeded original expectations. Felicia dedicated time to conduct research investigating the drug's anti-cancer properties and how to increase its ability to kill cancer cells. Five years earlier, the Division of Cancer Research at the National Health Research Institutes conducted the Phase I clinical trial of this drug in Taiwan. Although the drug was not as effective as anticipated, it did give the Taiwanese medical community experience in clinical trials. Felicia pursued excellence in all her roles, that of a wife, mother, and teacher. To say Felicia was a person who always sought perfection is by no means an exaggeration.

    I have often thought about what might be a suitable word to describe Felicia. In Taiwan, the term "Superwoman" is often used, but this refers only to her attitude towards her work. It does not describe her outstanding accomplishment in her family life. Were this book written by Felicia, it would have probably been focused primarily on her lifelong fight against cancer, serving only as an inspiration to cancer patients and their families. She certainly would not have written much about her own strengths. Felicia's success in simultaneously raising a happy family and building a successful career can serve as an example to women all over the country. A common saying these days that describes Felicia would be: "Brave, dedicated and committed women are the most beautiful."

The author of this essay is a member of Academia Sinica.

Preface III

An Outstanding Researcher of All Time
Min Wu

With the increased scientific exchange between researchers across the Strait, I had the good fortune of becoming acquainted with Professor Felicia Chen. Although the occasions when we met were infrequent, she still made a great impression on me. Once, when I was serving as the director of the life science division at the National Natural Sciences Foundation, I invited her to Beijing to participate in a conference. She gave a brief introduction to Academia Sinica including its organizational structure, operational budget, and research projects. She made a great impression on everyone and narrowed the distance between researchers across the Strait.

While Professor Chen was presenting her report, she was energetic and her thought process was extremely quick; it was impossible to see and discern that she was afflicted with cancer. I later read in an Academia Sinica publication that due to the recurrence and spread of cancer, Professor Chen had not only undergone numerous chemotherapy treatments, but had also traveled to the United States to receive the latest treatment involving high dose chemotherapy and autologous bone marrow transplantation.

I have worked in oncology for a long time. Although what I do is basic research, I know well the kind of pain and loss that these treatments inflict on patients. Many patients are unwilling to endure even a single treatment, so I am in awe of the determination that Professor Chen demonstrated in enduring the incessantly numerous painful treatment sessions.

In the beginning of 1999, I saw Professor Chen participate in the Cross Straits Cell Biology Conference despite being ill. Though on the surface she appeared energetic as usual, she left the conference early. I then had a bad premonition, but still felt that she could conquer the illness. As a cancer researcher, I knew that despite the advances in medical treatments, there were still limitations. Professor Chen herself was an outstanding researcher, she must have had the same understanding, but most worthy of our respect was that her love of life paralleled her love of science. The ten over odd years that she fought against cancer were by no means easy.

Her enthusiasm for life and her esteemed image will not fade from my memory, and will be an encouragement for me to continue to work on the fight against cancer. In the future, I hope the day will come when cancer will no longer be able to plague a life as precious as this one; if there is such a time, then Professor Chen's efforts in the fight against cancer will not be in vain.

The author is an academician at the Chinese Academy of Medical Sciences.

Prologue I

A Book of Life

I hung up the phone, concluding a conversation with my children. They had just reproached me for not letting them know sooner when I fell ill and was hospitalized. This time I became ill suddenly without a warning. I had diarrhea five or six times in the night. When I woke up in the morning, I still had a slight fever, but I went to work as usual because there was an extremely important meeting that day. It didn't occur to me that by noon, I would be vomiting and experiencing diarrhea, a steep drop in blood pressure, and a high fever. I was immediately hospitalized with acute gastroenteritis as a result of infection.

While hospitalized I spiked a high fever, and though I was continually given nutrients intravenously through an IV drip, the extent of my water loss was so severe, I was unable to urinate for a whole day. The doctors were extremely worried and insisted that I stay in the hospital for at least four days, since a medical condition of such severity could potentially be life-threatening if not treated properly.

This was the first time since Felicia's passing that I had felt so close to illness. It served as yet another reminder of the fragility of human life. As a doctor, I knew that if I had been careless in the last couple of days, I could have lost my life. Those few days when I was hospitalized, with the IV drip inserted into my arm, the inside of my mouth burning and yet unable to drink a single drop, I felt that I understood even more completely what Felicia must have felt on the hospital bed. The physical discomfort I experienced those few days was nothing compared to the pain of Felicia's long, protracted battle against cancer; my little distress paled into insignificance by comparison to Felicia's suffering. But even so, from my hospital bed, I had the disheartening realization that if even ordinary people are unable to hold their fate in their own hands, how a cancer patient like Felicia could do it then?

After leaving the hospital, I was sternly admonished by my children, who had managed to hear news of my sickness despite being an ocean away. That day happened to be the deadline for me to submit the draft of Felicia's biography. It had already been two years since Felicia passed away; the publication date of the book coincided with the night before the second anniversary of Felicia's passing. Time had flown by quickly. I wanted to say to Felicia that she was my greatest source of strength for those last two years. Continuing her research and writing her biography gave me the strength I needed to pick myself up and start over during a time of loss and desolation. I felt I had to cherish the remaining years of my life even more so that I could carry on her legacy. In the midst of my recollections, I realized that life was short, ephemeral but if one were able to produce something of value, the significance could be eternal.

Felicia was a scientist who researched on anti-cancer drugs, and she herself had the misfortune of suffering from cancer. During her thirteen-year struggle against cancer, Felicia endured the pain of fifty-three chemotherapy treatments, including the strongest high dose chemotherapy accompanied by autologous bone marrow transplantation. As a patient, she never shirked from the most difficult treatments, instead, she worked even more diligently and energetically in the laboratory in the spirit of a true scientist. She performed her dual roles as scientist and patient with great compassion, and wrote her chapters of life with eternal spirit — that of determination, love, and gratitude. This is Felicia's language; it is also her legacy which I wish to portray in writing this biography.

Felicia departed from this world at the age of sixty. Her time on Earth was so short, I have difficulty accepting her passing, especially since she always seemed to have a stronger physical constitution than me. This was also the reason why we were so shocked and saddened when we found out that she was afflicted with cancer.

But we had to face the challenge of the disease. Furthermore, in our hearts we knew that Felicia would have to live with cancer for the rest of her life. As a scientist who researched on anti-cancer drugs, how could she not know? Oh yes, she knew a great deal about the anguish of living with cancer, but she loved her family and her research, and was not willing to give in easily to the vicious disease. Felicia mustered unfathomable determination and strength of mind to meet the attack of cancer. Though deep down in her heart, Felicia knew this battle could never be won, she kept on fighting until the last day. What a brave life warrior! She was the most exceptional individual I have ever met.

In the last two years of her thirteen-year fight against cancer, Felicia went public about her dual identity as scientist and patient, and attempted to disseminate correct information about the fight against cancer. Aside from the media attention she received, there were also publishers who wanted to publish her biography. I thought it was a great idea, and continually mentioned to her that she should organize her materials as soon as possible to enable a publisher to draft a plan. Although Felicia always said that she would, she never actually worked on it.

I knew what she was thinking; Felicia always thought that she had not yet won the war. If she were to write an autobiography, she would prefer to wait until she had conquered the cancer; she thought only then would the autobiography be meaningful. Sadly, however, she was unable to live until that day.

So after Felicia passed away, what I wanted to do for her most was to finish this biography. Who has ever successfully evaded death? No one can avoid reaching life's end. The mental energy alone that Felicia put into her battle reflects her triumph over it, to say nothing of the time she committed fighting it. The vicious disease never exhausted her determination to fight. Besides battling it physically, Felicia displayed incredible determination to give meaning to her life. In that respect, cancer could never defeat her.

This is the reason why Felicia will always occupy a place in my heart and why I decided to undertake her biography. To me, this is a book of life, a passion for life which Felicia told through her own life. She never stepped back from appreciating life, because she was full of love for the world. Besides her love for our family, she loved her friends, enjoyed her research, and gave even much more of her heart to those who suffered from cancer like her. I have learned a great deal from Felicia, and her selfless love is what I admire most.

In order to write her biography, our whole family retraced the path we took to get to this point, setting foot in places all over the United States including Cleveland, New York, Long Island, Bethesda, and Ithaca. We were able to meet up with old friends and colleagues and interview them, and because Felicia gave our whole family memories of love, we were able to let go of the pain and hurt, return nostalgically to the past, and face the future with gratitude.

Taking an analogy of the family's "journey of life" as "longitude" and Felicia's life as "latitude," this book chronicles the time from her childhood up until when she passed away at the age of sixty. I have recorded in detail her unusual fight against cancer and the story of our family. From the time that Felicia and I met, to the time of our separation in the realms of *yin* and *yang*, we were together for forty-two years. Felicia was the most important part of my life. Besides raising our three children David, Faith, and Albert, we were both partners in work and partners in life. During the times when Felicia struggled against cancer, we faced the disease together, joining hands and holding on firmly until the very last moment. So when I say that this is a book of life, it is, in fact, not only about Felicia's life, but also about our lives together.

I finished writing this book on Mid-Autumn Festival in the year 2000. That night I ascended Dajianshan by myself. There were many couples appreciating the night scenery. Though I was there alone, I did not feel lonely, because in my heart, Felicia was always there with me. It was a comfort to me that I could finish this biography for Felicia and climb the Dajianshan for her. The sentiment was the same when I took Faith to make an ascent to the Koxinga Temple at Waishuangxi. Then I told Faith: when Mom was sick, she had wanted to climb it but was unable to do so; now we were doing it for her, she would surely be very happy.

Although the deadline for the book was last year's Mid-Autumn Festival, I wanted to make it even more polished and perfect, so I revised and edited it, and another year elapsed. I did not expect that the publication date would be two years after Felicia had departed. Though time inevitably passes, my feelings remain as deep as before. My only wish is that in revising and finetuning this biography, I am able to express everything that I felt for Felicia.

This time, my sudden illness caused me to realize even more acutely life's unpredictable nature — how circumstances beyond one's control occur every day. Since we are unable to prevent the unpredictables or foresee our future, it is even more important to live for the present and treasure every moment of our lives. In our attempts to comprehend the known and the unknown, we must persist with sincerity and in faith, just like the way Felicia faced her illness. Because in her heart she always preserved every single ounce of faith that she was able to survive the most difficult treatments.

Now the value of Felicia's life has already become a part of my heart. I believe that if Felicia knew that I had finished her biography, she would let out her carefree laughter and pat me on the back. Oh, yes! When I think of Felicia, how thankful I am to her. Only because of her could my life have been so enriching. She enabled me to learn the beauty of excellence and determination in life, and to realize the glory of perseverance in face of difficult challenges and the unexpected. Had it not been Felicia, how could I experience such depth of emotions?

I hope this biography can offer an inspiration and a source of strength to people who encounter difficulty, disappointment, and pain in life, and empower them to recapture their faith and calmly face the ebbs and flows of life. Furthermore, I would like to offer this book to people whose hearts are full of love, because love is the fountainhead from which sprang Felicia's strength and unflinching determination. If the words in this book can achieve this purpose, then that is enough.

Thinking of Felicia, I dedicate this book to all who treasure life.

Cheng-Wen (Ken) Wu
July 2001

Prologue II

Touching More Lives

The year was 2001, hailing the beginning of a new millennium. That year was also the launch of the first Chinese edition of the biography on Felicia. And, reverberating is the word that aptly describes the reaction of Taiwanese readers and book industry to the book. Indeed, Felicia's uplifting, scintillating life story as an acclaimed cancer researcher who was unfortunately diagnosed with cancer, and her 13 long years of relentless battling with cancer gave great inspirations to many cancer patients. The extraordinary life of Felicia, her perspective and the philosophy she lived by will best exemplify the human spirit that all of us — the general public and those who are afflicted by cancer — can learn and uphold. In 2006, a second re-print of the Chinese edition was thus published, by a different publisher then.

For 23 years, Felicia and I committed ourselves to conducting scientific research in the United States — the very land on which we established our career and built our family. Through the years and along the way, we had many friends and colleagues in the scientific community who knew about Felicia's illness, her valiant fight against the cancer, and her passion for life. On learning that the Chinese edition of Felicia's biography had been published, our friends are earnestly hoping that there would be an English edition of the book in the near future.

My friends from the international scientific community are not the only ones who would like to lay their hands on this English edition. Even my children, who were all born and educated in the United States, are prospective readers. Given their American education, reading their Mom's biography in the Chinese edition proved to be quite a challenge for them. The earnest anticipation to accomplish the English translation of the biography has thus blossomed into the deepest hope in my heart.

To manage the English translation work and the publication of the biography, at an uninterrupted pace and solely on my own, is no easy feat, what with my busy day-to-day schedule in overseeing the administrative affairs of the institution and conducting research. Fortunately, through a friend's referral, Ms Annie Chen became my first original collaborating translator for the English edition. Annie's strong command in both the English and Chinese languages is a birthright due to her Chinese heritage and her American upbringing. She had spent almost a year of "word-smithing" to craft and mold the English translation of the biography to shape. Thereafter, my three children lent their time and effort to cross-check the fact and content, and recommend amendments, whereas I took the watchdog role of supervising and approving the changes that were made, and spent another year to make several rounds of re-writing. Finally, the preliminary draft in English was completed.

Meanwhile, I was in an aggressive search for a suitable book publisher. As the biography is an English publication, it is difficult to find the right bookseller and publisher in Taiwan that has an extensive and established distribution channel worldwide. Furthermore, based on the fact that both Felicia and I are scientists, we hope to tap on the expertise and resources of a scientific publisher with strong distribution network to academic and scientific organizations to achieve a targeted readership and the desired positioning for the biography.

Eventually, by sheer good chance and help of a close friend, we found World Scientific Publishing Co Pte Ltd which assigned Ms Ho Wei Ling, from its professional team of editors, to work alongside with us. Her astute acumen for words came into play in this biography — every single word and phrase was reflected upon and refined to draw out the essence and emotions portrayed in the biography, while adhering closely to the context of the original Chinese edition. Collaborating with Wei Ling was a two-way consultative and interactive experience with a slew of e-mail exchanges, and what culminated is a fresh injection of life in the English edition of this biography, and its successful publication.

Felicia's last thirteen years of her life journey was a relentless battle against cancer. She underwent fifty-three chemotherapy sessions, including the high dose chemotherapy and autologous bone marrow transplantation (BMT), all of which were torturous experiences analogous to painful physical inflictions of turbulent floods and vicious fire. However, in her constant tug-of-war struggles with the critical disease, Felicia fought and forged on with her strong willpower and her passion for life. It was a journey that read like an epic poem interwoven with bloods and tears — if you read and reach the end of her biography, you will feel intensity of her vitality and her strong desire to live.

Modern medicine advances by leaps and bounds. Cancer treatment, however, is still an arduous and endlessly long process. It is a irrefutable fact that cancer patients have to endure painful therapy regimen, but learning to cope with the disease mentally and psychologically by adjusting one's mindset and recognizing the inherent self-value and self-worth one has is extremely important. In fact, this explains the altruistic objective — of deeper significance and impact — of publishing Felicia's biography in the English edition. By sharing Felicia's story, I hope to take a step further to encourage cancer patients and their families from all over the world to confront cancer with tenacious grit and a "never-give-up" attitude, which, besides the essential treatment, are the absolute and most powerful weapons in the battle against cancer.

This would put across the background of the launch of Felicia's biography in the English edition. Up there in Heaven, Felicia will certainly feel rejoiced to know that her biography in English edition will continue to inspire and make a difference in the lives of many cancer patients worldwide.

Cheng-Wen (Ken) Wu
August 2009

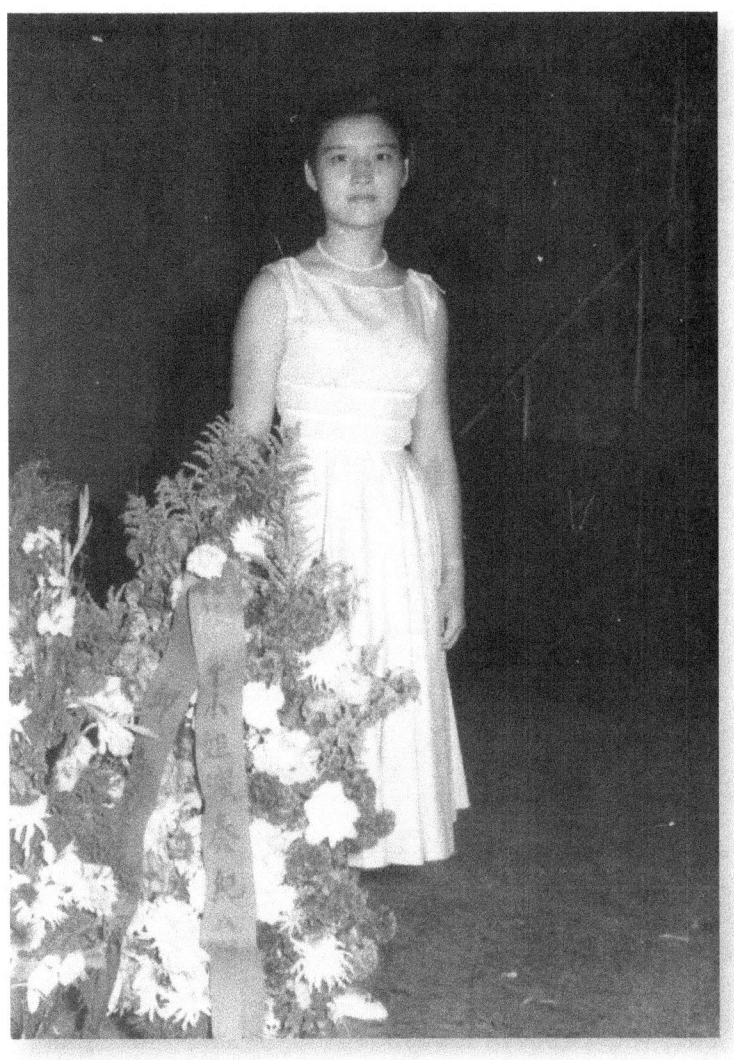

Ever the embodiment of the five tenets of excellence of education (morals, intellect, physique, team spirit, and aesthetics), Felicia performs a repertoire on the piano at her high school graduation.

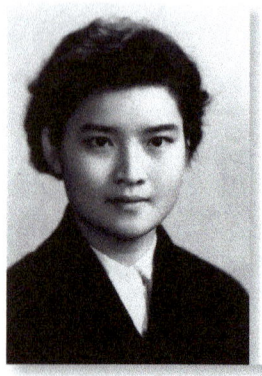 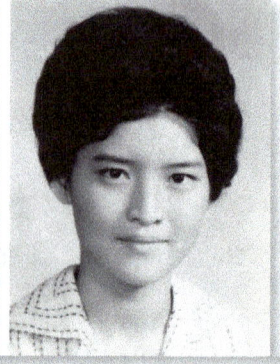 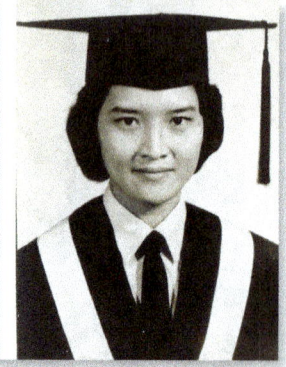

Felicia during her university years.
Left: Felicia in the second year; **center:** Felicia's first perm;
right: Felicia in university graduation gown.

Felicia takes a trip to the lake while pursuing a Master's degree at the University of Minnesota.

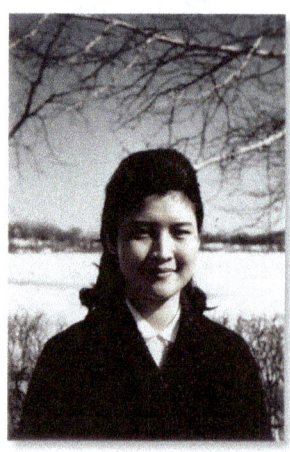

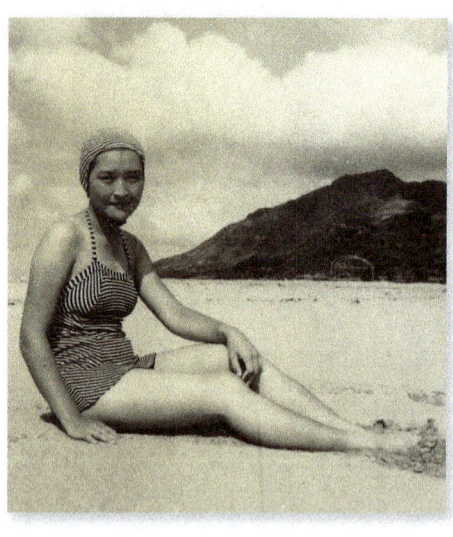

Felicia loves traveling and outdoor activities; she is also an excellent swimmer.

Felicia inside the laboratory at the University of Minnesota. She wears the laboratory coat which I gave her.

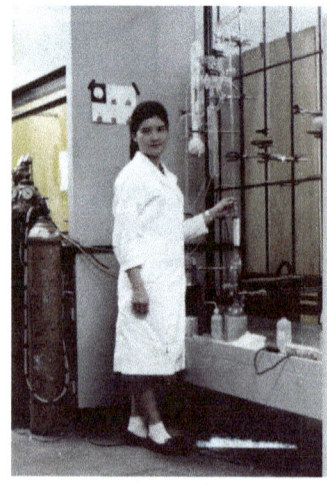

We tie the knot on
November 10, 1963.

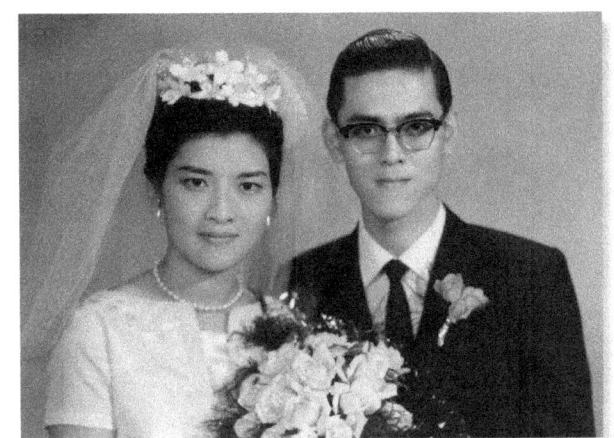

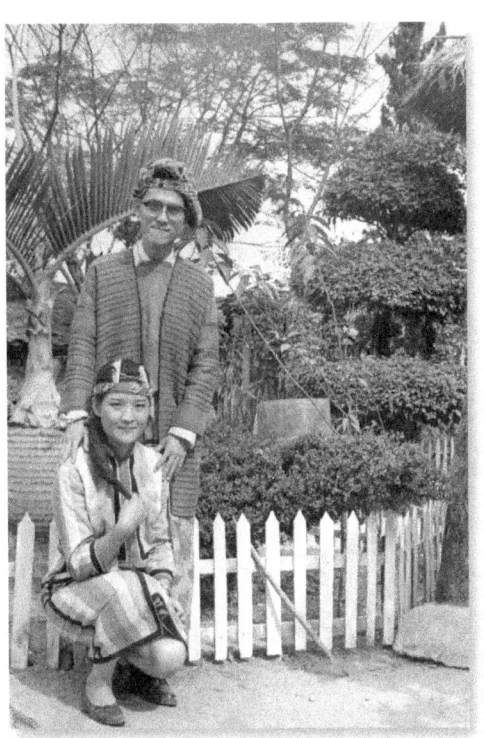

Our honeymoon
at the Sun Moon Lake.

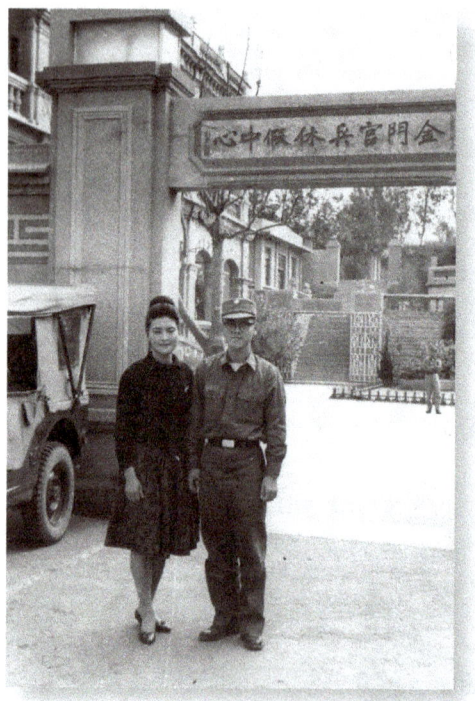

I am fulfilling my military duties at Kinmen, and Felicia comes to visit me. Twenty years later, the local residents could still remember the incidence.

Felicia and my elder sister join the Glorious Star Choir and are thus given the opportunity to visit the military base on Kinmen Island.

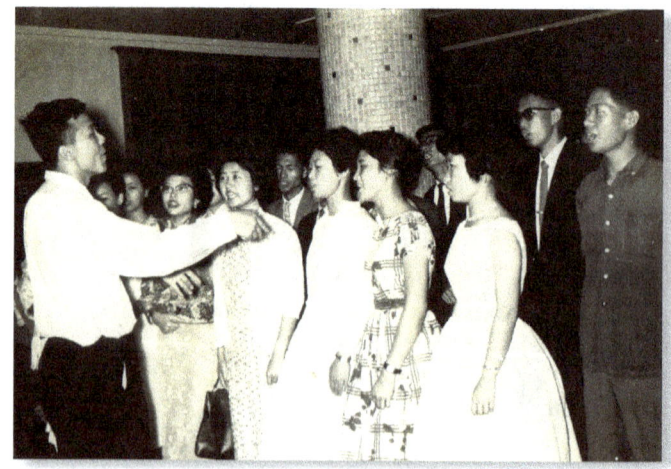

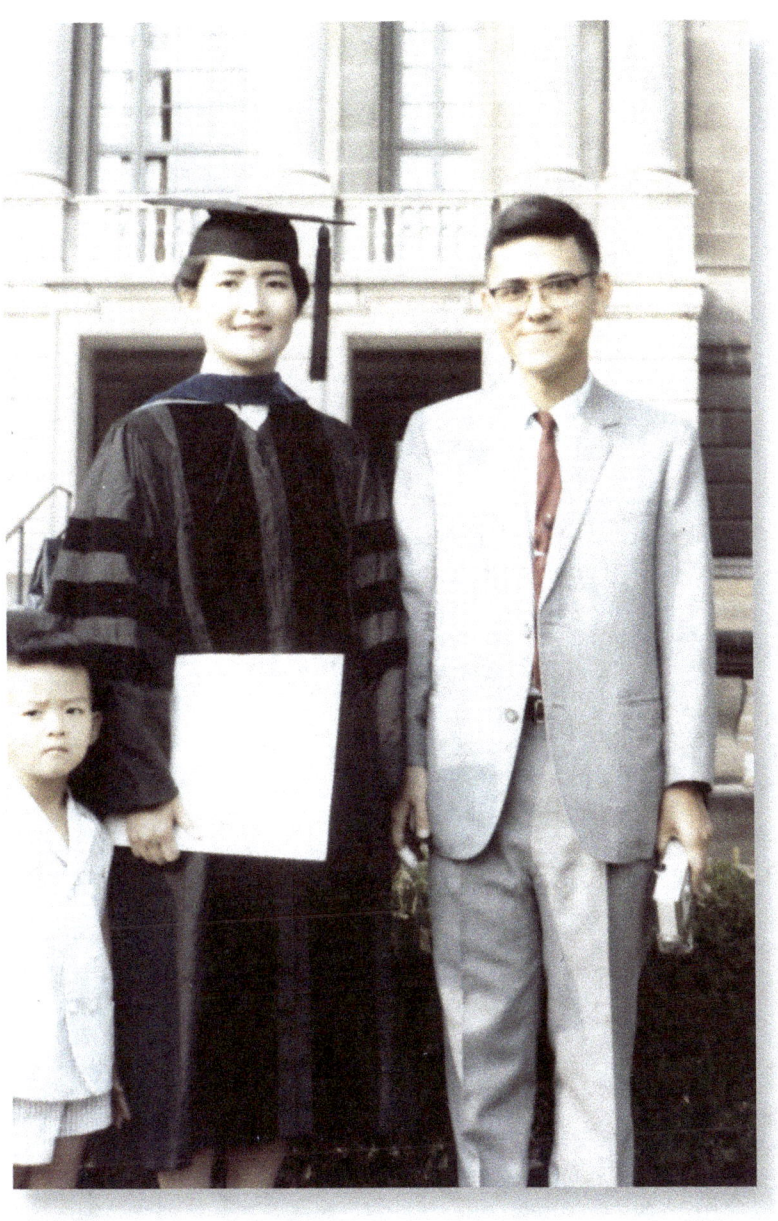

Our son David and I share Felicia's joy in this family portrait taken when she is awarded her Ph.D.

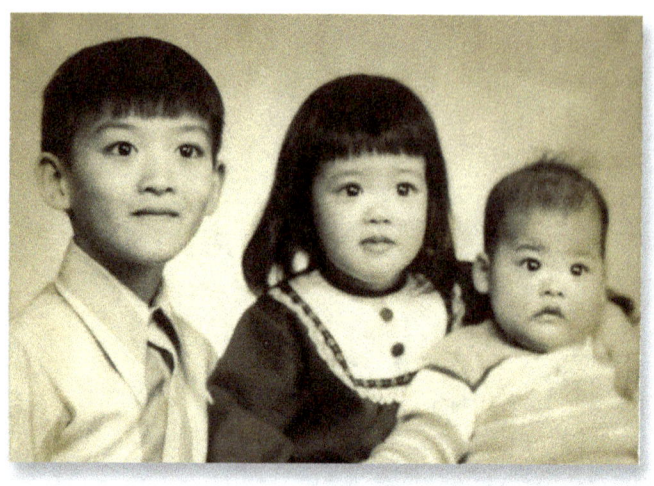

Our three cute, adorable children.
From left to right: David, Faith and Albert.

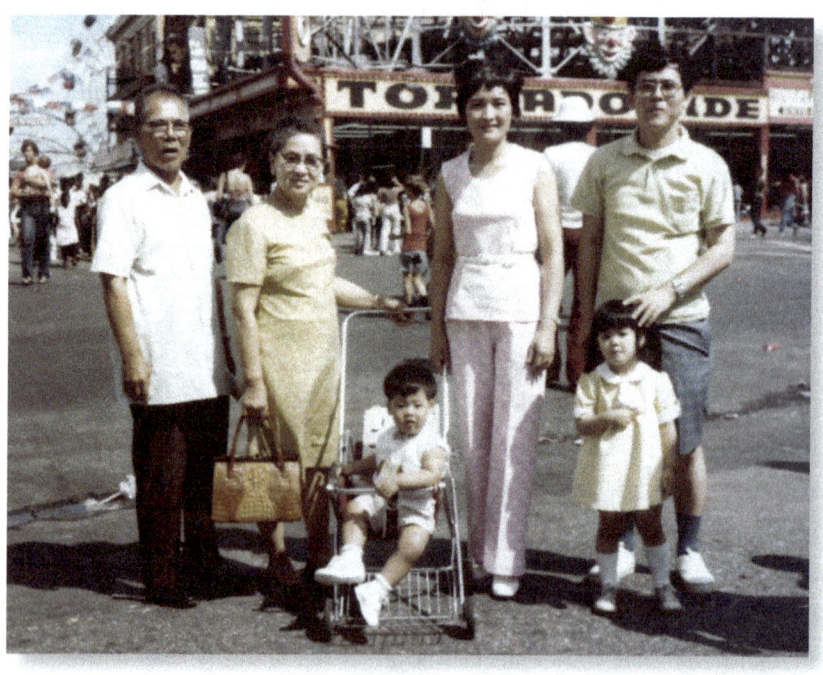

My parents visit and live with us in the United States.
We have beautiful memories of our travels together as a whole family.

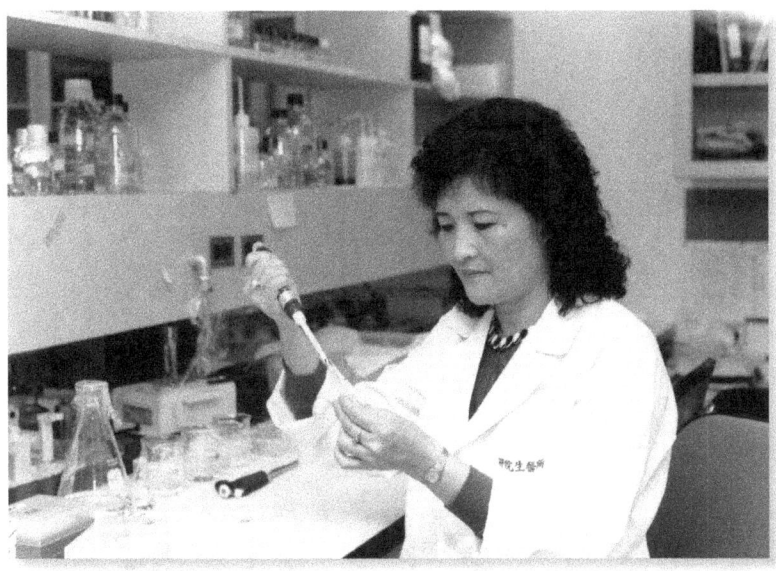

Felicia conducting experiments in the laboratory at
the Institute of Biomedical Sciences.

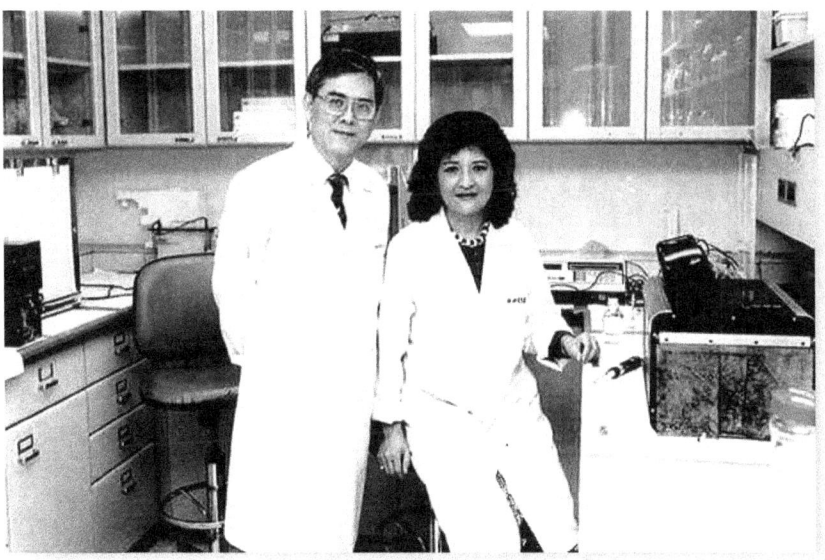

Felicia and I decide to return to Taiwan together and do our part to contribute to the establishment of a strong foundation for scientific research.

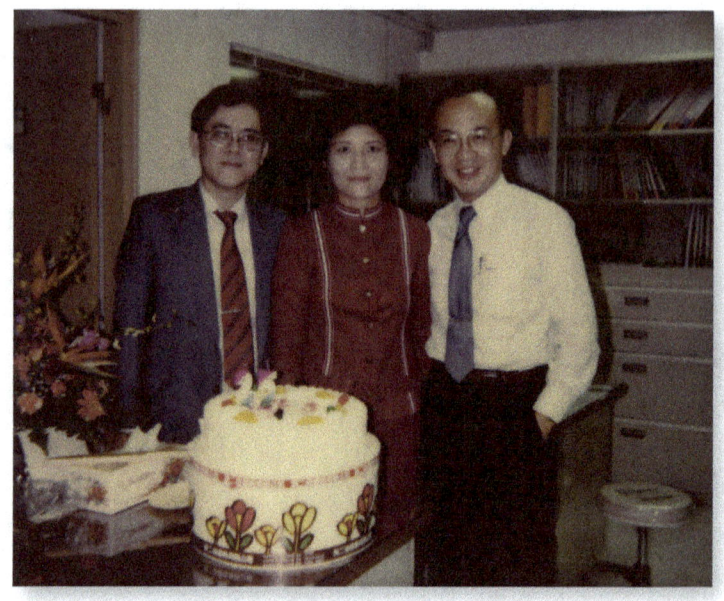

We return to Taiwan, our motherland. Shu Chien stands next to Felicia in this photo taken at the Academia Sinica.

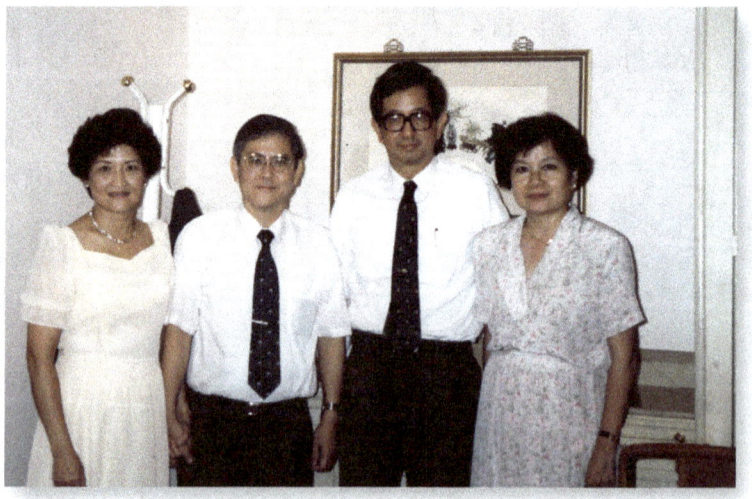

Dr. Yuan-Tseh Lee and his wife, who are also back in Taiwan recently.

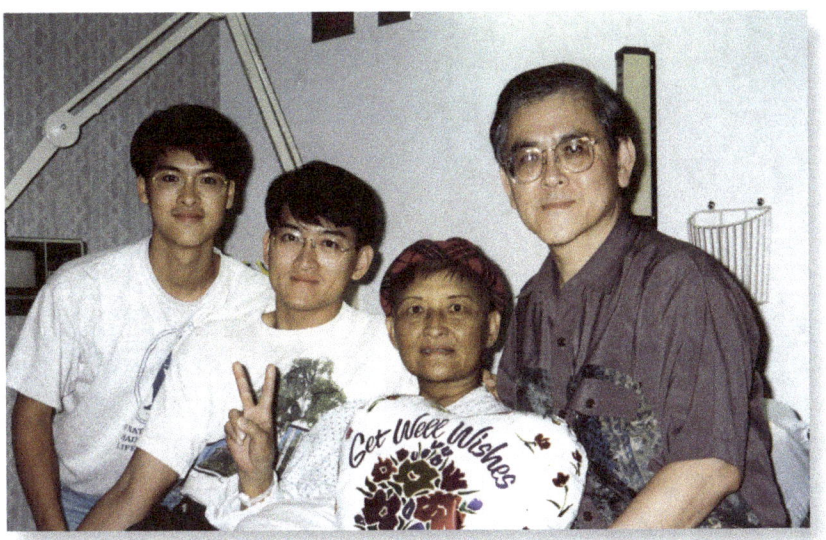

When Felicia undergoes high dose chemotherapy at the NIH, she experiences severe side effects, causing all her hair to fall out overnight and her face to turn dark and dull in tone as if she has been fed with poison.

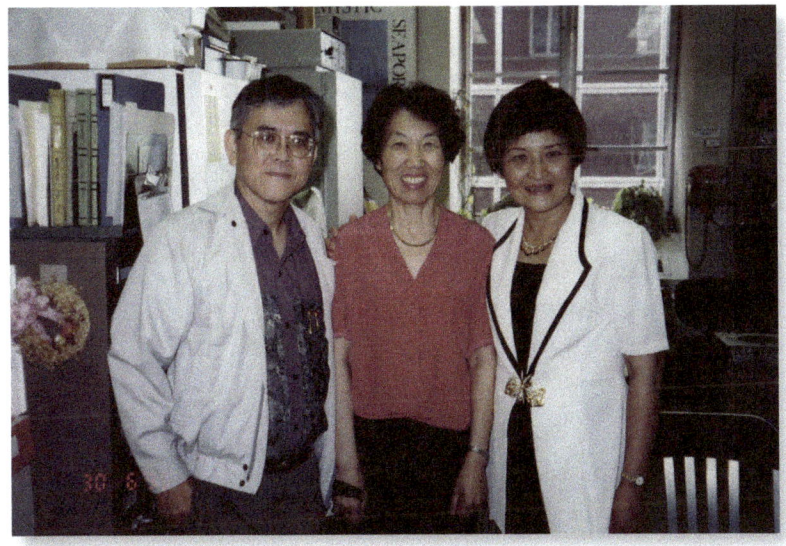

Dr. Jacqueline Peng-Wang (center) is a tremendous help to Felicia in her struggle against cancer.

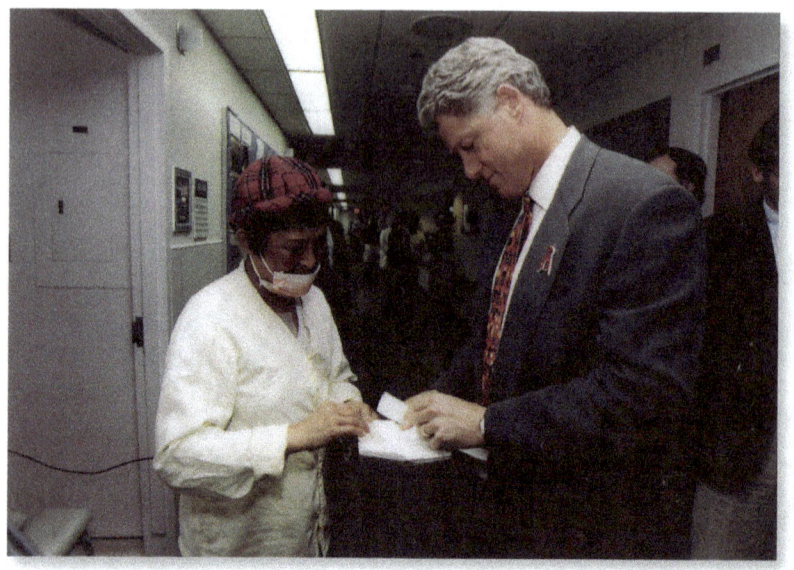

Former United States President Bill Clinton comes to visit his friend at the cancer center at the NIH. Felicia takes the opportunity to meet him and have a photograph taken with him. Thereafter, he sent a card wishing her well every Christmas.

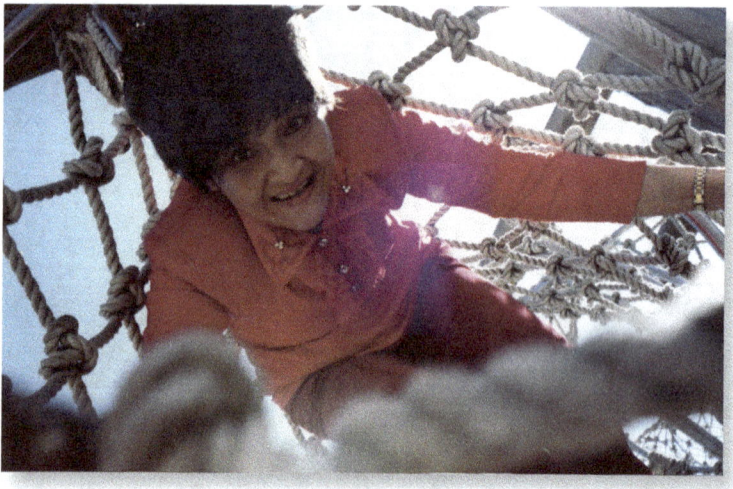

Felicia participates actively and enthusiastically in outdoor activities not long after receiving high dose chemotherapy and autologous bone marrow transplantation.

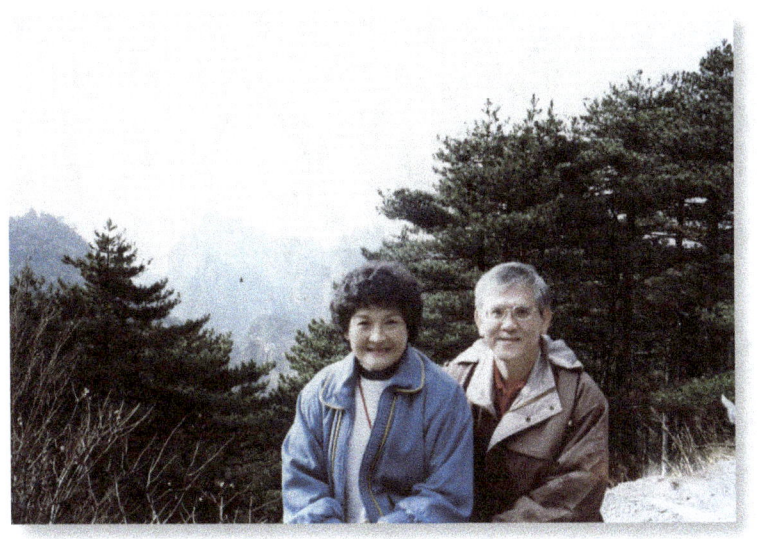

Though weakened as a result of the numerous high dose chemotherapy treatments, Felicia succeeds nevertheless in climbing the Yellow Mountain (Mount Huangshan).

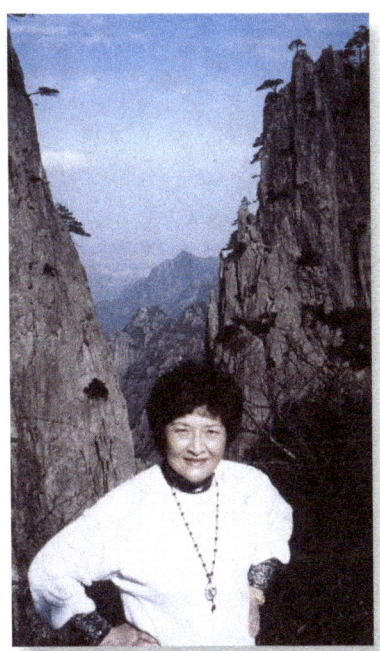

This picture of an ebullient Felicia at Yellow Mountain symbolizes and accentuates her optimistic spirit and proactive attitude as an eternal fighter.

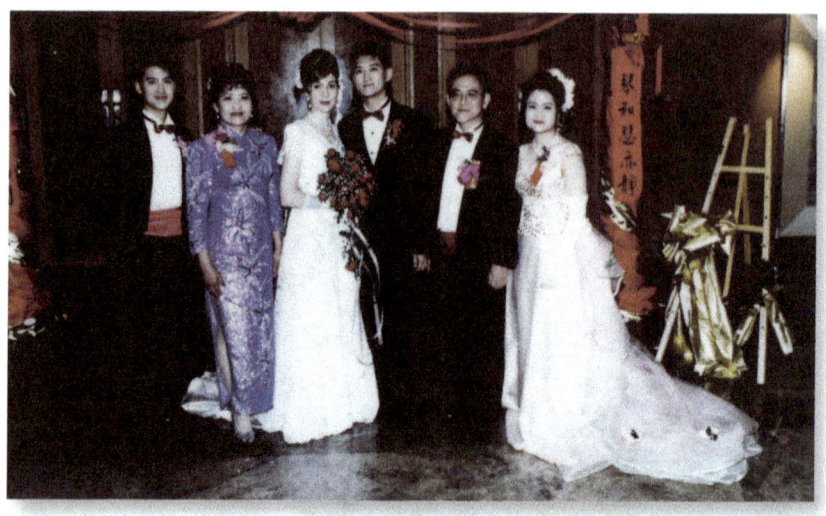

Our eldest son David and Christelle marry;
the entire family poses for the family portrait.

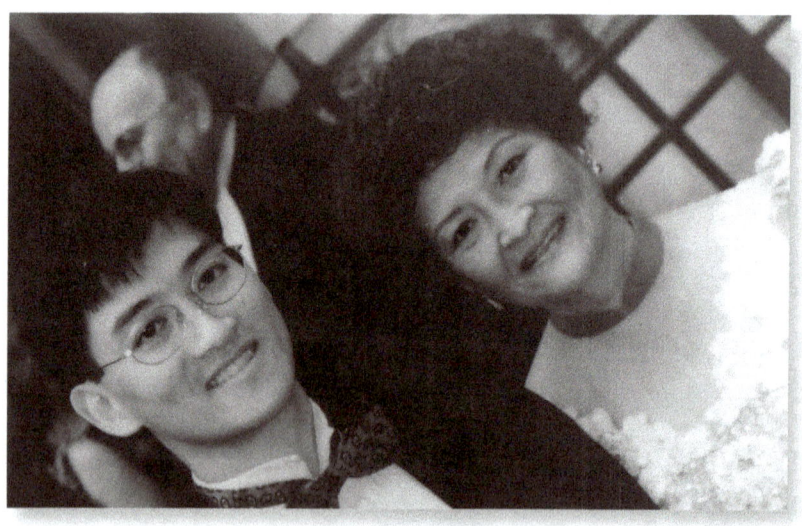

Though critically stricken with cancer, Felicia travels to France
to attend David's wedding.

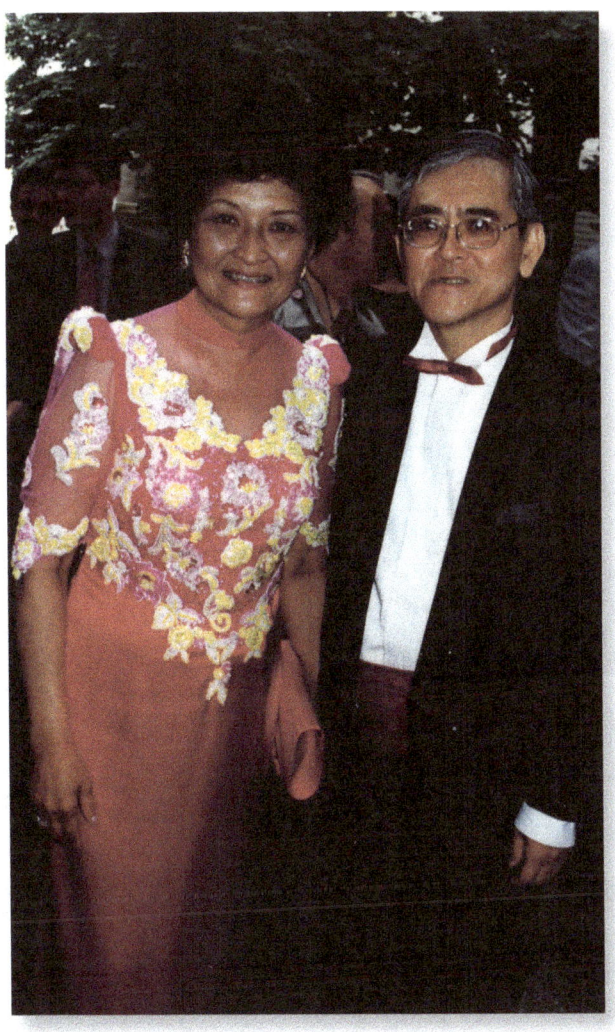

Although, at first, Felicia's physicians do not permit her to attend David's wedding in France, Felicia has her mind set on it. At the wedding, she appears energetic and resplendent in her red *chi-pao* (the Chinese dress), but her energy dissipates as soon as she is onboard the flight home.

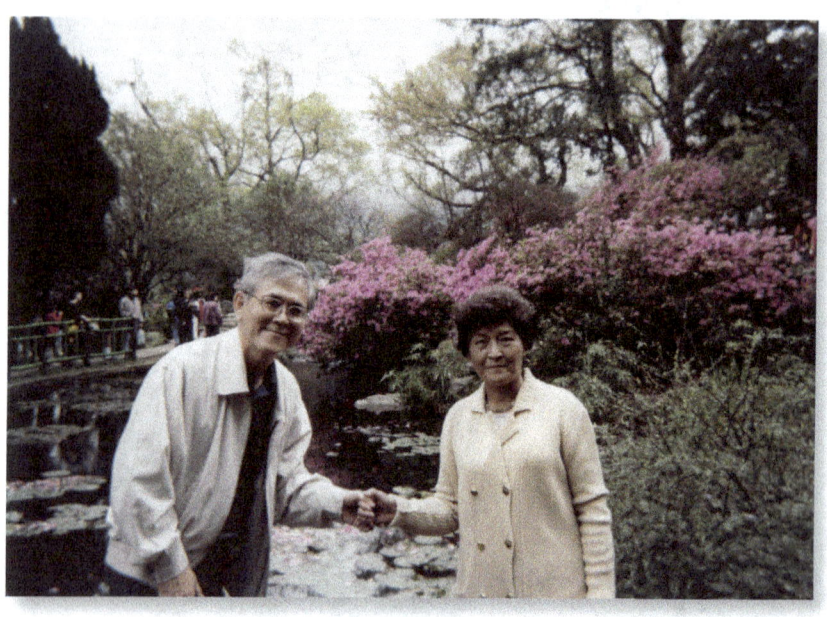

A trip to the Yangmingshan in 1999 to admire and appreciate the springtime flower bloom. Felicia's time is coming to an end.

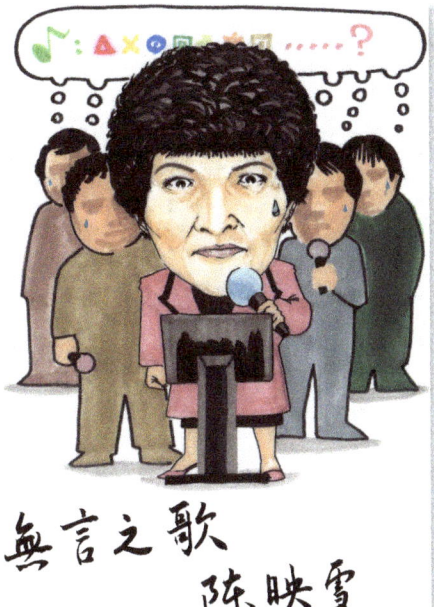

無言之歌
陈映雪

Wu, Felicia

For the discovery

that, to be a leader, one have to lead by example. So, by all means join her in whatever endeavor when she leads by the couragous way she battle with cancer (or the Cancer group), but when she try to lead by inviting you to sings in Karaoki, excuse youself politely.

This is a cartoon caricature of Felicia drawn by a laboratory colleague, captivating the lively and effervescent personality of Felicia.

Even on her hospital bed, Felicia continues to work industriously and with dedication. The notes depicted here are her instructions she wrote to her laboratory staff just before her passing.

Introduction

Days of Youth

As I contemplate Felicia's life, I marvel at how constant and steadfast she was. From the beginning to the end, her hopes and dreams were consistently the same. Sometimes, she was so earnest, it hurt to see. When I think of how in the last stages of her cancer, she was still unwilling to waste a single moment of her life, working as if the hospital were her office... This trait of hers was evident from the days when Felicia and I were just classmates and friends.

Life Abroad

Despite Felicia's outstanding contributions to scientific research, she experienced a great deal of unfair treatment simply by virtue of the fact that she was an Asian woman. However, she faced all of these obstacles with an iron will and dealt with them one by one, never once admitting defeat. The most difficult war that Felicia ever waged was that against breast cancer. As her closest companion, I walked alongside her every step of the way. The emotional pain that she experienced in this journey is one that is certainly difficult to put into words.

Transition Period

Felicia's love for her family enabled her to stand up, face difficult treatments one at a time and survive many close brushes with death. The Felicia that I saw took full advantage of the life that she was given, fueled herself with love, and succeeded in helping many other fellow cancer victims. Her determination enabled her to battle against cancer, and what is more, to fight for her life for thirteen years.

Fighting Cancer

Felicia was both a scientist who researched on anti-cancer drugs and a patient who knew the pain of cancer treatment. In the laboratory, she always made the utmost effort in her research; she was hopeful that she would be able to obtain results that could offer people a cure for cancer. If high dose chemotherapy and autologous bone marrow transplantation together could be a potential cure for cancer, she was willing to offer herself as a trial. Besides curing her own cancer, she might be able to serve as an example of a successful treatment case.

Fighting to the End

Before closing the coffin lid, I caressed Felicia's cold face and gently kissed her lips. My eyes brimmed with tears. The transparent coffin cover now separated Felicia and me. The children cried silently and tears fell from their eyes. There were tears running all over my face as well. Felicia was really gone. Heaven knew even in the last moment Felicia had not given up. In this lifetime, she had really lived her life wholeheartedly, but now she was ready to embark on a new journey. I would never see her again; she and I could only meet in our dreams.

SECTION I

DAYS OF YOUTH

1

Precocious from the Start

Memories are like a set of puzzle pieces that enable us to reassemble our past, and the pieces that reside in our memory are the remnants that stand as a testament to our past. A full, enriching life can never be erased from our memory, because it is the "song of life" that every person writes. My memories of Felicia are deep and indelible. To me, these recollections and the various phases of her life are a set of puzzle pieces that tell her story.

I know now what Felicia and I shared is more than a life as husband and wife; we were partners in our careers, friends with mutual trust in each other, and lifelong companions in quest of ideals and dreams. I was fortunate to be able to share this life with Felicia; it has truly been a life journey that we both treasured. Today, as always, I think of her, and an incessant flood of memories comes to mind. Now, I attempt to write about Felicia's life, so that her heart, desires, and extraordinary life will continue to burn brightly.

This story spins like a long river; the image in the water is that of Felicia. Years have flown by like the sun's rays reflecting off the water. But now, I draw the scene back to the year when Felicia was born.

Felicia and I are products of the post-colonial Taiwan; she was born in the year 1939. The years thereafter were a turbulent and tumultuous period in Taiwan's history, and during those times, Felicia grew up in a unique household.

Memories of the White Terror Era

In the year 1950, traces of the Japanese Occupation still lingered in the air of the lush green city of Taipei. Men clad in working pants walked around in wooden sandals; tension permeated in the air. Though the Japanese had left, those who had lived during the Japanese colonial period, try as they might, could not become accustomed to the new government. Tension gripped every street and every lane.

"The Law Office of Yi-Song Chen" on Nanjing West Road was firmly locked, as the well-known civil rights lawyer and his eldest son had temporarily gone into hiding. Yi-Song Chen's wife Ti-Yen was with the other younger children — Jing-Ren, Ying-Hsiueh (Felicia), and Hsi-Kuan. She stood at the window looking out, surveying the Taipei landscape bathed in the soft, warm glow of the waning sun.

Ti-Yen, who grew up during the Japanese Occupation period, was the eldest daughter of Yun-Nian Yen of the Keelung Yens, one of the five most distinguished families in Taiwan. She was a woman with an unconventional education, holding a degree from the Kyoto Women's University in Japan. In addition to the advantage of having grown up in a wealthy household, Ti-Yen was blessed with a wholesome spirit, level head, and iron will. Her poise and dignity not only immediately gave a clue to her privileged background, but also shaped her unique approach of raising children. Ying-Hsiueh was her eldest daughter. Even though Felicia had two elder brothers, in her mother's eyes she was always the eldest daughter — being the most reliable and able to take on responsibility. As the years passed, it became apparent that Felicia came to take after her mother in many ways.

Felicia's memories of her nursery school years during the White Terror era were somewhat hazy, but she said her mother was always tense, alert, and watchful, ready to do whatever was necessary to protect her children. This particular memory stayed firmly etched in her mind throughout her whole life.

One evening, a ferocious clamor was heard from outside the window. It sounded suspiciously like an explosion. Felicia turned her head towards the direction of the sound. She saw a ball of flame akin to a torch ready to fly apart at any moment. Her mother forbade the children to venture outside. The smoke outside the window suddenly rose, and the second child,

Jing-Ren, noticed that the house of the doctor living at the end of the lane had suddenly caught fire. The children were all fear-stricken. Their mother Ti-Yen simply gazed fixedly in that direction with intense anxiety in her eyes.

Because Ti-Yen left her family to study overseas in Kyoto while she was extremely young, she not only became one of the few women of her time to have the opportunity to receive higher education, she also developed a sense of independence. As her husband and eldest son had gone into hiding, she knew that if something were to happen to her family, it would be her perseverance to save the situation regardless of the fact that she was a woman.

As Felicia was only a first grader at the time, this fragment of the family history was told by the second child, Jing-Ren. School was cancelled for a couple of days due to the instability of the times. Though still young, Felicia was blessed with acute perception and a keen sense of awareness. This made her childhood memories of the White Terror era extremely clear and vivid. Felicia did not have much interest in politics, but she had great love for her homeland and her country; that was also one of the strongest reasons she supported my decision to return to Taiwan later in our lives. During the White Terror era, Felicia, who was still young, was kept safe and secure under the wings of her loving mother Ti-Yen. But the chaos on the streets outside, the haunting silence of the people behind closed doors — all the details of that afternoon would stay firmly imprinted in her heart.

Strict Father, Doting Mother

Felicia's father, Yi-Song Chen, was from Luodong in Ilan County; he graduated from the Tokyo University with a degree in law. While studying at the Okayama High School No. 6 during the Japanese colonial period, he responded to the call of famous anti-Japanese activists Xian-Tang Lin and Pei-Huo Tsai and joined the movements they organized. At school, he founded the Okayama Taiwanese Student Union and collected signatures of students studying abroad in Japan to support the anti-Japanese movement in Taiwan. To do this during the Japanese colonial period, Yi-Song Chen had to have a great deal of courage. Yi-Song Chen first displayed this valiant spirit during his teenage years through his advocacy for freedom and democracy. He demonstrated sympathy for the weak and the disempowered, embraced socialist ideals, and fought for these political ideals his entire life. It is evident that Felicia inherited her father's fighting spirit.

According to Yi-Song Chen's account of the Japanese colonial period in *The Taiwanese Spirit under the Flag of the Sun* (Yi-Song Chen's Recollections Vol. 1, Taiwan Publishing House), the Chen and Yen households were vastly different in their backgrounds. The Keelung-based Yens started off in the mining industry. Yun-Nian Yen and Guo-Nian Yen founded the Tai-Yang Mining Company. At its peak they exported coal to Japan. At the end of the Second World War, the second generation Yens operated Tai-Yang Enterprises, with Ti-Yen's older brother Chin-Hsien Yen at the helm. The company engaged in shipping, coal mining, metals, machinery, and various other industries. Tai-Yang Enterprises dominated the market for sixty years. It was not until oil became an important source of fuel that caused the subsequent decline in demand of coal that the conglomerate gradually lost its leadership position.

The Keelung Yens were an industrious, hard-working family who valued education. When Ti-Yen went to Japan to study, she lived a simple life of the bare minimum that was completely devoid of luxury, though at the time, the Yens were at their peak in terms of wealth. It was precisely because Ti-Yen was exposed to a life of austerity at a young age that she developed an iron will as well as the ability to endure suffering. Although she was originally a delicate and vulnerable young girl, life in Japan gradually galvanized a hardened spirit to emerge from her soft inner self — a spirit undaunted by the possibility of failure.

Because of Yi-Song Chen's passion for politics and his busy law practice, Ti-Yen's dedication to her children's education and upbringing left a strong impression on Felicia and her siblings. Hence, the emotional bond between the six siblings and their mother was also extremely strong.

As far as the children were concerned, their mother Ti-Yen was the center of their world. In the summertime, she would round up all the children and take them to the Yen family home in Keelung. There, Felicia, her siblings, and cousins would go with Ti-Yen to the seaside to swim. That was their most beautiful memory — playing enthusiastically in the sea by the rocky shore under the clear blue sky. Mother taught them to float in the water and swim; afterwards the whole family laid on the beach and sunned themselves until their skin turned red. Laughter was the most indelible memory of their childhoods. Thus, although their father seemed austere at times and the children felt a degree of estrangement from him, their mother's overflowing love and tenderness more than made up for it.

When they were young, everyone would gather together after dinner when their mother had finished clearing the table, and she would tell stories of her life in Japan. The children would, in turn, reflect upon their own experiences and share their dreams. The warm glow of the lamp seemed tinted with their mother's love. Felicia's younger brother Hsi-Kuan spoke nostalgically of those innocent and carefree years during which the siblings basked in the glow of their mother's love and smile. If not for the enormous changes outside their home, perhaps the children would still not know anything other than the love in their home. But the chaos of the world outside had reached startling proportions.

Fortunately, the tense atmosphere in Taipei gradually settled down, and their father and eldest brother returned home. The charred remains of the doctor's home on Nanjing West Road still stood as a silent testament to a chaotic era, but at least Father was busier than ever before…

Gaining Admission into Taipei First Girls' High School

In her early years, Felicia was the epitome of a model daughter — obedient, clear-headed, intelligent, and fun-loving. She would by no means be a cause of worry to her father and mother. Even as a young child, she was extremely self-disciplined and displayed great talent, especially in academics. This left a great impression on her siblings even to the present day.

Mother's unique style wielded an enormous influence on Felicia. The women's university that Ti-Yen attended in Japan produced well-educated women of eminence. Ti-Yen and her fellow classmates were taught how to cook, hold the fort at home, and instill family obligations with a sense of refinement and elegance, and, that was reflected particularly in flower arrangement. Ti-Yen excelled in all these subjects, but perhaps the most noteworthy talent is that she was also an excellent athlete.

Ti-Yen studied piano and flower arrangement since young, but swimming and tennis were activities that differentiated her from other children.

Felicia spent countless happy childhood moments with Mother and her elder brothers swimming, playing ping-pong and riding bicycle. Felicia's active and fun-loving nature was undoubtedly due to her mother's influence. Playtime asides, Ti-Yen also kept a close eye on the children's studies. On this account, Felicia never gave her mother any cause for worry.

Felicia attended Peng Lai Elementary School as a child. After graduating second in her class, she passed the entrance examinations for Taipei First Girls' Junior High School. When elder brother Chi-Ching took her to register, Felicia was the first student to complete all the enrollment paperwork. Felicia excitedly told her older brother that it was a very good beginning. Little Felicia broke into a smile — so pure that her smile resembled a lotus flower that had just bloomed. To this day, her elder brother still remembers that moment vividly as if it had occurred yesterday.

Felicia's diligence, strength of mind and penchant for pursuit in perfection reflected her upbringing in a unique household. Throughout her life, her thought, speech, and conduct remained pure and unadulterated; her character stayed simple and wholesome. The years passed by like a dream, the world was ever changing. Needless to say, as a child, Felicia was unaware of what obstacles lay before her, but armed with the talents she developed during her growing-up years with her family, what she achieved on the life journey ahead of her would stir the astonishment and admiration of all.

Pursuit of Excellence and Perfection in Studies

At the start of junior high school, Felicia demonstrated her relentless pursuit for perfection. The younger of her two elder brothers, Jing-Ren, was older than her by three years. When they were children, the two of them slept on a large bed. If Felicia did not understand her homework, Jing-Ren was always the first to help her. When she was six, Felicia started taking piano lessons. Ti-Yen was Felicia's first piano teacher. The piano in their home was her parents' present to their daughter when Ti-Yen married. Felicia was the first child to practice the piano diligently; all the other children, including Jing-Ren, avoided the piano after just one or two lessons. But Felicia was different. Whatever the subject was, she always studied diligently and continued what she began until she attained a level of excellence.

By junior high school, coursework became more difficult. Every day after school, Felicia disciplined herself to finish her homework first, then took a short nap to re-charge. After waking up refreshed, she would continue to revise her studies and prepare for the next day's lessons. This would go on until the wee hours of the night. On cold winter evenings, when her brothers and sisters would already be in their warm cozy bedrooms playing, Felicia would still be at her desk, engrossed in her studies without a moment's regret for not being able to join her siblings.

The next day, after getting up at dawn and completing her morning ritual in the bathroom, Felicia would sit down at the piano and begin playing. The crystal-clear melodic tones from the piano were Felicia's gift to her entire family; around that time, enticing aromas would already be wafting from the kitchen. Felicia's siblings would all sit around the kitchen table and enjoy the music quietly. Only when the music stopped would everyone begin the breakfast.

The siblings rode to school together on their bicycles. Felicia got ready for school faster than her brothers and sisters; she was usually the first one out in the garden waiting for her elder brothers. Although it was only a matter of minutes, she would pull out her book naturally and, still standing next to her bicycle, read as she waited. Thus, Felicia's spirit for keen competition and conscientiousness enabled her to finish six years of secondary school with an unsurpassable record.

Jing-Ren and Hsi-Kuan often said that although Felicia was not the most intelligent among the siblings, she was undoubtedly the most industrious. In addition, Jing-Ren said that there was once when he was explaining a physics problem to her, she cried because she could not comprehend his answer right away. The principles of motion stayed on her mind for days until she finally understood the concepts, and only then was she able to relax. This was Jing-Ren's strongest recollection of Felicia's serious attitude towards everything. As far as I could see, Felicia's determination and iron will remained unchanged throughout her life. At forty-eight years of age, Felicia developed cancer and fought for thirteen years. Those thirteen long years that included fifty-three chemotherapy sessions took an emotional and physical toll on her, but her spirit remained strong until the very end. This was Felicia, my lifetime companion.

Six Years of Perfect Attendance

Felicia's talent was evident during her first year at Taipei First Girls' Junior High School. She played the piano, her grades were impeccable, and she took first place in track and field. In volleyball, softball, and the athletics, she was virtually unbeatable, and school principal Hsue-Chu Jiang started to notice her.

Without a doubt, Felicia's love for sports was due to her mother's influence. In piano-playing as well, her mother was her first teacher who inspired her love for music. The hardworking, serious and competitive spirit that coursed through her veins was undoubtedly the attributes passed on to her by her parents. All of her life, Felicia had the greatest devotion to her mother and the greatest respect for her father. Her privileged childhood, and especially her mother's tireless concern and guidance, motivated Felicia to regard academic goals and self-accomplishment as one.

Though she was busy pitting in numerous competitions, participating in activities of all sorts, and practicing the piano, Felicia's grades topped her class without a doubt. Her teachers could not stop praising her. In addition, Felicia got along well with all her classmates, not only because she was a model student, but also for the fact that she was a warm-hearted and sincere class leader. Having passed the third year of junior high school, the forever smiling, warm-hearted Felicia entered Taipei First Girls' Senior High School.

Felicia's secondary school life was enriching and fulfilling. She had no regrets, other than her father's increasingly busy schedule which further widened the distance between him and his children.

In college, Felicia and I already knew each other. One day she came over while I was organizing pictures. Noticing the Taipei City Junior High Model Students commemorative photograph in my hand, she exclaimed, startled, that she too was in this picture. We spotted our faces in the picture, looked at each other, and smiled. In the years thereafter I have often thought that it was then that I knew the two of us were meant to be together. We felt a common bond between us; we pledged loyalty to each other and started a family together. Fate, love, and faithfulness — not one element was missing in our relationship. Felicia and I began based on a single picture, perhaps this was our fate. But in fact, this was not the only thing we had in common. Felicia and I were similar in many ways. We were blessed for the fact that our parents guided us to work hard in school, and that we did not have to struggle through our childhood. Although our family backgrounds were extremely different, there were similarities in our parents' care and parenting, that we grew up happily. Felicia's and my parents were optimistic and active people. These similarities were common guiding principles for Felicia and me to build a home and to share our lives together, year after year.

In high school, Felicia's performance was even more outstanding, and Principal Jiang grew extremely fond of her. Hsue-Chu Jiang was known for being an open-minded albeit strict educator. For example, she did not believe that students should bury their heads in their books; she believed true excellence meant apart from standing out academically, one should also participate actively in extracurricular activities, be morally upright, and excel in sports. Excelling on all fronts is by no means an easy task. But Felicia was exactly the ultimate model of a well-rounded student, so Principal Jiang viewed her with special regard.

In her third year high school, Felicia was busy as always. When the school choir entered competitions, Felicia went along with them. She also became a member of the school volleyball, softball, and track and field teams. Of course she would never let her grades slip, and thus her third year was both busy and fulfilling.

Felicia's two sisters, Wan-Chan and Shing-Yin, remember that their older sister often came home from school tired from some sports competition. The age gap between the youngest sister Shing-Yin and Felicia was eight years. Shing-Yin, who was still quite young at the time, would hop onto her older sister's back and massage her with her feet. Sometimes her older sister would fall asleep due to exhaustion, but Shing-Yin's two feet would continue to drum up and down her back. The memory of massaging the back of her older sister remains forever ingrained in Shing-Yin's mind.

Felicia loved sports and music, but she never once let her exemplary grades falter and drop. In the three years of high school, Felicia never once skipped class, arrived late, or left early. Adding on the three years of perfect attendance from her junior high, Felicia's six-year secondary school attendance record is one that is not easily emulated.

Winning First Prize in a Cycling Race

Felicia had some great stories from her high school years. Shing-Yin and Jing-Ren remember that she wanted to represent Taipei First Girls' High School in the All-Taiwan High School Bicycle Race. Her mother was terribly concerned about her participation in this race because, in her opinion, whenever a group of young people participated in any competition, a thousand things could go wrong. In addition, in those days, bicycles were primarily used as a mode of transportation and not for exercise, cyclists did not wear protective gear which is a mandatory safeguard today. Should an accident occur, that would definitely be a cause of worry. Therefore Felicia's mother reminded her that she must ride slowly and carefully, and not vie for the first place. But that, of course, was not what Felicia was thinking.

She and her older brother Jing-Ren went through all that she needed to do during the competition in order to win. Jing-Ren thought that although Felicia was neither the tallest nor the strongest among the competitors, she possessed excessively great patience and strong determination, hence, as long as she wanted to win the competition, there had to be a way. Jing-Ren advised Felicia to look for a bicycle with large wheels. At that time, the bicycles that girls rode usually had 24-inch or 26-inch wheels. If Felicia was brave enough to ride a men's 28-inch bicycle, Jing-Ren thought she should have a good shot at winning. Older brother and younger sister made their plans on the sly; Mother, of course, was unaware that on the racing day, her daughter fearlessly entered the competition on a men's bicycle.

Since that was the first time China Youth Corps had organized an All-Taiwan Bicycle Race, none of the competitors really had any experience. All the young people at the race simply rushed forward when they heard the whistle blow. Felicia, however, started off slowly and found herself at the end of the pack. She gradually accelerated by relaxing her whole body, focused her attention, and slowly lowered her head. By this time, the others were already at the sprinting stage of the race. However, the cyclists, who were at the head of the pack, had been pushing themselves far too early in the race, and were already drenched in sweat and exhaustion. Felicia knew it was time to make her move.

One lone rider gradually pulled ahead of the pack; she lowered her head and leaned her body forward. The huge bicycle and her little body seemed grossly mismatched, but she certainly was fast. In an instant, she pulled away from the pack. The weary competitors that she left behind huffed and puffed, but could not muster the strength to catch up, so they could only watch as Felicia flew by.

This last stretch gave Felicia the chance to win the championship for Taipei First Girls' High School to the great astonishment of her mother Ti-Yen.

Happy to Help Others

Though Felicia had a privileged family background, she never allowed this to be a cause to be arrogant. At that time, the standard of living in all average household was meager and the living conditions cold and bare; few families could afford to support their children past high school. Felicia had a schoolmate Shi-Jin Tsao with whom she got along very well; the two always did their homework together after school and a deep friendship developed between them. Unfortunately, Shi-Jin Tsao was one of those children whose family situation could not afford them to continue their schooling past high school.

Seeing all her classmates prepare for the college entrance exam, Shi-Jin Tsao became extremely depressed. Felicia, who had graduated first in her class, was guaranteed admission to National Taiwan University without having to take the entrance examination. She patiently comforted Shi-Jin Tsao, offering her constant encouragement, "As long as one has a special skill and continues to work hard, there will always be a foothold for him or her in the society." This statement had a profound and lasting influence on Shi-Jin Tsao's life; henceforth, whenever she encountered any circumstance that left her frustrated or upset, she would think of Felicia's words. Now Shi-Jin Tsao has a successful career, and a happy family. She believes that Felicia is the friend who had the most influence in her life.

Throughout her life, Felicia's warm, helpful nature never waned and changed which was what people appreciated about her most. Her personality beamed like the sun, eternally radiating warmth — and she was always eager to share her thoughts with others and offer assuring words and encouragement to those who were depressed or frustrated with life. Her hope was that everyone could always be diligent, perseverant, and live life to the fullest. One could always see she was brimming with the exuberance of life and the flourish of love for others.

The Future Looks Bright

Taipei First Girls' High School had an award to encourage the balanced cultivation of five values in the morals, intellect, physique, team spirit and aesthetics domains. Students who were awarded this scholarship were certainly model students; without a doubt, excelling in all five areas was not easy. Yet Felicia made it on the list throughout the twelve terms while she was at Taipei First Girls' High School, an unprecedented feat in the school's history.

In recognition of her six years of perfect attendance, when Felicia graduated from high school in 1957, Principal Jiang showered her with praises and presented her with a gold medal made specially for her. On the graduation day, Principal Jiang told Felicia as she handed her the medal that she must wear it on her wedding day.

It was a difficult period for the country economically at that time, and to have a medal made was indeed expensive, so this medal held special meaning for Principal Jiang. Not only did she pin great hopes for Felicia, she also adored her. Felicia, on her part, was determined not to let her principal down. So, the instant when Principal Jiang conferred the medal on this student whom she had particularly high expectations of, was an unforgettable and beautiful moment for both of them.

Bidding goodbye to her childhood, Felicia was prepared to step out and embrace the vast world — that is, the university. She was already making plans; she wanted to follow in her brother's footsteps and major in chemistry at the National Taiwan University.

While the moonlight shines upon the balcony, time and the moonbeam linger… Our aspirations, the aspiration of the young intellectuals of the fifties era, were simple and traditional. We nurtured dreams in our hearts. We thought that as long as we studied hard, the beautiful world which seemed so foreign and distant would actually not be far away at all. We believed that as long as we worked hard, remained focused, and continued to learn and grow, we would be able to overcome any difficulties that lay ahead of us.

Felicia thought the same way too. The lush green and the sunshine vibrance of the summer day outside the window were like Felicia's heart — filled with romantic realism and overflowing with warmth. Though everything she wanted was still not within her grasp, she was reaching out and the world was already responding to her aspirations. "I'm going to start university now," she thought. "I have to work even harder."

There seemed to be a plenitude of plans buried in Felicia's heart. She was prepared to take in and absorb vast reservoir of knowledge from the wide expanse of the academic world. She had no way to foresee that we would meet for the first time, though of course at the time, neither did I.

2

Meeting and Getting to Know Each Other

Looking back, I realize that it has already been over forty years. I think of Master Yi Hong's song, "Farewell", which Felicia and I often sang together after we came to know each other well: "Outside the garden, along the old path, the fresh fragrance of grass pervades under the bright blue sky, the night wind whistles as it blows and ruffles the willows, the soft rays of the sun shine on the mountains as dusk falls. The heaven, the earth, knowing that they are separate and apart…" We would stroll on the grass turf admiring the beautiful landscape that lay before us, with our own voices in accompaniment with the nature's symphony. After Felicia left, her melodious voice, so uniquely hers and in its full richness of emotion, often resonates in my head. This song brought us back to our younger days, and our courtship days. In my mind, these memories are as fresh as the day when it happens.

First Meeting

To me, that was my first most memorable day in my life. I was at my house waiting for my classmate Shiao-Lei Yu; that day both of us had decided to go to Taipei First Girls' High School where the college entrance exam was being held. We planned to serve drinks to our classmates from

National Taiwan Normal University (NTNU) Affiliated High School during the breaktime in between their exam.

It was July 28, 1957. Shiao-Lei and I rode our bikes happily to Taipei First Girls' High School. It was a perfect sunny day — not a trace of cloud in the bright blue sky. The weather seemed to reflect our good mood — we knew our admission to National Taiwan University was secure without taking the entrance exam.

I graduated top from the NTNU Affiliated High School and was thus guaranteed admission to National Taiwan University. I originally chose electrical engineering as my major, but later switched to medicine. Shiao-Lei was guaranteed admission to National Taiwan University's School of Civil Engineering. We were close friends and we would often talk deep into the night before heading home.

Upon arrival at Taipei First Girls' High School, we proceeded to the counter where students test-takers were reporting their attendance. The area around the counter was extremely busy; students were milling everywhere, so we waited until they had all entered the examination room. Shiao-Lei and I looked at the bright sun and could not help but feel sticky due to the humidity of the air that engulfed us. Our minds were preoccupied with the students inside taking their exams. After the examination they would certainly get thirsty, so we strode back to the counter to find out if we could borrow a kettle.

In front of me stood a girl with large eyes, a wide smile, and shiny black hair, in a grass-green colored blouse and long black skirt. Her beautiful skin, bright eyes and cheery, friendly smile gave us the impression that she was very nice and approachable.

We asked the girl at the counter where we could borrow a tea kettle. The bright-eyed girl carried out her role as a school host perfectly; she took us to the school lounge, where there was a teapot that we could use. After filling it up, we brought it to the counter, where students could have a drink to refresh during the break. After the break, when all the students rushed back into the examination room, Shiao-Lei and I had some free time, so we took a leisurely stroll around the campus.

As that was the first time we entered a girls' school, we were a little curious; scrutinizing in all directions — up, down, left and right — we took in all the sights around us. Just inside the main entrance, there was a long corridor. Above us as we looked up on the wall, we saw the words, "Hall of Fame," on the bulletin board. Above the list was an enlarged photograph of a pretty, smiling girl. "Hey, that's the girl who just lent us the tea kettle," Shiao-Lei and I exclaimed at the same time. The caption indicated "Felicia Chen" below the picture. "So *she's* Felicia Chen." We were both a little surprised, because the name was not at all unfamiliar to us and our classmates.

At that time, the NTNU Affiliated High School Twelfth Grade Honors Science Class No. 2 had a physics teacher named Shu-Chin Chang who did relief teaching at Taipei First Girls' High School and had taught Felicia during that occasion. The teacher would sometimes talk about Taipei First Girls' High School and a consistently high achiever student named Felicia Chen was mentioned. Besides being a model student year after year, she had served as a class leader for six straight years. Her grades were invariably the top and highest in her class in all subjects — even music and sports — and it was virtually impossible for anyone to surpass her performance. So the students of Honors Science Class No. 2 knew there was an outstanding student at Taipei First Girls' High School named Felicia Chen.

After the examination, we had to return the kettle, naturally. Shiao-Lei and I took the teapot over to the counter and said to the girl, "You're Felicia Chen; our teacher has mentioned about you before." It just happened, we ended up introducing ourselves, and thus the examination center and teapot became the serendipitous events that brought us together.

The first impression that I had of Felicia, besides her talents and intellect, she was also forthright, generous, and not at all coquettish. In that day and age, people were generally still quite conservative and girls were extremely shy, so Felicia really stood out among them. She certainly made heads turn and caught people's attention. Young people in that conservative era were simple and unsophisticated. The day I met Felicia, only one thought occurred to me: "So she is the famous Felicia Chen." Then I thought happily there would be one more friend with whom I could exchange academic knowledge.

The second day at the examination center, we took advantage of our free time to make conversations again. I told Felicia that I had graduated in first position from the NTNU Affiliated High School and was guaranteed admission to National Taiwan University's electrical engineering program. Since Felicia had graduated top from Taipei First Girls' High School and was guaranteed admission as a chemistry major, we were sure to be schoolmates. Her father, Yi-Song Chen, was CEO of Taiwan's first rubber company, Hou-Sheng Rubber Company; her older brother was studying chemical engineering and had plans to study abroad. Felicia chose chemistry because she wanted to help develop and expand the family business. We had a great time chatting at the examination center, so we exchanged our home addresses and telephone numbers, and promised to get in touch during summer vacation.

To many students, July 28, 1957, meant a frantic scribbling on paper, and a desperate battle to the finish line. For Felicia and me, this serendipitous encounter under the brilliant sunshine rays was to lead to immeasurable happiness. Of course, for all our youthful simplicity and innocence at that time, the thought never occurred to us.

Bashful Feelings of Youth

Though it was not love at first sight, we enjoyed our conversation immensely during that two days when we first became acquainted. When Felicia and I reminisced those moments, tenderness and sweet emotion still swarmed and overwhelmed us. Fate is fate; as youngsters we were unable to express our feelings clearly. All we knew was that studying together, discussing our future hopes and dreams together, was purely an exchange of aspirations and enrichment of our hearts and souls. However, the seed of affection was planted and naturally sprang forth.

Not long after, I rode my bicycle to Felicia's house for a visit. She lived on Ning Bo West Street; in the 1960s' Taipei, the area was considered an upper-class residential district. Both sides of the street were lined with lush green plants, and the neighborhood permeated a strong cultural ambience and character. Felicia's family owned a two-story house of Western architectural design. The garden landscaping was elegant and refined; adjourning her house was what at that time the Philippines Embassy. To ride from my home on He-Ping West Road in Wanhua to Ning Bo West Street took only ten minutes. I had already telephoned and made an appointment to meet Felicia at her house that afternoon.

It was the first time I had ever been in such a splendidly-decorated living room. It was bright and clean; an elegant flower arrangement adorned the coffee table, covered in exquisite white lace. Everything about the house was meticulous and detailed, bestowing an air of a scholarly and majestic household. Felicia's mother went into the kitchen and made tea for us. The two of us sat on the sofa, enjoyed the tea and proceeded to have a lively converstaion about what college life would be like.

Felicia and I had very diverse interests. For example, I was an avid reader, your stereotypical "bookworm." I read books of all genres; thus science, philosophy, literature and yes, even Felicia's beloved chemistry, were subjects which I was well-versed in. With her, I could enjoy the pleasure of an intellectual conversation. Felicia would talk animatedly about the music and sports she loved. She exuded warmth; as soon as you started a conversation with her, she would continue enthusiastically about it to no end. Summer days were hot and humid, endless conversations with Felicia about everything under the sun was an enjoyable activity to pass the time. It was those afternoon chats that Felicia and I developed a strong bond and friendship, which later became the foundation for our future relationship.

A piano concert offered me the first glimpse of the wide breadth of Felicia's talents. Before entering university, Felicia held a concert; she had learned diligently with her teacher Tsi-Mei Kao for many years, when she already built a strong foundation in music. That was my first time to hear her play. How elegant, how spirited, and how refined! In Felicia's own words, the music that she loved was like flying horses — it could take her thoughts and mood on journey far and wide. I believe people who love music are emotionally more expressive, more sincere and unadulterated than those who do not. I saw this characteristic in Felicia — music has accentuated her warm-heartedness, and sentimentality.

When school started, Felicia and I became part of a group of cyclists who wove in and out on both sides of the willow-lined streets. I rode from Wanhua to West Ning Bo Street, where Felicia would always wait for me, and then off we rode to school together. During the first year of college, there were many compulsory classes as required of all students; the classes that Felicia and I shared in common were Calculus, English, Chinese, "Three People's Principles," and military training, so we had substantial quality time together.

As we had many common classes, it was only natural that we studied together in the library, and prepared for our exams together. Felicia was extremely hardworking, but that did not mean that every subject was a breeze to her. Calculus gave her the most trouble; every time we had a calculus exam, I had to spend more time coaching her in the subject. There was one occasion, we had made plans to revise calculus at her house in preparation for the examination the next day, but something unexpected cropped up and I was delayed. By the time I made it to Felicia's house, it was already eight or nine in the evening. To my surprise, as soon as Felicia saw me, she started crying. She had waited anxiously the entire day, and she came to the conclusion that I had forgotten our appointment, which then set her on a panic mode of the impending exam. My presence made her both happy and eager to get started on the preparation immediately.

Another incident which left a strong impression on me is that Felicia often said she was not a good essay writer and she envied classmates who could write well. I told her how, when I was younger, a teacher made us write a peice of composition every week to improve our writing skills. And if she was willing, I could come up with a topic for her to write every week and then edit for her. Imagine my surprise when she actually did turn in her essays to me every week.

These two little incidents crystallized my thoughts about Felicia's life — how she had always been perseverant from the beginning to the end. She was never careless about anything; she never wasted a single minute of her life. At times my heart ached to see her so serious, so conscientious in her approach towards life. Looking back on the days when she was hospitalized toward the end of her battle with cancer, she still treated the hospital room like her office, as she industriously corrected the student papers and planned her research with enthusiasm. For every minute she had, she would find some way to squeeze out an extra ten seconds; she was unwilling to while her time away. This unique characteristic left a strong impression on me from the time we became classmates.

During our first year of college, we read Russell's selected writings on Einstein's theory of relativity. We became quite curious, and were, in a way, full of hopes about time, space, eternity, and future. Whenever Felicia participated in athletic competitions or track meets, I would always be at the track sidelines cheering her on. During vacations, we would take our younger siblings to the beach to camp. At night, all of us, young and old alike, would gather around the campfire and sing. Everyone had a smile on his or her face. The excitement turned up a notch with each lapping roll of the waves. When exams came, we would wait until the last minute and then "embrace Buddha's feet in our hour of need." Yet somehow we managed, and understood and enjoyed the subjects that we were studying.

The Experience of Loneliness at Our First Separation

During the summer vacation after the freshman year, Felicia went to Yilan Prefecture and stayed at her cousin's house for two weeks. When she came back, I went to meet her at the train station. Though it had only been two weeks, life without Felicia for even just a brief moment seemed empty. Those two weeks, I experienced loneliness for the first time.

That day, the train station was extremely busy. In the midst of chaos and thick crowd, I finally spotted Felicia's silhouette. Fifteen days of swimming under the sun had given her a darker skin complexion, but to me, she looked healthier than ever. When Felicia saw me, she too was exceptionally happy. Though it had only been a fortnight, we both had endless things that we wanted to tell each other. Felicia held onto me as I walked my bicycle, and we strolled from Taipei Train Station through throngs of crowd down to Xi-Men Ding. Felicia was animated as usual, her crystal-clear, cheery voice relating to me how she had a great time swimming and chasing the waves at Yilan. I listened with rapt admiration, and thought happily, "Felicia's back." I felt so joyful that I wanted to whistle a tune at that instant.

It took fifteen days of separation for us to realize that our lives were already inextricably intertwined. Then as we walked along the streets of Taipei, our hearts and thoughts seemed as though they were floating every second of every minute. It was such a sweet feeling. Felicia's youthful and lively face, especially when she was in pensive thoughts, certainly moved me. We strolled leisurely to Wan-Guo Theatre. Felicia loved Japanese food, and next to Wan-Guo Theatre was a Japanese restaurant called "Mei Guan Yuan" (which literally means the "Beautiful Garden") where we shared an exquisite meal. Felicia drank beer for the first time, and savored the sashimi that she loved so much. Though she was not accustomed to drinking beer, she loved to try new things which she found fresh and exciting.

After our meal, we went outside under the star-filled sky. Felicia was feeling a bit woozy from the beer. Even though she only had a small glass, slight headache set in, and her legs felt as if they couldn't support her. Thinking that she probably needed some fresh air, we decided to walk home. She felt her stomach churning when we began our walk; by the time we reached a garden, she couldn't endure it any longer and threw up.

I was a little worried as I rode my bicycle and took Felicia home. In my heart I blamed myself, wondering why I had ordered beer. That night I tossed and turned, constantly worrying about Felicia's condition. The next day, I bolted to her house at the first available moment to call on Felicia and inquire after her condition.

Felicia was in the study. Standing with her back to the door, her hair fell softly over her shoulders like silk, cascading down like a waterfall, shimmering like stars. I couldn't stop myself from touching her hair. Felicia turned her head and her gaze fell on me. Her eyes were bright and deep-set. In them I could read the peaks and valleys of our emotion in our hearts.

That beautiful moment brought the two of us even closer.

Thirty years after, on the day of our wedding anniversary, Felicia had become extremely ill, but she had not forgotten the times we shared together in our youth. We fixed a date to visit "Beautiful Garden" and relive our past. In the midst of the lively and energetic din from the young crowd, "Beautiful Garden" looked as if it had always been. Its appearance had not changed, although it did show some pleasant signs of aging. The restaurant seemed a little out of place in an area such as Xi-Men Ding that is a hang-out place for young Generation Xers. However, this is the place which bore witness to the start of our lifetime journey together — the "Beautiful Garden" stands the test of time and destiny and nothing can change its existence.

Inseparable Like Shadows

At the beginning of our second year at university, I switched my major from electrical engineering to medicine. Changing majors meant attending classes that I had to make up for the first year course in medicine, and particularly because I switched to medicine, the prerequisites and requirements were rather extensive. Felicia and I were already known as the school sweethearts. We went to school together and went home together; Felicia was my best study buddy. Studies aside, during our leisure time, we were always together.

Felicia loved outdoor activities, and although I was nowhere near as active and energetic as Felicia, I do enjoy nature. Our off-school days were times when we fully wielded our athletic abilities. Once, we walked along the North Coast of Taiwan. Carrying water bottles and light snacks, we left at dawn, took public transport from Taipei to Jinshan, and started on foot from there. We walked the entire distance from Jinshan to Keelung.

Under the perfect blue sky and golden sun, with the rolling green hills and weathered, sandy cliffs as our only companions, we walked the whole day, singing as we went. Felicia's voice was crystal-clear and melodious, and our happy laughter and singing accompanied us through the winding, narrow mountain roads.

> Her robe flows like a cloud, her face beautiful like a flower;
> Her balcony, glimmering with the bright spring dew,
> Is either the summit of the earth's Jade Mountain
> Or the moon-edged roof of paradise.
>
> There's a perfume stealing dew from a stem of red blossom,
> And a mist, through the heart, from the magical Hill of Wu,
> The palaces of China have never known such beauty,
> Not even Flying Swallow with all her glittering garments.
>
> Lovely now together, his lady and his flowers
> Lighten forever the Emperor's eye,
> As he listens to the sighing of the far spring wind
> Where she leans on a railing in the Aloe Pavilion.
>
> (Source: 300 Tang Poems, University of Virginia Library Chinese Text Initiative)

Felicia and I sang word for word every phrase of Li Bai's *A Song of Pure Happiness*. In our youth, we enjoyed every minute of our days to the fullest, there was never an idle moment. We walked the entire day till sunset, only then we took the train home physically exhausted, but mentally fulfilled and contented. On that chilly evening, we gazed at the stars that were glittering like lanterns outside the train window and we experienced an ethereal sensation — one that could cure ten thousands woes and set us free.

Anxieties in the Midst of Love

In school we were known as a couple; our love for each other was pure like water. Though we were in love, we still studied hard to prepare for examinations, and I went to Felicia's house as before. I played with her younger brothers and sisters, and her mother was always cordial towards me. In the beginning, of course, her parents were completely unaware of our blossoming feelings, however, by the third year of university, Felicia's mother found out.

Her eldest brother had already gone to the United States for further study; at that moment, her second brother Jing-Ren was also making plans to go abroad. Felicia was already in her third year of college; in a year's time, she too would begin making plans. Her mother Ti-Yen was a little worried that Felicia might change her mind at the last minute due to an emotional attachment.

Felicia's parents were both from distinguished families of prominent status, so they would naturally be concerned about whom their eldest daughter was dating. Her mother Ti-Yen happened to have a relative in Wanhua, so she took the opportunity to find out a little more about my family background.

My father's hometown was Yingge. He was originally apprenticed to my grandfather to learn pottery, but decided that there was not much of a future in pottery, and so he moved to Taipei and managed to get an education. In all his life my father had worked extremely hard. He, together with my mother, managed to raise the seven of us by selling mainly coal. He erected a five-story house in Wanhua. He had always wanted me to study medicine and hoped that someday I would build a practice in his house at Wanhua. That was the reason why I changed my major to medicine, but I regret that I was not able to realize his dream.

Of course, someone of an ordinary, humble family background from Wanhua was not Felicia's mother's idea of what makes an ideal son-in-law material, but fortunately, her mother was also a very logical and open-minded person. She only hoped that Felicia would not throw out a well-thought-out plan simply for a fleeting moment of young love. One day, I unexpectedly received a telephone call from Felicia's father asking me to meet him.

I was already quite close and familiar with Felicia's family, but Felicia's father was seldom at home, hence, I never really had an opportunity to get to know him. My impression of him was that he was an idealistic lawyer with a firm, unwavering character and a stern countenance that rarely broke into laughter or even a conversation. It dawned to me that the first time I was to speak with him, the subject would be about Felicia going abroad.

Her father Yi-Song Chen had a wealth of experiences in life, and therefore he had a fairly sophisticated way of thinking. He did not request for a split-up between Felicia and I; he just hoped that we would allow our feelings for each other to cool down for some time, and that I would not stand in the way of Felicia going abroad.

In the context of Taiwan in the 1960s, going overseas was certainly no easy task. At that time, the government was still experiencing many problems in its relationship with the mainland China, and the economy was tightly controlled. The lives of most people were simple and devoid of luxury. And of course, during such times, traveling overseas was also tightly regulated by the government. Furthermore, considering the fact that an average person could hardly afford the price of a round-trip plane ticket, studying abroad really was an option open only to children of the upper class.

As Felicia's mother and father had both left the country and studied abroad in their younger days, both were rather cosmopolitan and worldly-wise. They hoped that their children would also have the best possible education, and to them, that would mean studying abroad. Thus, it was understandable that they would not allow anything to get in the way.

After speaking with Felicia's mother and father, we were naturally all in amicable agreement. I, too, did not want Felicia to take a false step with regard to her education as a result of our feelings for each other.

In addition, I was confident that the separation would not put a strain to our relationship.

That was perhaps a ripple in our otherwise simple and naïve relationship during our university years. Because of the understanding between Felicia's father and me, I visited Felicia's house less often during my third and fourth year at university. Also, I started to spend a great deal of my time in the laboratory from my third year onwards, so the time we had together was invariably more spread apart. But we still studied for exams together, and Felicia would make time to come to my house. My parents liked her a great deal, but in our hearts we both knew that as soon as she graduated, she would have to go far away. Sometimes my thought would dwell on her impending departure and I then became overwhelmed with depression.

Inseparable, we were together for three years, from day to night. We started out as classmates, but gradually from two individuals, we united and gelled as one. We were together almost every single moment of our university years — we experienced the euphoria of shining in our studies and doing research together. This built the basis of an understanding that enabled us to jointly establish our academic careers. And thus, our common interest in the academia played an extremely important role in bringing us together.

These were the reasons why I did not believe Felicia's further study in overseas would change our feelings for each other. We had, by that time, already established a mutual trust, which was as solid as a rock. She knew this clearly, and I knew this.

3

Lifelong Mutual Commitment

Though I am already over sixty, I still look back at every single memory ever so fondly. No one can avoid birth, aging, illness, and death. Time, regardless of how long a duration, has lapsed, the death of the person closest and dearest to you will always hurt like a fresh wound.

The feelings I had for Felicia will always remain, partly because she entered into and became an inseparable part of my life, and largely for the heartfelt fact that when she went abroad, she fulfilled her promise and came back to me. I have never forgotten this simple true act of love.

Separated But for a Better Tomorrow in Future

We reached our last year at university, and I was busier than before. Despite the heavy study workload in medical school, the laboratory research I was doing progressed extremely well. At that time, like a newborn colt unafraid of anything, I shouldered as much school load as I could and withstood the stress that came with it. I was extremely busy, and Felicia also did not have a minute to spare; aside from studying with me, she had to make preparation for her departure to overseas. The time that we would be separated drew closer with each passing day, but we continued to build our common dream.

We harbored so much hopes for the future: after getting married, we hoped to work together, travel the world together, do research and publish papers jointly, and to raise high-achieving and morally upright children. When one is young, it is inevitable to be naïve and romantic, but the wondrous thing is that those faraway dreams actually came true for us.

In 1965, we left the country and went to Case Western Reserve University in Cleveland, Ohio, to do our doctoral studies. We were a twenty-four-hour couple virtually, be it studying, doing research, or in everyday life; we even later ended up in the same laboratory and supported each other in our scientific careers. And by virtue of our careers, our family had the opportunities to set foot in many different countries.

We even achieved the goal that Felicia and I set during our university days — to publish papers under the names, "Wu & Wu." In total, we wrote over thirty papers together; one of them, "Role of Intrinsic Metal in RNA Polymerase from *E. coli*: *In Vivo* Substitution of Tightly Bound Zinc with Cobalt," has already been cited over two hundred times in scientific papers all over the world. In over twenty years in the United States, Felicia published over eighty papers. Because her research on the role of zinc in gene transcription was way ahead of its time, she won acclaims and the affirmation of the international scientific community. In 1990, we edited an anthology of research papers, published by Raven Press, entitled, *The Structure and Function of Nucleic Acids and Proteins*. That was the culmination of our thirty years of research together.

Reminiscing, I marvel that after three decades of experience in academia and a lifetime dedicated to diligent research and raising children, we were never tired of taking on new intellectual challenges. And to think of this sentiment actually began from nothing but from the shared idealistic and romantic dream of two young individuals.

All our fellow classmates knew Felicia would graduate that year and leave for the United States. I was enrolled in a seven-year medical school and would not be due to graduate until a few more years later. My well-meaning classmates all advised me not to let go of Felicia to leave the country. Someone with as much talent and intelligence as Felicia was sure to have many avenues opening up before her; thus the possibility that her life would take new directions was high indeed. Furthermore, leaving the country was no easy task and a chance hard to come by, hence, many who left chose not to return.

Yet I could not allow my own self-interest to diminish and obstruct Felicia's enthusiastic quest for greater knowledge. Though it broke my heart to do so, I encouraged her to leave my warm embrace, venture abroad and experience the liberal academic and research atmosphere overseas. During her senior year, we treasured the little time we had remaining, we constructed our dreams of the future, and we learnt English diligently. In other words, we were making preparation for our future together. We thought naïvely that as long as we could get through those two years of separation, we would once again be reunited and stay together forever.

Because of the immense trust and love that Felicia and I shared, the thought of separation did not fill us with anxiety or dread. Rather, we turned our focus to look ahead in the same direction with great anticipation of the future home we would build and the dreams we would fulfill together.

A Trip Together Before Farewell

The fourth year of college flew by quickly. At that time, Felicia often experienced moments of uncertainty — she would question herself whether she should wait until we got married in order to leave the country together. However, I thought of the three years of university studies that I still had left, marriage would have to wait until I graduated. From my point of view, this would actually be the most appropriate time for her to leave the country. Of course, these discussions were only between Felicia and me; our parents knew nothing of our plans. Her parents, especially, were enthusiastic about her upcoming journey and did everything they could to help her get ready.

Just before graduation, I went along with Felicia on her class graduation trip around the island. During our second year in college, Felicia and I had talked of circumnavigating the island someday to appreciate the beautiful nature of our motherland. We looked forward to holding hands and sharing our thoughts as we held in our sight the rocky mountain slopes of Hualien and Taidong, the night view of Suao Fishing Port, and the pristine water of the Cheng Ching Lake lined with slender willow trees. The trip was to finally become a reality. Hence, you can imagine our excitement.

Once upon a time, when I was still in high school, I set off to cycle the entire island by myself. As I watched the vast expanse of land unfold before me, the feeling of relaxation and freedom intoxicated and filled in me. When evening fell, I pitched a tent and built a campfire to keep away the nocturnal critters. As I sat by the fire, I wrote my journal, laid down on my back and gazed at the stars. The journey was like an adventure. When I told Felicia about it, she said she too would like to take a trip around the island sometime. Though the graduation trip would not be a camping experience in the wilderness, it was still a rare opportunity to see the island once more before she left. But most importantly, that would be an experience we could share together.

At Taroko Gorge, we gawked at the magnificent stone cliffs and traced the outline of the peaks that pierced into the sky. The spectacle was truly a masterpiece carved out of the earth by Mother Nature. One could not help but kneel and cry out in awe in front of the majestic peaks that surged straight up from the gorge. Felicia and I held hands, we were happy to be at Taroko together. We trekked to the Eastern Coast from Taroko Gorge. We finally spotted fishing boats on the water of Suao Fishing Port, illuminated in the evening lights. We strolled along the pier, hand-in-hand. The boats lining on two sides of the banks seemed like chess pieces poised for battle. After the slow walk, we lounged relaxingly by the waterside, and enjoyed the light waft of moist, salty sea breeze upon our skin and the scent of the sea that refreshingly greeted our noses. Finally, we had a satisfying sumptuous meal, complete with beer, at a deli near the waterside. Soon, we felt a tingling sense of intoxication from the sheer beauty of the evening.

For a finishing touch, we returned to Taipei and wrapped up our graduation trip with a stroll through Yangmingshan National Park. We were intimately familiar with a stretch of road which we often walked in the past. The trip, which Felicia and I particularly treasured, brought us even closer, because of the imminent separation that lay ahead of us.

I went with Felicia's parents to send her off at the airport, she kept looking back at me as if to say, "In two years' time, I'll be back." I was choked with melancholy, but at the same time, I had complete confidence and faith that our feelings for each other could stand the test of separation. Just before she left, I gave Felicia a diary hoping that she would write her stories and experiences abroad, so that I too could share and partake in her experiences.

Father-in-Law Becomes a Friend for Life

When I had night shifts at the hospital, Felicia's father Yi-Song Chen would occasionally visit to chat. He was an extremely interesting person to talk to and was vocal with his political opinions. There was one night when he came with the intention of voicing out his political views to me.

Prior to Felicia's departure, her parents had been worried that I would put up an opposition; thus, there was naturally some tension between us. But knowing the fact that I did not express any objection, her parents actually became friendlier towards me than ever before. In fact, after Felicia left, her father came to the hospital more often to chat with me.

At that time, though we were technically not yet father and son-in-law, the feeling and bonding already existed between us. Yi-Song Chen was well-versed in a wide variety of topics; he could discuss anything under the sun from politics to philosophy, history and even literature, reveling in his passion for all genres. That evening, he came to tell me that he was planning to run for the mayor of Taipei City.

In 1964, Yi-Song Chen, Yu-Shu Kao, and Bai-Lian Chou were contesting against each other in the election. The chances of Yi-Song Chen being elected were almost non-existent; the Nationalist Party had initially pooled all their resources together to get party member Bai-Lian Chou elected, but midway through the campaign, they changed their position and rallied their support behind Yu-Shu Kao. The circumstances that happened in the election made Yi-Song Chen's mission a near impossibility. I have a great deal of respect for Yi-Song Chen's persistence in the endeavor despite knowing the fact that a defeat would adversely affect his law practice.

Because of my fluency in both Mandarin Chinese and Taiwanese, I became an interpreter at the pre-election debates. I also took on the responsibility to write some of Yi-Song Chen's campaign materials. As long as I was off my duty hour at the hospital, I would accompany Yi-Song Chen, carrying nothing but a water bottle as he hastily visited one place after another delivering speeches. He spoke one sentence, and next I would interpret one sentence. Working under the tense political climate at the time, I too had developed a sense of fearlessness. But I knew from the start that Felicia's father would lose. The results were announced. As expected, the number of votes Yi-Song Chen received was extremely low.

His financial status then was wobbly and unstable, hence, it was inevitable that this defeat brought upon him considerable damage.

This episode, however, brought Felicia's parents and me closer in a way that we could never have foreseen and imagined. When we discussed her father's political endeavors through letters, Felicia and I felt a tinge of happiness that we had never experienced before. Ironically, the separation bore positive outcomes as Felicia's parents had accepted and welcomed me into their family. As for me, I felt blessed to have another elder I could regard as both my mentor and friend, and with whom I had developed a lifelong connection.

One Heart Spanning Across Two Lands

Those two years, Felicia would write at least once a week relating to me her life, research, and studies in Minnesota. In 1962, Felicia was admitted to the department of chemistry at the University of Minnesota specializing in organic chemistry. She chose University of Minnesota because her older brother Chi-Ching was pursuing doctoral studies there at that time. Felicia's family naturally hoped that the siblings could watch out for each other. The other reason that Felicia chose University of Minnesota was its stellar reputation in the field of chemistry.

Felicia had always been very studious. From the outset, her goal was to complete her graduate studies in the shortest possible time so that she could return home and get married; thus, Felicia was more motivated in her studies than other students. Her professor, Dr. Edward Leete, was a world-renowned academic. He was not only very demanding of his students, but was also full of vibrant energy as an academician. He had the habit of running in early dawn and would invite the doctoral students and postdoctoral fellows working in his laboratory to join him. In the beginning, everyone was enthusiastic, but in the end only Felicia persisted to do the daily morning run. Her inner strength amazed those around her. Because of her never-give-up attitude, Dr. Leete heaped endless praises on her for her patience and stamina.

While in Minnesota, Felicia had a full schedule every day. On top of her busy routine of doing research in the laboratory, going to classes, and discussing her dissertation with her professor, she still found time to run every morning, write at least one or two letters to me every week, and participate in extra-curricular activities. Athletically inclined since young, Felicia enjoyed horseback riding, golf and tennis — all of which, she had mastered competencies and skills. Those days, women rarely engaged in these sports, but Felicia and her older brothers Chi-Ching and Jing-Ren, who occasionally traveled from Texas to visit her, would engage in the sports with her.

Chi-Ching remembers back then, young men around Felicia were enamoured with her youth, natural beauty and fun-loving spirit, but Felicia was not the least interested. She told all her secret admirers that she already had a wonderful boyfriend, and she would return to Taiwan and marry him after completing her Master's degree.

Our letters to each other were largely devoted to exchange of our thoughts about the research work we did. I began work at a laboratory in Taiwan; Felicia started her research career in the United States. Our affection, though in hibernation during that period, was passionately expressed in our letters and in anticipation of our reunion in the not-too-distant future. Our love was like a gust of wind: when stirred, the momentum was unstoppable. That two years was a test to our relationship laden with earnest expectation. Separation and longing could be a painful experience, but we felt that it was worth the wait knowing the future would be a life together of mutual love and support.

I have a brown lambswool overcoat which I have worn for thirty, perhaps even forty years. Felicia sent me this coat from Minnesota in 1963. She scrimped and saved in order to pay for it. During the time of material scarcity in Taiwan, the coat was deemed as an expensive item, but the love and thoughtfulness of the woman who bought it were priceless to me. Whenever I put on the coat to keep myself warm during the winter seasons abroad, I would remember our younger days and our ocean-deep affection. The coat accompanies me till this very day.

Becoming a Family, Finally

Felicia appeared amidst the dense crowd of people at Taipei Songshan Airport — with her long hair falling over her shoulders, and her infectious smile on her face. My whole family, Felicia's family were there, and, of course, including me. I looked longingly at Felicia who was standing right in front of us. At long last, she had returned.

Without a moment of hesitation, Felicia took my hands and smiled widely, aglow with affection; her lovely eyes glistening with jubilance and excitement. She looked tanner. Two weeks before returning to Taiwan, she visited all of America's most famous colleges, and gathered informational materials for our future journey there to pursue further studies. While doing the college exploratory trip, she had the opportunity to do some sightseeing, so when she arrived home, her complexion was bronzed with a healthy shade of copper.

Felicia returned to Taiwan in September 1964. We were engaged on October 20 and got married on November 10. Two lovers had finally entered the holy sacrament of marriage. Our hearts brimmed with joy and love for each other. Our engagement followed the practices of Taiwanese customary traditions which include seeking permission from our parents, savoring the engagement cookies, drinking the ceremonial tea, and exchanging red packets. The engagement ring for Felicia was commissioned by her parents as a commemoration to Felicia's fulfilment of promise to return to Taiwan and her faithful commitment to love. This engagement ring also symbolized our everlasting and unchanging love for each other.

Alas, July 18, 1999 was the most heartbreaking day in my life. Felicia's condition became critical and she had to be transferred to the intensive care unit, the nurse removed Felicia's engagement ring and handed it to me. Felicia's sudden departure struck me unprepared, and I was not quite myself. It was not until the next day when I returned home exhausted after settling various procedural matters at the hospital, that I put the ring away in a drawer. After Felicia's funeral, when I went to look for the ring, I was shocked to discover that I could no longer find it. Until today, the loss causes me great distress. To some people, a ring is merely a representation of marriage, but to me, it is a divine vow of a lifelong commitment and trust. Every time I think of the ring, I sink into abysmal grief.

The witness of our wedding was former Taipei City mayor San-Lian Wu; at that time, he was the chairman of the Wu Clan Association as well as a well-respected senior in the Taiwanese political arena. Introducing Felicia as the bride was her uncle Huo-Yau Wei, then Dean of the National

Taiwan University Medical School. The wedding was held at Chungshan Hall, a venue considered the grandest at that time. Bound by marriage, Felicia and I were finally ready to step forward hand-in-hand to realize our common dream — to create a home which embodies not only romantic love, but also parental love and universal kindness. We would share the joy of raising our little ones together and fill the house with boundless love and warmth. I have no regrets because Felicia had been a wonderful wife and devoted mother throughout her life.

After we got married, Felicia worked as a special assistant in the biochemistry department of the United States Naval Medical Research Unit No. 2 in Taipei. Her primary responsibility was to collect information on the genetic mutation of red blood cells. Her workplace was located at what is presently known as the Jing-Fu Building at the National Taiwan University Hospital where I was completing my final term of internship, hence, we commuted by scooter to and from work together, much to the envy of all our friends.

Military Service at Kinmen

Felicia and I once again faced separation after our wedding. As newlyweds, we were joined at the hip, as if we were stuck together inseparably. I knew that upon graduation from the medical school, I had to be conscripted to fulfill my military service. However, I would never imagine in what was considered as random allocation and placement, I would be posted to Kinmen, an offshore island also known as Quemoy near mainland China. Felicia was deeply saddened to know that I had to go so far away, as we were just married for half a year. What's more, at that time, the relationship across the strait between Kinmen and China was extremely tense, with skirmishes breaking out from time to time. During that period, what all parents in Taiwan feared most was that their son would be conscripted to Kinmen. Unfortunately, I happened to be one of the so-called "lucky" ones, so to speak.

Felicia accompanied me to Kaohsiung where I would travel by sea across the Taiwan Strait to Kinmen. We were reluctant and could not bear to leave each other. I joined the other new conscripts and entered a vessel cabin for the first time in my life. The cabin was dark and humid; I had the faintest idea that the wind and waves in the open sea would be so strong and ferocious. In my mind, Kinmen marks a significant phase in my life, and in Felicia's life as well. Many years later, our family visited the island, albeit as tourists. However, upon arrival on that embattled island as a new conscript, all I could think of was to take good care of myself for the sake of my family and Felicia.

At Kinmen, I served as a medical officer in Division 26 of the Medical Corps. Other than being in charge of the health condition of the soldiers in that division, I was also responsible for providing medical care to the three thousand civilians living in Kinshi Base, located on the western part of Kinmen. A watchtower atop a mountain was where the soldiers stayed. The Base Medical Office soldiers, however, stayed at a private Siheyuan[1] residence. I was stationed at the Base Medical Office where the civilians came under my care. Because I was the only certified doctor at Kinshi Base, I was treated with the respect usually garnered by a superior officer.

Felicia desperately wanted to come and see me, so she and my older sister Yue-Mei joined the Glorious Star Choir, knowing that the choir would travel to Kinmen in a couple of months' time to entertain the troops. I was in Kinmen for four or five months when I received Felicia's letter saying that she and my older sister were coming soon. I was astounded and in awe; I had had no idea that she would go to such great length and effort to come and visit me.

Meeting Felicia and my older sister, finally, greatly uplifted my spirits. The thought that they braved the turbulent times in Kinmen without fear to come here deeply touched my heart. Being surrounded by many people who loved and cared for me was a fortunate thing and a consolation to me, despite being away in Kinmen. That day, as I listened to the Glorious Star Choir perform uplifting renditions of various patriotic songs, while immersed in Felicia's and my older sister's radiant smiles, I was incredibly moved.

After the Glorious Star Choir performed, they immediately departed and returned to Taiwan. Felicia, however, stayed behind to accompany me.

---

[1] The term Siheyuan literally means a "four-sided enclosed courtyard." It refers to a traditional Chinese architectural style in which a courtyard is formed by houses flanking on all four sides and surrounded by enclosure walls.

Strictly speaking, this was against the rules and regulations of Kinmen Base, but my friend Colonel Chu helped me obtain the permission for her to stay. At first, the permission granted was only for one evening, but as luck would have it, we experienced five straight days of bad weather during which it was not safe for planes to take off or land, so Felicia was able to extend her stay. Well, that just goes to show that no matter how much one plans things out, Mother Nature always intervenes.

Felicia and I stayed at the Siheyuan. She came along with me to the medical office to understand my work with the patients there. The Kinmen people are extremely warm-hearted. Knowing that Felicia had come to visit, they gave us fish and eggs, which were rare luxuries for a soldier. With the food, the soldiers whipped up a delicious meal that was imbued with the warmth of friendship of the Kinmen people.

Kinmen was a place that was inaccessible to the ordinary Taiwanese folks. Colonel Chu knew that Felicia and I rarely had the opportunity to be together, so he generously assigned a soldier to take us around the island in a jeep. I could still remember that this sincere and friendly soldier's name was Chun-Hsiong Chen.

Those five days were like our honeymoon. We took the jeep and traveled to the point on Kinmen Island that faces directly opposite to the city of Xiamen on the mainland. Through the binoculars, we could see the streets of Xiamen, as well as students of the Xiamen University playing basketball in the far distance. Geographically, the cross-strait distance seems close-by like the thin, fine line of the horizon but a vast ocean of difference separates the two. A feeling of sadness welled up within us as we looked through the binoculars.

Memories of Kinmen

It was twenty-five years later, in 1990. Felicia and I returned to Taiwan, and we were working at the Institute of Biomedical Sciences in Academia Sinica. At a meeting, I happened to bump into General Cheng-Ping Ma, the then Chief of the Bureau of the Medical Corps. It came naturally without thinking, I rattled off my memories of my military service at Kinmen. He replied heartily that I should go back to visit, for the island had changed a great deal. Felicia and I were immediately excited by the idea, and our three children, David, Faith, and Albert, who had heard so many stories of Kinmen during their growing up years, found the excitement contagious. Since all our three children happened to be in Taiwan, it seemed that was an opportune time for us to visit the island together. We decided on a three-day trip to Kinmen. General Ma made all the arrangements and took us on a tour of the island himself.

During the trip, I found the island clean, the sky clear, and the land green and lush. There was an orderliness about the place. The tension on the streets with frequent sight of soldiers in their military greens two decades earlier had disappeared. The island seemed to have returned to its sparkle, reclaiming its original beauty as an island and small town. Felicia and I hoped to be able to re-visit the old, familiar spots, and be reunited with old friends.

General Ma met us on the plane. A quarter of a century later since we were last there, we realized Kinshi had become a different place. Felicia and I went around to look for the old movie theatre and pool hall, but we were unable to find them at first. We were a little disappointed, but we did not give up. We asked the people there for directions, and finally, as we roamed and wandered off farther and longer, we found the old movie theatre hidden among the newer, and more modern buildings. The movie theatre had apparently closed down for quite some time. Adjourning to the movie theatre was the Siheyuan residence which had previously served as the Base Medical Office.

Our knock at the door was answered by a woman in her sixties; as soon as she saw me, she exclaimed, "Dr. Wu, you've returned! And your wife, did she come with you?" Her words brought tears to my eyes; two-and-a-half decades had flown by, she could still remember a young medical officer being stationed here, as well as his wife who traveled far to visit him. This old woman said I had saved her life once when I was stationed there. I had long forgotten, but she never forgot that. Felicia was moved to tears. The old lady showed us a picture of Felicia and me. We were touched.

That evening, we stayed at a guest quarter in Kinmen and spent the whole evening reminiscing and recounting old stories with the old friends in the village who came to visit us. They said I was remembered fondly as a medical officer who took good care of the well-being of the villagers, and saved quite a number of lives. However, deeply etched in the memories of the villagers about me was — at a time when any ordinary folks from Taiwan were not allowed to travel to Kinmen, and obtaining a travel permission was virtually impossible — Felicia overcame all obstacles and found a way to travel to Kinmen.

Felicia and I looked at each other and smiled. For over two decades together as a couple we had weathered many ups and downs in life together, including my military service days which happened eons ago. Kinmen inadvertently became a testament to our relationship and enduring love. At this point, our children were able to witness this moving reunion, and understand the path that their mother and father had trodden together in their lives.

Our connection to Kinmen in fact extended to both sides of the Taiwan Strait. In 1990, we traveled together to participate in the Asian Pacific Cell Biology Conference in Shanghai. Among the participants was well-known Chinese cell biologist De-Yao Wang, who was then teaching at Xiamen University. He invited us to visit Taiwan Research Institute of the Xiamen University, and we gratefully accepted.

Seen through a set of binoculars two decades earlier, Xiamen, to us, was a fantasy world. We now stood on the rooftop of Xiamen University's Taiwan Research Institute, and over the edge, we looked afar. The sight of Kinmen unfolded before us. Twenty-five years when well water does not intrude the river water, political affairs have a way of working out. Not only had we both aged, the cross-strait relations had also changed dramatically. Back then, Felicia and I were recently married — only half a year. The call of duty to protect our country culminated to our separation. Undeterred by the unpredictable conditions in Kinmen, Felicia tried every avenue and found a way to visit me. The fruition of our happy reunion was our another unforgettable piece of memory that strengthened our bonding.

We held up our binoculars. The hand of the copper statue of Cheng-Gong Cheng (also known as Koxinga) in Kinmen points toward China; on the Xiamen side, another majestic copper statue of Cheng-Gong Cheng faces toward Taiwan. The two coasts across the strait have unwittingly come together. Felicia and I would never have thought that the day would come when we would have the opportunity to stand across the coast once again and hold hands, and admire the horizon and gaze out over Kinmen.

Many changes took place over those twenty years. To say nothing of the politics, life in itself within such a span of time already has its ups and downs. Our family hit its nadir when news of Felicia's illness broke. But she was always brave; no matter what happened, she never furrowed her eyebrows. As her companion who went through the ordeal with her, I knew that despite her optimism and openness, there lurked a bleak and dark abyss of hopelessness deep in the recesses of her heart that she occasionally fell into, and hid away from us. As a scientist, Felicia fully understood in entirety the reality and all the possibilities her condition would bring; as an individual who cherished her life, she was forced to come to terms with the fact that she would lose it within a known quantifiable period of time. Felicia's ability to deal with such immense burden was beyond us and our imagination.

Time stands witness to the trials and tribulations of life, tracing and tracking our past like marks of goose claws in the snow. What is life? Perhaps we do not know what the next turn will bring and how high the next wave we will have to surmount, but with Felicia around, there is hope and love in life. The Kinmen-Xiamen relation in that twenty-five years zipped by like a snap of one's fingers in the vast boundless universe. To us, Felicia and I, regardless of which coast we are on, which corner of the earth we stand, or whatever space, time and dimension we end up in, we remain inseparable and our existence, though temporal, will live in eternity. I am convinced that up in the Heaven, Felicia's radiant soul agrees with me.

4

Studying Abroad

Till today, I still think of the smile of Felicia, her thirst for new things and knowledge, and her enthusiasm to take on fresh challenges. While I was serving my military duties in Kinmen, Felicia worked at the United States Navy Medical Research Unit No. 2. She would ride my 50 cc scooter to commute to work. The scooter was a fashionable mode of transport on the streets of Taipei in the 1960s; furthermore, to see a pretty, young girl speeding by on one was an extremely rare sight. The impression and image that she could have conjured bring a smile to me.

We had many great dreams for our future such as traveling abroad together to study and establishing our mark in the academia. Felicia was always the motivator to propel our dreams forward. During that period when I was in Kinmen, she would be busy researching on the prerequisites for scholarships, admissions applications and the like. By the time I completed the military service, Felicia had already taken care of virtually everything that was needed for us to study abroad.

In the end, we chose to go to Case Western Reserve University because its biochemistry department was ranked among the top ten in the United States, and also because it was the only school that offered scholarships to both of us. Taiwan underwent an economic recession at that time, thus, only the more affluent families could afford to send their children to schools in the United States. In addition, Felicia's second elder brother Jing-Ren was in Cleveland, and we would have someone to look and watch out for. Our decision was made, and we set off to pursue our dreams.

A Mountain of Obstacles to Get Out of the Country Again

My father-in-law, Yi-Song Chen, had a unique way of doing things. During the White Terror era, he ran for the city mayor post and challenged the government's authority. Although the government treated him with leniency, he was in the blacklist. When Felicia was doing her Master's degree in the United States, she came into contact with various parties which opposed against the Taiwan's political situation at the time, and knowing that she was the daughter of the famous human rights lawyer, Yi-Song Chen, the dissidents would occasionally send her propaganda material. Even though Felicia had no particular interest in politics, the political message somewhat aroused her curiosity.

She wanted to share this literature with me, but feared the tensions of the political climate, so she tore out the page of the material and used it to wrap some photographs that she was going to send me. That particular package never reached me. She, of course, did not bring it up after that, thinking that it was a closed case.

When we received our admissions letters, we rushed to apply for our exit visas. I received mine immediately, but for some reasons, Felicia did not receive hers. As the start of school term was fast approaching, we began to worry.

In the 1960s, the government did not make public their policy on immigration control, but we did know that the Taiwan Garrison Headquarters handled all applications for exit and entry into the country. After pursuing the issue, we found out that Felicia's application had reached the Taiwan Garrison Headquarters, but the paper trail stopped there. We asked around to see if we could find out why. One of my superiors at Kinmen said that if we were to pay a token sum of money the paperwork would go through, and he also heard from someone inside the Taiwan Garrison Headquarters that NT$10,000 would be sufficient. That was a large sum of money during those days, but on seeing that we were determined to study in the United States, my parents offered to give us the full amount. But all that was for nothing, the money went down the drain and we still did not hear anything about Felicia's application.

We were unwilling to give up. We wrote a letter to the Taiwan Garrison Headquarters inquiring into the matter. They sent a response, which simply stated, "Request denied." We had exhausted all the methods we could think of, and there was only a week left before the school term began. I had to go, but what about Felicia? What were we to do? We were at a loss, especially since Felicia was already pregnant!

The First Child That We Lost

Actually, this was Felicia's second pregnancy — our second baby. Our first baby Long-Sheng was born during my service in Kinmen, but unfortunately he died not long after. Felicia and I often told our three children about their elder brother. Although our only impression of him was his cheeks, large doleful eyes, and his weak, soft whimper due to the injury he sustained at childbirth, we still loved him dearly.

Felicia was healthy throughout her first pregnancy; we had no idea that something was amiss. She had prenatal examinations on a regular basis, but none of these examinations revealed that the baby was in the breech position. It was not until she had been sent to the hospital and the baby would not come out that we discovered that something was really wrong.

At that moment, the doctor sought us out for a discussion; we had two choices. The first was Caesarean section. The disadvantage of Caesarean section was that if Felicia were to have another child, the child would also have to be delivered the same way, and in addition, she could only have at most two children. Thirty years ago, medicine was not as advanced as today; Caesarean sections were considered high-risk operations. Thus, on top of the disadvantage that she would only be able to have two children, the operation itself might pose a risk to Felicia's life.

Our alternative option was birth through natural methods. Felicia would have to endure even greater pain and stronger contractions. Although natural birth would be excruciatingly painful, there was a ninety-five percent chance of success. After discussion, Felicia decided that with a ninety-five percent chance of success, natural birth was the obvious choice. Felicia was already in tremendous pain, but she thought as long as it was possible to have natural childbirth, she would endure the pain and avoid having the Caesarean birth.

Giving birth to a child who is not in the normal head-down position is very difficult. The doctor must use both hands to find a way to rotate the baby around, while at the same time worrying that the umbilical cord might coil itself around the baby and cause him or her to suffocate. Felicia pushed with all her might, her entire body broke out in so much sweat that it seemed as if she had been drenched in a rainstorm, but despite all her efforts, the baby could not come out. Finally, worried that the baby might suffocate, the doctor used a pair of forceps to pull the baby out.

When Long-Sheng was born, his cry was soft like a cat, weak and fragile; his two large eyes seemed to glisten, but pain was evident in his eyes. His eyes darted around the room for a while and then closed. Though Felicia's strength was spent, she still held the baby, giving her all — her endearing motherly love and warmth — to her baby. But the tongs and the force applied had been much too strong; the newborn baby's brain had already been damaged!

The doctor shook his head regretfully and immediately sent the child to the infant care room. I looked at Felicia's face, exhausted and void of expression. I was concerned about the health of both Felicia and the baby. I named the baby Long-Sheng (which meant "Dragon Voice"), the second character taking the meaning of voice. Little did we expect that Long-Sheng's sojourn in this world could be so transient, before we could wait to hear him make a "roaring" impact, the very next afternoon, he passed away.

Felicia was terribly saddened. After her discharge from the hospital, she stayed inside the room and refused to come out, crying continuously the whole time. I comforted her by saying that though Long-Sheng's early death was unfortunate to us, it was a fortunate thing to him because a child who is mentally handicapped will meet with more difficulties and obstacles in the course of his life compared to a normal child. At that time, I did my best to bring solace to Felicia. At night, I would take her to Long-Shan Temple to grab a bite to eat, tease her to make her smile, and tell her that, soon, we would have another child. I did everything I could think of to help her forget her pain and cheer her up.

That was the first difficult and painful period in Felicia's life. I hoped she could have another child soon, to ease the pain of the loss of her first child, and to abate the loneliness she faced due to her separation from Long-Sheng.

The Garrison Headquarters Incident

Felicia became pregnant again while we were applying for schools. We could hardly believe our eyes when we received the letter from the Taiwan Garrison Headquarters. How could I leave my wife all by herself, not to mention our precious unborn baby — the crystallizaiton of our love? Classes had already begun, and we really could not wait any longer.

Felicia was naturally concerned, but she urged me to go ahead without her, insisting that she would think of a way for us to be together. I knew she was saying that just to comfort me and motivate me to go because she didn't want me to miss the classes. I knew distinctly that if she could not get the permission to leave the country this time, she would likely never be able to study abroad again. How grossly unfair! She had given up the opportunity of continuing to remain in the U.S. to get a Ph.D. because of me. Without hesitation, she came all the way back to Taiwan in order to marry me. If her study plans were cut short because of our marriage, I would never be able to forgive myself.

Two nights before my departure, I tossed and turned and was unable to sleep. Facing Felicia and her baby bump, I resolved that I must find a way to keep our family together at all cost — Felicia and I and our own flesh and blood, we must not be separated in two continents again.

The night before I was to leave the country, I mustered up the courage to visit the second-in-command in Taiwan Garrison Headquarters at his residence. Lifting my finger, I pressed the doorbell. From within the high walls, an extremely gruff voice barked, "Who's there?" That voice sounded like a guard.

The then second-in-command at Taiwan Garrison Headquarters was a man named Li-Bo Lee; he happened to be the father of one of my junior high school classmates, Ben-Tang Lee. I went to Ben-Tang Lee's house once during my junior high school day, so I knew his father was an important figure at the Taiwan Garrison Headquarters. Unfortunately, Ben-Tang Lee was already in overseas then, and we thus gradually lost contact. Nevertheless, that was the last resort I could think of to help Felicia and the unborn child in her womb.

Although the guard's voice was not at all friendly, I replied in a firm, loud voice, "I am Ben-Tang Lee's junior high school classmate Cheng-Wen Wu. I know Ben-Tang Lee is out of the country, but I have come to speak to Uncle Lee." Still, the guard refused to open the door, but luckily for me, Ben-Tang Lee's younger sister knew me and heard my voice from inside the house. She told the guard, "Wait, he's my elder brother's classmate." Then, she opened the door herself and took me inside. I then saw Li-Bo Lee, the second-in-command of the Taiwan Garrison Headquarters.

A little to my surprise, Li-Bo Lee asked me in a friendly tone what the matter was. I could still remember the scene. I explained, "Uncle Lee, I have exhausted every possible option I could think of to obtain permission for my wife to study abroad, and I'm at the end of my tether. I have come here today hoping to know the reason why my wife's application has been denied." Then I told him that Felicia's application had been held up at the Taiwan Garrison Headquarters and her father was Yi-Song Chen, but she had never participated in any political movements. Furthermore, she was already married, therefore it was not possible for her to involve in her father's political matters.

I explained to him how Felicia had given up the opportunity to continue her studies to come back so that we could marry, and now it was she who was not able to leave the country. Going through all these, the most frustrating part was that I really had no idea why her application did not go through at the Taiwan Garrison Headquarters.

"Tomorrow I'll be leaving the country, so tonight I come here to request for your help. I can't bear the thought that Felicia came back and sacrificed her future because of me." Those were my parting words to Li-Bo Lee. After that, he simply nodded his head and promised that he would look into the matter.

I left for the Case Western Reserve University the next morning. The whole family including Felicia came to see me off. My heart was full of mixed emotions. I couldn't bear to leave both my parents and parents-in-law, and I couldn't bear to leave my wife who was heavy with a child. I was extremely worried that if there was really no way for Felicia to leave, we would be separated once again. The clouds outside the aircraft window seemed thick and heavy like a silk tapestry, and the sound of the engines whirred like an owl in flight. Though I should be happy to finally embark on an eye-opening journey of the academic world ahead of me, without Felicia, all seemed lost.

Miracle happened. Not long after I arrived in Cleveland, I received a letter from Felicia stating that the Taiwan Garrison Headquarters had already contacted her about coming in for an interview. The situation had turned optimistic. One week later when Felicia arrived in Cleveland, she told me the root of the problem was the propaganda material which she used to wrap the pictures that were meant to be sent to me. The Taiwan Garrison Headquarters had labeled her a pro-independence activist because of that.

Gaining Entry into the United States

Felicia left the country to study abroad for a second time, and the "Garrison Headquarters Incident" became albeit a small episode of her life story. Truth be told, when Felicia came back the first time to get married, we already knew that to leave the country together to study abroad would not be an easy task. At that time, Taiwan and the United States still maintained diplomatic relations, so the American embassy made the final decision on whether Taiwanese citizens could enter the United States. If an immigration officer had any hunch that a foreigner might harbor the intention of staying in the United States permanently, the officer would deny the visa application. I didn't encounter any problem because I left the country alone, but Felicia encountered problems because the United States government did not view too favorably at married couples leaving the country together. The chance that they would decide to stay in America and not return to Taiwan was much higher.

Therefore, before leaving the country, I wrote a letter to the American ambassador to Taiwan to enquire whether the United States law stipulate a couple could not enter the United States at the same time to study. I had never thought the ambassador would actually reply my letter, but he did, stating that the United States has no such law. Before my departure, I left the ambassador's letter of reply with Felicia and told her that if she received approval from the Taiwan Garrison Headquarters, she should give this letter to the immigration officer at the embassy when she went to apply for her visa.

Unfortunately, when Felicia went to obtain the stamp of visa, she ended up coming face-to-face with a stern-looking immigration officer. He said in a gruff, ill-tempered tone, "I can't grant you a visa because your husband is already in the United States." Composed and unruffled, Felicia took out the letter in which the ambassador expressed his opinion on the matter. The immigration officer looked stunned for a moment. He could have thought that Felicia was well-connected and perhaps a personal friend of the ambassador. Since he did not dare to go against the wishes of his superior, Felicia was granted her visa without further trouble.

The final challenge was getting past the customs officers, who would have the final word. At that time Felicia was already five months pregnant. Customs clearance was most likely not going to be easy. But luckily, when she entered the United States, it was already the beginning of November; Cleveland showed the first signs of winter, and the weather was extremely cold. Felicia managed to hide her baby bump under her heavy winter coat. When her second elder brother Jing-Ren and I finally saw her at the airport lounge, we both heaved a huge sigh of relief. At that point of time, classes had already been in session for a month.

As this episode of Felicia's story clearly demonstrates, in the 1960s it was not easy for any citizens to travel out of Taiwan. We were just ordinary folks, a couple passionately in love, with boundless hopes for the academic world before us. At that time in Taiwan, a doctor who graduated from the medical school was guaranteed both money and respect. My father also wished I would start a medical practice at home. But that was not what Felicia and I wanted. Our dream was to explore the various fields of knowledge. What we experienced in those days were challenges and difficulties that were inconceivable to the young people today — in pursuit of our ideals, we inevitably disappointed our parents for not being able to fulfill their expectation of us, and Felicia's second trip out of the country was full of adversities and obstacles.

But she had finally succeeded. We were separated for a month. More than ever, we understood how imperative it was for us not to be separated again.

After leaving the country, we would continue to encounter difficulties in academia as well as in our everyday life, but as long as we were together, we were ready to overcome any obstacles that stood in our way.

Seated in elder brother Jing-Ren's car, the world outside was draped in a hazy fog and the temperature, bitterly cold. Felicia held my hand and snuggled up to me, settling into my embrace. I put on the large overcoat which she gave me. Though the passing scenery of the world outside the car window seemed boundless and remotely alien, it was the world we saw in our dreams. As we embraced, we felt warmth despite the cold and frost.

We were separated for only a month, but our hearts were filled with unspeakable longing for each other. The feeling of home and our soon-to-be-born child kept us together. We had created another little life. This reality led us to the understanding that life is navigated by the two forces of love and responsibility. Our lives bore testimony to this belief.

Financially Struggling but Fearless of Hardships

When we first arrived in the United States, we only had two hundred dollars to our name. My father bought Felicia and me two air tickets and gave us two hundred dollars; we had to rely on ourselves for the rest of our academic and living expenses. Felicia and I would each receive a scholarship of two hundred dollars a month. Half of my scholarship would be used to pay the rent; the other half I would have to send home. So at the outset, all my scholarship was already accounted for; Felicia's scholarship of two hundred dollars was all that we had to live on each month.

At the Case Western Reserve University, Felicia continued to study chemistry, and I went to the biochemistry department at the medical school. During the first half of the year we had lots of homework, especially since I had to make up for the physical chemistry classes which I had not taken back in my college days. Because Felicia had to juggle school and the preparation for motherhood, she had a particularly tough time. Just as the first semester concluded, Felicia gave birth to our eldest son. In the bitter winter cold against a backdrop of pure white snow, David was born into the welcoming arms of two financially struggling but delighted parents. The child we waited in earnest anticipation had finally arrived.

After nursing the baby for just two weeks, classes started again. Felicia had not yet completely recovered from the childbirth. In addition, our little son David had jaundice when he was born, so we had to take him to the hospital every day to have his blood checked. The snow penetrated our warm clothing, and chilled our skin as we made our way through the bitter cold wind. Felicia and I took slow, measured steps as we carried our little David, taking care not to slip on the wet and slippery snow. The walk to the hospital took at least forty minutes. The cold was unbearable even to us adults, let alone our little newborn son, David.

I was worried that the numbing cold would freeze and take a toll on David, so I took out the two hundred dollars that my father gave us and our entire savings, which was another two hundred dollars, and bought an old, cranky car. Jing-Ren taught me how to drive. The first time I took the car out on the road, it swerved and traced the shape of an S in the snow. Even parking by the side of the road was difficult. But for the sake of David and Felicia, who had not yet returned to her full strength after her child delivery, I forced myself to take the old car out on the road.

When classes started again, Felicia requested to be allowed to take fewer courses so that she would have time to take care of David. Unfortunately, the school replied that should Felicia take a lighter course load, her scholarship would be revoked. At that time, Felicia's scholarship was our family's only source of income, since my scholarship went to support my family back in Taiwan and pay our rent in Cleveland. If Felicia's scholarship were to be revoked, then we would have trouble supporting ourselves.

Felicia pondered the situation for a long time, she finally gritted her teeth and decided to continue to go to class. Since there were only the two of us taking care of David, we figured out a plan to take turns to watch him. Felicia would look after him the first half of the night; she would then get up at dawn to go to class. I would watch him the second half of the night, and go to class after half-past nine. For common classes, just one of us would need to attend and take notes. We would then discuss the material together at home. If we had different classes during the same time slot, we had to find someone to babysit David. We were accustomed to studying together during our undergraduate days, though this study arrangement was difficult and challenging, it was still manageable.

We could get by our classes with this arrangement, but on days when we had examinations, we had to find someone to babysit David for the entire day. Usually we would put up a posting the week before our exams to look for a babysitter.

Little David Accompanies His Struggling Parents

In the days thereafter, there were two incidents that subsequently became our frequent fodder for conversation about David's care. The first incident happened on the day of an examination, we went to the babysitter's house, rang the bell for over ten minutes, but there was no answer. Apparently, she had forgotten. We frantically called all our classmates, desperately trying to find someone to look after David. When we finally found someone, took David to meet the babysitter, and rushed to the test location, we only had thirty minutes left to complete the test.

Another incident caused Felicia a great deal of heartache. It happened on an exam day, we took David along with four bottles of milk to the designated babysitter's house at the crack of dawn. The babysitter opened the door, looking bleary-eyed like she had just been roused out of her sleep. We were deeply concerned, but decided to trust her. So after putting David down on the sofa and thanking the babysitter profusely, we hurried over to the exam venue.

It was already half-past five in the evening after we finished the examination. Felicia went home to prepare dinner, and I hurried over to fetch David home. I arrived at the babysitter's front door, I could hear the faint, plaintive cries of a baby from within. The crying started and stopped, as if the baby wanted to cry but was unable to. I was furious. I pressed the doorbell repeatedly, but I still ended up waiting for ten minutes before the babysitter, hair tousled and eyes still heavy with sleep, came to answer the door. When she saw me, she still had the nerve to ask in surprise, "Why are you back so early? Isn't it only noon?"

Enraged, I strode into the house without a word and spotted David on the couch crying his heart out. The four bottles of milk that Felicia had filled that morning still stood on the coffee table. Our child had had neither a single drop of milk nor water for the entire day. My heart broke. Without exchanging a word, I held David up and walked out of the door.

When I reached home and Felicia caught sight of David, she immediately broke out in tears. She held him close to her, and whispered to David that she was sorry, her voice was filled with deep remorse that only a parent is capable of feeling it. And how would I not feel the same way? Looking at David, I just hoped that I could graduate soon and never to put our beloved young son to any discomfort and inconvenience.

When David was born, we went through the most difficult period that we would encounter in the United States. Not only did we have to devote our energies to schoolwork, we also had to survive and live by with only two hundred dollars a month. After David was born, we were so tight financially that our clothes were practically worn-out with holes at the elbows. Felicia was able to nurse David for three months, but because she had to attend classes, there was no way for her to breastfeed him at regular intervals, so he had to drink milk prepared from infant formula powder. However, we didn't even have the money to buy milk powder.

David's milk came from the donations of the children's ward of hospitals. Every month, manufacturers of milk powder would donate their product to hospitals which would then distribute free of charge to needy households with young children. Felicia and I were two such recipients. Every month we went to the hospital and took home a carton of milk powder, which became the means of David's sustenance.

There goes a line in a famous poem by Yuan-Zhen: "The impoverished couple faces a hundred difficulties and achieves little in life." Felicia and I didn't think that way; our dream was to leave the country, pursue further education, raise a family, and create a home filled with love and warmth. We knew that we would have to endure countless difficult times, but we believed these struggles would only strengthen our family and our mutual bonds. Only upon looking back did we realize the difficulties that we went through. But they did not seem so difficult then. Fortunately for us, as time flew, our love continued to flourish, and in the midst of all our struggles, our family bonding grew stronger as well. Thus, the hardships toughened us and enabled our rare and precious love to shine through brighter than before.

A year later, Felicia and I had the good fortune of meeting a wonderful person who took care of David and became to this day someone whom David still remembers fondly as "Yuan Mama."

This lady's husband was from mainland China. He was a doctor, and his name was Song-Ling Yuan. Dr. Yuan was unable to practice medicine in the United States; he could only be an assistant in the medical laboratory because he had no license to work in the United States. Other than living on their savings, they would occasionally take on odd jobs to supplement their income.

We met Mrs. Yuan near the school. She understood the difficulties that we two poor students encountered and was quick to lend a helping hand. She took care of David and only charged a dollar a day; this was how much we used to pay per hour to babysitters who took care of David on our exam days. Mrs. Yuan was really warm-hearted; she only accepted the dollar as a token of goodwill. But what moved us most is that she truly loved and doted on David, and treated him as she would like her own grandson. Thus, Felicia and I paid thirty dollars every month for David's care and for peace of mind. Knowing that David was in good hands, we could finally concentrate on our studies. Felicia often said that without Mrs. Yuan, she wondered whether she would ever be able to graduate.

Support from Both the School and Home

Felicia's doctoral dissertation was on organic chemistry as before. Her dissertation advisor was a highly esteemed organic chemistry professor, J. Eric Nordlander. He was full of admiration for Felicia's capabilities and always encouraged her to develop further academically. Dr. Nordlander passed away due to cancer at a young age while at his prime. Thinking of him makes one sigh and wonder if God was perhaps jealous of his offspring and wielded retribution, or whether Lord purposefully chose the same fate for both teacher and student. Her entire life, Felicia dedicated herself completely to her field of academic expertise; she did not allow herself to slack for even a single moment. Besides those years of relentless fight against cancer, I marvel at how she managed to struggle tirelessly in every aspect of her life as I reflect upon the drive and persistence she demonstrated as an academic.

My doctoral dissertation advisor, David Goldthwait, still goes strong and healthy to this day. To me, he is both a father and a teacher. I owe him a great deal for what I have been able to achieve academically.

My doctoral dissertation was on RNA polymerase in bacteria. Before me, there was another student who had been working on the project for two years, but had not been unable to isolate the enzyme. Within the span of half a year after taking over the project, I succeeded in isolating the enzyme from the bacteria several times. This also meant that I had to stay in the laboratory and go without sleep for days on end. Each time after the enzymes were separated from the bacteria, I would have to stay until three or four o'clock in the morning to work. Once I had finished, I would give a call to Felicia, and she would fetch me home in the car.

In fact, Felicia provided the support necessary for me to complete the research for my dissertation. While I was in the laboratory, she was at home taking care of our child; at night, she would come and drive me home regardless of the time and whether she was already in bed when I called. Although not tangibly visible to those around us, the burden she shouldered was truly heavy. From the start, Felicia's and my academic careers were inextricably intertwined. Without her support and encouragement, we would not have enjoyed our joint achievements.

Three years passed by. Day after day, it was a repeated cycle of classes, experiments, examinations, dissertation writing and child care. But in the midst of our arduous struggle, we could still taste sweetness. Somehow, the everyday experiences we shared added up and became the wellspring of emotional strength for our family. Various stories of our time in Cleveland became our family's treasure of eternal memories.

The Lunch Boxes — Twenty-Three Years of Gastronomic Delight

For twenty-three years in the United States, I had a lunch box waiting for me every day at noon; there was not a single day that I went without one. Sometimes when I was busy in the laboratory, Felicia would prepare two meals. Besides being a top-notch scientist, she fulfilled the roles of wife and mother in perfect synchrony. I was always amazed by her passion and energy.

At Case Western Reserve University, we would always have teacher and student discussions at the laboratory during lunch time. I would usually heat my food on the steamer in the laboratory, and the delicious aroma filled the whole room. While my other colleagues had their apple or sandwich for lunch, mine was a complete meal that came with hot soup as well. Soon, my colleagues' curiosity bowled them over, and they asked to have a taste of my food. Thereafter, they were won over and praised Felicia's cooking to no end.

My other story that has to do with lunch boxes concerns the nostalgia for one's homeland and cuisine. There was a Japanese American professor by the name of Warwick Sakami from my department; he was born and raised in the United States. During the Second World War, he served in the military and fought for the United States in Europe. Quite to his surprise and outrage, when the United States declared war on Japan, the government threw him in a concentration camp. After the war, he immigrated to Japan and was again aghast when the Japanese treated him as a foreigner. With no country to call his own, he finally moved back to the United States. That was the depressing plight faced by many of the descendants of immigrants!

On evenings when I had to work late in the laboratory, Felicia would prepare an extra lunch box; at times, it would be sushi. Conducting experiments was the occasion when everyone, including Professor Sakami, would have to stay late. When he saw that I had sushi, an expression that spoke of envy and pain at the same time flashed across his face. Once he remarked that it had been an extremely long time since he last tasted his mother's Japanese food. His mother had passed away quite some time ago, and he had married an Italian American wife who did not know how to make sushi. With teary eyes, Professor Sakami remarked, "My mother made these for me when I was little." Deeply moved, I, of course, invited him to share the food Felicia had prepared for me.

For twenty-three years, the everyday meals we had at home were traditional Chinese food, except on Friday nights, when we would prepare a Western meal together. During vacations, we would go on outings as a whole family and enjoy both Asian and Western cuisines. With regard to cuisine and culinary skills, Felicia was certainly able to satisfy the entire family, especially for someone from Wanhua,[1] like myself. On this account

---

[1] Though the neighborhood of Wanhua is no longer as bustling as in days of yore, the abundance of traditional snacks in the area bears the rich legacy of its former glory.

I never have any woes or grievances; Professor Sakami, unfortunately, has not met with the same good fortune.

Sweetness Through Tough Times as Foreign Students

The difficulties we experienced as overseas students provided us with anecdotes which we could still recall distinctly as if they had occurred just yesterday. The old, beat-up car that I bought for four hundred dollars lasted for only half a year. The story begins when Felicia and I arrived at Atlantic City to attend a scientific conference. On the way home it was sunny and there was a pleasant breeze. At that time Felicia had just got her driver's license and wanted quite badly to drive. Seeing that the weather was clear, I allowed Felicia to take the wheel.

We took the freeway that goes around the mountains in Pennsylvania and as we made it through the halfway mark, a strong wind suddenly picked up. The sky turned dark, and it started to rain heavily. On the other side of the windshield hovered a large and ominous patch of blackish gray. Felicia panicked and slammed on the brakes. As a result, the car spun 360 degrees and rammed into a guardrail. The car flipped over, was bent completely out of shape, and became an irrecoverable wreck. Fortunately for us, aside from being thrown and jolted heavily against the insides of the car, we walked away without any major injuries.

After the ferocious wind and raging rain subsided, we waited in the valley until a freight truck came along. The truck driver helped us call for help, and then the police arrived and called for a tow truck, which took another forty minutes. We were towed to a town so small that it could not be found on a map. I could still remember the name of the town — Shipenburg. Only a few houses and one nondescript and disorderly car garage stood in the vicinity. The mechanic took one look at our banged up car and shook his head emphatically.

I asked, "How much to fix the car?" He looked again at the car and then finally said, "Six hundred dollars." Oh, my God! This old car only cost us four hundred dollars. How could we pay six hundred dollars to have it fixed? Where would we get the six hundred dollars? "If we were to sell it to you, how much would we get in return?" The mechanic furrowed his brows and said, "At most fifty dollars."

Felicia and I looked at each other. We had no choice but to sell the wrecked car. It was already dark. Of the fifty dollars, we had to fork out twenty dollars to stay for the night at the only motel in town, and the remaining thirty dollars was just enough to pay for our ride home on the Greyhound bus. Thus, I ended up selling our first car for a paltry sum of fifty dollars just half a year after owning it. After that, Felicia and I had to walk to school or to the groceries, until we saved up enough money to buy a second used car a year later.

When we were students, life was hard and we practically lived on bread and water. When we needed furniture or new clothes, we would go to the Salvation Army. We picked up second-hand clothes, second-hand furniture, and our first television set was a used set as well. That old television set was as heavy as an elephant. The two of us carried it up to our fifth floor apartment. We turned it on. The black screen came on with an image of fuzzy patterns of black and white dots, but nevertheless we watched it with fascination. Every Wednesday night, Felicia would go and buy groceries. David and I would wait at home, watching television programs. Even to this day, David remembers watching shows on that television set.

Whether it was our studies, raising David, or just living our daily life, every day seemed filled with a multitude of different tasks. We were poor, but we had infinite hopes and we shouldered the responsibility of raising our child. We devoted ourselves completely to our laboratory and class work, exam preparation, and dissertation writing. That three years, I know not whether it was our patience and fortitude that finally paid off, or whether it was the heart and passion that fueled Felicia and me in our pursuits, but we finally graduated.

With the goal of completing our doctorates behind us, we started to make more plans. David was already three years old. The two of us began wondering, "When should we have a second child?"

SECTION II

LIFE ABROAD

5

Memories of Studying Abroad

Over thirty years later, in order to write Felicia's biography, my children and I returned together to the Case Western Reserve University. Felicia's advisor had already passed away. My advisor, Professor Goldthwait, had retired but was still healthy. That evening, our flight arrived an hour late. But when we finally disembarked and entered the waiting area, we immediately saw the gentle-faced eighty-year-old professor sitting in the lounge, waiting patiently. We were touched by his presence there to welcome us all.

We embarked on this trip so that my children could retrace the path Felicia and I had taken and relive some of those experiences, event by event, episode by episode. This time, Felicia was not with us, and there was no dazzling snowfall outside the airport, but the events thirty years earlier seemed but happened a moment ago. I told David, "This is the beginning of our family's time in the United States; this was also the hardest period of our lives." I rode in my professor's car; my children followed behind us in another car. Outside the window, the green landscape zipped past in a blur. I was eager to show the children the laboratories where Felicia and I used to work, the old apartment building where we once lived, and the roads that Felicia and I previously walked. Although I was always unsure whether these memories would resurface, as we sped along gush of flashbacks were already flooding my head — before me was the image of Felicia more than thirty years earlier.

The next morning, Professor Goldthwait and my family visited the university grounds. It was still March, and the air in early dawn was bitterly cold. Faith predicted it would snow in the afternoon. I recalled the day that Felicia and I had our final examination, and we carried David with us at the crack of dawn looking for a babysitter. Oh! In the blink of an eye, thirty years flashed past! Why is it that today I am alone without Felicia? Why is it that I have returned to Cleveland in spring to recapture my memory of Felicia, to the laboratory where I savored the lunch box prepared lovingly by her every day? And where are our footprints? Even though Felicia has already left us and traces of her life may have faded over time, I still hope my children could understand this chapter of her story.

Fulfilling Filial Duties

That spring when we were due to receive our doctorates was also the time we were preparing to have our second child and celebrate David's third birthday. I had already been separated from my parents for three years. The desire to see them was constantly on my mind, so I fervently hoped that they would attend our graduation. All preparations were carried out with the greatest delight, especially those in anticipation of our second child.

But we did not expect Felicia to have an ectopic pregnancy. Felicia had an incredibly high threshold for pain, but the pain was so agonizing that she could not tolerate it. My medical training and instinct told me instantly what the problem was, and I sent her directly to the hospital. The doctor confirmed my diagnosis: an ectopic pregnancy that required immediate surgery. Immediate surgery! That was yet another thorn that pricked us, impoverished students — the student health insurance did not cover prenatal care. I took one look at Felicia's pained and pale white face, hurried back to school, and told Professor Goldthwait about Felicia's condition, and I borrowed five hundred dollars from our department with him acting as the guarantor. Then I rushed back to the hospital. Felicia's surgery got through thanks to that sum of borrowed money.

Felicia needed rest after the surgery. It went without saying that her dissertation defense and graduation examinations all had to be pushed back, so I received my doctorate half a year earlier than Felicia. Not long after Felicia underwent surgery, my parents came to the United States.

I was ecstatic to see both my parents. Felicia could tell how I was feeling, and though she had not quite fully recovered, she still tried to fulfill her responsibilities as a daughter-in-law, including looking after David and taking care of the household chores. Everything that needed to be done, she selflessly tried to do all by herself.

After I completed my doctorate, I had some leisure time on hand before the graduation ceremony. It was the first time my parents had left Taiwan; they were extremely curious about this vast country called the United States and hoped that their son would take them around to see more of the country. I wanted to show my parents the United States, but money was always a concern. We were still extremely poor; we had to borrow more money to cover Felicia's medical expenses after her surgery. My parents, of course, did not know anything about our financial situation.

In addition, Felicia was recovering after surgery, she still required someone to look after her, so I was hesitant to leave her alone. Felicia sensed my hesitation and encouraged me to take my parents out. Thus, I borrowed another five hundred dollars to take my parents and David on a two-week trip, leaving Felicia at home to recuperate on her own. I would never forget this generous act of sacrifice on her part. Those two weeks, Felicia single-handedly tended to her own wounds so that I could entertain and take care of my parents.

The Accident of a Crushed Finger

After the graduation ceremony, my mentor Professor Goldthwait organized a little cocktail party for Felicia and me. He realized that the apartment we lived in was quite small, and that made it even smaller when my parents put up with us. So he invited our whole family over to his house. Upon receiving our doctorates, we were able to secure postgraduate research positions at Cornell University with Professor Goldthwait's assistance.

The graduation cocktail party was held at Professor Goldthwait's house, and he and his wife covered all the expenses. They invited members of the department, friends, and teachers. Altogether there were forty, perhaps fifty people. Taking with us, David and my parents, who were curious about anything and everything related to the United States, we all piled into the old car which was hitched to a trailer packed with all of our family belongings and furniture, and drove off to the teacher's house. This was because we planned to move to Cornell University directly afterward.

Felicia and I had finally graduated. After three years, it seemed we had reached the end of a long, arduous struggle. Since we had weathered the ups and downs together, our family bond was unbreakable. The multitude of factors weighed heavily on us to reach this extremely difficult decision, but after careful deliberation, we decided to stay in the United States.

My professor helped persuade my parents to accept this decision, explaining to them that we could not apply the knowledge that we had learned to the fullest in Taiwan. At that time, with access to promising employment prospects, my parents could come live with us in the United States, and we could also gradually return all the money we had borrowed from the department.

That night at the cocktail party, I was relaxed, carefree, and extremely optimistic about the future. Felicia was as radiant as a lotus flower. Although her ectopic pregnancy had forced her to delay the completion of her doctorate by half a year, she was on the verge of completion. Those hectic moments in the laboratory, those late nights of burying ourselves in the messy stacks of papers at the study desk, in front of David's cradle, or outside on cold, snowy evenings, we had sown seeds for our future, one kernel at a time, during those three years of ongoing struggle and hardship. That night saw the fruition of our efforts.

The next morning, the sky was clear and there was not a cloud in sight. We thought my parents had not yet had an opportunity to see the Cleveland downtown since they arrived, so we decided to round up the whole family and make a trip.

We did not need the trailer that was attached to the back of our car, so my father and I attempted to unhitch it. Professor Goldthwait had already left his house for the university. Neither my father nor I had the experience of unhitching a trailer, but my father was able to pull apart the large pin using some tools. He tried to set the trailer on the floor, as he was doing so, the weight of the heavy furniture inside caused the trailer to start to tip precariously. The trailer seemed to come crashing down on my father's hand any moment, so I panicked and immediately stretched out my hand to help him. But the trailer continued to slip, and it landed directly on my right index finger. The top half of my fingertip was crushed, and blood spurted out from the wound like a fountain gone awry.

My father saw my face twisted in pain and he let out an agonized cry. Mother and Felicia heard him and they rushed toward us. As soon as they saw what happened, they started wailing and hastened to help my father pull my hand out from underneath the trailer. Felicia held my hand sobbing, and attempted in vain to stop the bleeding with a handkerchief. She then drove me to the hospital at breakneck speed while I attempted to endure the pain and reassure everyone that I would be fine.

In the afternoon, thirty years later, the three children and I went to the professor's house. Just as Faith had predicted, it started snowing. I remember it was snowing on the day of the accident. Rain layered with soft snowflakes fell incessantly against the windshield. I reminded David to drive carefully because the road was slippery. That was typical of the wet, cold weather in Cleveland during spring; it was the weather that Felicia and I had endured for three consecutive years. The road which we had walked to take David to the hospital was the same as before.

The professor's front yard was where we had unhitched the trailer from the car. The injury to my finger and Felicia's tears seemed as vivid as yesterday. The professor talked on and on, of this trip's purpose, and of every aspect of Felicia's life. At that moment, the snow outside whirled and swirled as it fell, and the trees and rooftops were all covered in sparkling silver.

The children all knew how my index finger was hurt, but it never seemed to them as real as the day when we visited the professor's house, where the accident happened. This trip enabled them to understand better where their roots lay. If it were not for Felicia, my children and I would not have made this long trip back. She made this happen for the whole family to relive the events of the past. Towards evening on the way back to the professor's home, we saw the beautiful crystalline snowflakes dancing in step with the rain. It was a little like Felicia's dancing silhouette, which even now still resides deep in my heart.

It certainly did snow a great deal that night!

The Road to Cornell University

My finger continued to ache for over ten years. Eventually the skin around the fingernail grew into a large, thick cornified callus. That finger caused my mother, father, and Felicia shed so much tears. In life, a sudden change can happen any point of time. But as long as one has the comforts of a home and the love of a family, then how one faces and deals with the disappointment and frustration in life is entirely different.

The injury to my finger and the agony that Felicia was to experience later in her life are in no way comparable. However, I know Felicia's determination, resilience, and even her optimism were all due to the mutual dependence and trust in our family. She was able to steel herself and continue her journey on that long, hard road because we always trusted and encouraged one another. I sometimes flip through the photo albums that Felicia had put together so carefully. Even in the final months before she passed away, she was always full of smiles, her face emanating a blissful happiness. Life had to be that way, so that there would be no regrets.

The trailer took our whole family — my father and mother, David, Felicia, and me — down the road towards Cornell University. My hand was wrapped in a bandage since it was still bleeding slightly. I drove the car, and Felicia took care of our three-year-old David and my parents, who had never been on such a long car trip before. Aside from Professor Goldthwait's strong recommendation, we had chosen to do postgraduate research at Cornell University in order to steer forward our dream of building our academic careers together.

The Cornell University campus, located in Ithaca, New York, is one of the most beautiful in the United States. Because of its high northern latitude geographically, winters are long, sometimes lasting till as late as May.

When we arrived in Ithaca, it was approaching autumn in the year 1969. Though the sound of the wind whistling through the trees sent a foreboding of the imminent arrival of a frigid winter, the bright colors of the autumn foliage warmed the soul. The beautiful array of colors lightened and brightened our hearts and sent our spirits soaring. The picturesque Ithaca landscape was the site of many happy events; it was where Felicia and I raised our second child, Faith; the place where my father and mother had spent a year with us; and lastly, it was where our careers first took off.

As we hoped to be able to collaborate on various research projects, at Cornell we decided to switch disciplines to pursue each other's area of expertise. I entered the chemistry department to do my postdoctoral research, and Felicia was transferred to the biochemistry department.

My professor, Gordon Hammes, was well-known in the field of physical chemistry; Felicia's professor, Donald McCormick, specialized in enzymes and nutrition. Professor McCormick is currently still healthy and active. In the past, he always encouraged Felicia to spur her on in her research, and to this day he continues to speak of her exceptional achievements in the laboratory.

Doing Research at Cornell University

Molecular cell biology as a field of research took off in the 1970s. Because of our academic backgrounds, Felicia and I were well-equipped to excel in this field, and this was one reason we were able to establish a strong position for ourselves in American medical science. My dissertation topic at the Case Western Reserve University was "Studies on the RNA Polymerase involved in DNA-Dependent RNA Synthesis." In 1969, I had already discovered that there were two zinc ions tightly bound to RNA polymerase, but was unclear of their structure and function. This discovery had a great deal to do with the research that Felicia and I would be involved in the future. My purpose of coming to Cornell University to do postdoctoral research was to learn the new physico-chemical techniques used in enzyme research. This new technology would prove invaluable to me in my future research on the molecular mechanism of gene transcription.

Though not everyone is familiar with RNA, almost everyone has heard of DNA, the unit that controls genetic inheritance. Proteins are responsible for executing commands and performing biological functions as specified by DNA, and RNA is the messenger responsible for relating the orders from DNA to proteins.

To put it another way, DNA is a template of genetic information. RNA is constructed from this template in a process called gene transcription; RNA then passes the information it carries to proteins. An enzyme known as RNA polymerase is an integral part of the process of transcription. My research was to isolate this enzyme and elucidate its molecular mechanism.

Gene transcription includes a number of complicated steps which not only occur quite quickly, but are also extremely short in duration. At the time there was a Nobel Prize-winning scientist named Manfred Eigen who used a unique physico-chemical technique to record chemical reactions occurring in as short a span as one-millionth of a second. I set my sights on being able to use this technique in the future. However, for those of us living in the United States, Germany certainly seemed far and quite inaccessible. It would be extremely difficult for Felicia and me to travel to such faraway place to study this technique. As this technique had recently been introduced into the laboratory of Professor Gordon Hammes at Cornell University, we decided to go there so I could learn how to use and apply the technique. With this new technique, I could advance another step in the process of researching the molecular mechanism of gene transcription.

The focus of Felicia's research at Cornell University was the study of oxidative enzymes. Although my focus was different, we exchanged our fields of study, so our fields of interest were already merging. We stayed at Cornell University for about a year and a half, during which I wrote seven papers and Felicia, five. They were all published in leading scientific journals, and our standing and status in the scientific world had risen. But that was not all; Felicia became pregnant and gave birth to our second child, Faith. Our family life was warm and filled with contented joy.

Making Strides in the Academia Together

When we first arrived at Cornell University, we originally planned to be there for just a year and then move on to Yale University to do another year of postdoctoral research. For my research on gene transcription, I would need to ascertain the structural information in order to understand the molecular mechanisms. The fluorescence spectroscopy technique I was to learn at Yale would provide me with the means to do so. Professor Hammes thought it was odd that we would want to leave Cornell. I reminded him that the United States was experiencing the highest unemployment rate since the end of Vietnam War. There were many scientists who were not able to find employment. If Felicia and I had accumulated postdoctoral research experience at one or two more top schools, it would improve our chances of finding stable teaching positions in the future.

At that time I had only been in my professor's laboratory for three months, but my research was going well. I had begun my first paper and was preparing to publish it. Professor Hammes was quite pleased with my progress, so he said he hoped I would stay in his laboratory for two more years, and he would definitely help me obtain a position in the future. Felicia and I were quite happy with our research and life at Cornell, and my parents had also grown accustomed to their new surroundings. So we were, in fact, a bit hesitant to leave. Furthermore, Felicia was pregnant, and I did not want her to tire herself out with the process of moving, so we decided to stay at Cornell University.

But at the same time, I applied for several teaching positions at various universities around the country as suggested by Professor Hammes. Harvard University, Princeton University, and Albert Einstein College of Medicine all offered me assistant professorships, but I had not yet made a final decision.

Thus, enjoying all of these promising prospects as a postdoctoral researcher, strong support from my professors, and a warm and stable family life with Felicia enabled me to march forward and forge ahead dauntlessly in my scientific research endeavors.

One day a year later, Professor Hammes said to me that I had already accomplished a lot for him in his laboratory and asked me whether I still wanted to go to Yale. Faith was born not too long before, and Felicia had already recovered physically. My parents, homesick and not used to Ithaca's harsh cold winters, had returned to Taiwan. After discussing the matter, Felicia and I agreed that honing our skills at another top university before establishing our own laboratories was an opportunity not to be passed up, so we took up his suggestion gratefully.

At Cornell University, I studied enzyme kinetics using the fast-reaction technique, with the intention of applying it later to understand the complicated steps involved in gene transcription. There were two important breakthroughs — fast kinetics and structural analysis — in the field of research on molecular mechanisms. My reason for choosing to do a postdoctoral research at Yale was to study fluorescence spectroscopy at Professor Lubert Stryer's laboratory there, so I could apply it for structural analysis of macromolecules in gene transcription.

Before Professor Hammes' suggestion that we go to Yale, we had already decided that we would establish our laboratory at the Albert Einstein College of Medicine. At Einstein there was a professor by the name of Jerard Hurwitz who had conducted research on RNA polymerase for many years and was a leading authority in the field. I hoped I would be able to work closely with him and learn from him at the same time. At that time, I had already applied for a research grant from the National Institutes of Health (NIH). As soon as I received the funding for the grant, I would be able to take up a teaching position at the Albert Einstein College of Medicine.

I contacted Professor Lubert Stryer, a leading researcher in fluorescence spectroscopy at Yale and told him that I had decided to leave Cornell University, and that I wished to do research in his laboratory. I also informed him in advance that I would only be able to stay for six months to a year, because as soon as I received the grant from NIH, I would be expected to move on to the Albert Einstein College of Medicine to establish my own laboratory. Professor Stryer was understandably a little hesitant; after all, the time I would be available is considered too short to do meaningful, significant research. But he spoke on the telephone with Professor Hammes, who advised him, "If I were you, I would retain him as fast as I could." The next day Professor Stryer called me and requested that I come to Yale as soon as possible. At the same time, with Professor Stryer's help, Felicia acquired a research position in Professor James Coward's laboratory in the pharmacology department at Yale Medical School. Thus, her research focus was geared even closer to medical science.

David's Childhood

On the road, we passed by the nursery school which David had attended in Ithaca. He had long forgotten his first day in school — he could not understand anything that his teacher and the other children said, he cried all the way home, and told us that he did not want to go to school anymore. Before attending nursery school, David did not speak a word of English; at home we only spoke to him in our mother tongue. Both my parents also spoke to him in Taiwanese. That day in early March, Ithaca was covered with snow, as always; the soft beam of sunlight was unable to melt the snow that accumulated in cold springtime. The silvery spring snow glistened on the green grass like a spread of cover over it, radiating a healthy, vibrant glow. David's nursery school was situated at exactly the same place by the roadside. I asked the children to get out of the car and take a look.

David is taller than me by half a head. We took a picture together at the door of the nursery school; one of his hands rested on my shoulder. Behind us were large wizened trees; though their leaves had already withered, their trunks and branches surprisingly still stood tall. Springtime is a time of renewal — the land reawakens and new life springs from the earth. An assistant professor at the Colorado School of Mines, David is already thirty-three years old — an age when one's career would be on its fastest upward trajectory. Looking at him standing by my side, I think, only at times like this do I realize how much time has passed since those days at Cornell.

At that time, David cried and refused to go to school, but we insisted and sent a bawling and teary-faced David to school every morning. At three or four in the afternoon, Father would walk over to the nursery school himself to pick David up. Those were David's happiest moments, because he could finally speak to his grandfather in his mother tongue. The grandfather and grandson would hold hands and walk home together along the beautiful, mildly hilly path lined with verdant green trees. David still looks back fondly upon those happy times of sharing conversations with his grandfather in their mother tongue as they made their way back home.

Children adjust and adapt very quickly. Although the first couple of weeks of school saw David's resistance against going to school, in half a year's time even his dreams were in English. The period we spent at Cornell University was the time when our household transformed from one that was categorized as a "study abroad" family to "study and stay." Such is the process of putting down one's roots. Felicia's and my financial situation changed for the better; the research we did in the laboratory went smoothly; my father and mother lived with us; and our intelligent, charming and only daughter was born at Cornell. Although at that time we were merely postdoctoral researchers, our prospects in career and family were bright and rosy. Cornell was only a year and a half out of our lifetime, but it was the smoothest and most fulfilling period in our research careers.

Faith's Arrival into the World

Ever since she was little, Faith has been the Asian doll that everyone adores. Her angelic face and large, twinkling eyes reflect her sharp and intelligent mind. She was a pretty and playful child — very different in personality from her elder brother David, who is thoughtful and pensive. Faith was born when we were postdoctoral researchers at Cornell. After graduating from high school, she applied and was accepted into many top schools. But when Felicia accompanied Faith to visit the Cornell campus and Faith stood on the green lawn in front of the clock tower, she turned to her mother and told her that she had chosen Cornell.

Back at the Cornell campus, Faith narrated to me heartwarming stories, one at a time, of the time when Mom took her to enroll at college. According to Faith, she had a challenging and enriching time at Cornell where she was able to pursue her interests in politics, social sciences, music and the arts to the fullest.

Here in Cornell, Felicia and I raised Faith and advanced our academic careers. In our youth, we were energetic and motivated. As we walked to our old laboratories, my mind turned to Felicia. My heart and thoughts fluttered, and memories came back like tidal waves.

Ah! The Lover's Bridge is full of romantic stories. For example, if one kisses one's true love over the bridge during a full moon, then the lovers are destined to be together forever. Below the Lover's Bridge, the water flows swiftly, and there is no end to the romantic stories that our whole family can narrate and enjoy.

Faith and David's birthdays both fall on January 25. Both entered the world during the snow-filled season of the year. I remember the year when Faith was born was particularly cold. Snow was falling everywhere. On those cold winter evenings, the soft, airy flakes seemed to fly in every direction and fill the entire sky. It snowed heavily, I remember, and Father and I went out in the morning to dig the car buried underneath the snow, we found the snow had accumulated to almost the height of a one-story building.

Felicia's water broke in the middle of the night; at that time my parents had already gone back to Taiwan, tired of the cold in Ithaca. I entrusted David to the family of a high school classmate, Wen Lin, and in the middle of the snowy night, I took Felicia to the hospital to give birth to our second child. When Felicia accompanied Faith to Cornell University for registration, she took Faith specially to the hospital where she was born. Dusk had descended by the time the children and I arrived at the hospital. It was almost dark, and the lights shone dimly from the building. Faith walked towards the front of the hospital pensively. I recalled that night — as I drove the car to take Felicia to the hospital. The delivery went smoothly without any complications. Because Felicia was always healthy and strong, never had I thought that she would leave the world before me. Memories sometimes play tricks on us. Night had already fallen when we left Cornell University. I remembered the road that Felicia and I had taken. The events of the past seemed so fresh as if they had just occurred yesterday.

During those days at Cornell University doing postdoctoral research, along with her laboratory duties, Felicia played multiple roles of wife, mother, and daughter-in-law. However, no matter how smoothly everything went in the laboratory, every afternoon at five o'clock she would return home, prepare dinner and look after David and my parents. Even though the pregnancy took its toll on her body, she never once failed to fulfill her responsibilities.

At Cornell University, Felicia, together with the other laboratory fellows, and their advisor Professor Donald McCormick researched on flavinyl peptides and their role in the interaction of flavin and aromatic amino acids. Felicia's research performance was exceptional. Between 1970 and 1971, she published five papers in important biochemistry journals for which she was the leading author in four of them. In 1999, Professor McCormick still spoke enthusiastically of Felicia's achievements — albeit which happened thirty years earlier — at a conference he had organized in the States. To this day, Professor McCormick commends her for accomplishing so much on top of her multiple roles outside the workplace.

Our Time at Yale

It was not long after Faith was born that our whole family relocated to Yale University for a great start at one of America's foremost universities. At that time, we had already set our mind that our next stop would be New York's Albert Einstein College of Medicine, where we would establish our own laboratory. Thus, Yale University would serve as an excellent closure to our postdoctoral research experience.

Yale University is located in New Haven, Connecticut, a typical college town. Our son Albert graduated from the Yale University with a major in molecular biophysics and biochemistry. When Felicia and I returned to Taiwan, Albert was only fifteen. He spent his high school years at Taipei American School and became the first student from that school in many years to go on to Yale University. Because Felicia and I had been concerned about how he would adjust to his new environment, we were relieved and gratified to see him succeed.

When Albert returned to Taiwan from the United States, he had to make new friends and learn the ropes in an educational system that was vastly different from that of the United States. He went through a difficult period of adjustment. In addition, as originally intended at the time, we told him repeatedly we would be staying in Taiwan for only one year during our sabbatical leave.

But it is difficult to predict what life has in store. After returning to Taiwan, I decided to stay and establish the Institute of Biomedical Sciences at Academia Sinica. Many people said that giving up the prestigious positions in the United States and returning to serve the country was a form of self-sacrifice, but I believed that as long as it was my choice, then it was not so. Those who really made sacrifices were Felicia and my children. I can only take comfort in the knowledge that Felicia and the three children all supported my decision. Of course, most significantly, Felicia gave up the academic position and status that she had fought so hard for just to accompany me back to our country. The story of our family, including that of our children David, Faith, and Albert, is a page-turner of heart-warming and beautiful memories.

"Like the meeting of the seagulls and the waves, we meet and approach one another. The seagulls fly off, the waves ebb away and we, too, say farewell." These are lines in a poem by Bengali writer Rabindranath Tagore. Our time at Yale University was like the tide — gone in the blink of an eye. I feel the unpredictable nature of things in the world ever more keenly with the passage of time. Similarly, I also feel the same about the truth in the concepts of eternity and sincerity, especially when I re-examine Felicia's and my life. Tagore's poem expresses clearly life's meetings and partings and its endless changes. People inevitably seek constancy and routine in a world that is ever changing. I believe the significance of the so-called "eternity" lies in love; not just the love between husband and wife, but also the love of friends and family — from which one draws strength to weather the vicissitudes of life and pursue the ideal of everlastingness. Felicia was just the kind of person who would make eternal love a reality, and because of this, she lives forever in the memories of her family and friends.

We arrived at the lush green lawn of Yale University where I coached David how to ride a bicycle. Once, he accidentally fell off from his bicycle and broke his collarbone. I hurriedly took him to the hospital. This incident earned me Felicia's scolding for some time to come. Yale University was where David broke his ribs, Faith grew up as a cherubic baby, Albert spent intellectually challenging and stimulating years in college, and Felicia and I prepared for our lifetime of work in science. Yale University fills the page of our family's beautiful collection of memories.

Felicia entered Yale Medical School's pharmacology department. At Cornell University she did research on oxidative enzymes; at Yale, she would be conducting drug synthesis experiments. It was evident that Felicia was gradually executing her plan to pave the path for her academic career. After returning to Taiwan, Felicia conducted studies on anti-cancer drugs at the Institute of Biomedical Sciences in Academia Sinica. Some people assume that Felicia had an interest in cancer research because she herself suffered from it. In fact, far from it, that was not the case, as Felicia had been interested in the synthesis of anti-cancer drugs since her post-doctoral research years at Yale. Furthermore, she excelled in it. If both of us had not decided that we wanted to work together and build our careers together at the Albert Einstein College of Medicine, Felicia might have stayed on at Yale University. The university wanted her to stay on and assume a teaching position there. At that time, an Asian woman who earned the recognition from a top American educational institution was indeed quite an achievement.

Felicia focused on the synthesis of drugs; whereas I applied fluorescence spectroscopy to study rhodopsin's molecular structure, function, and reaction to light. In the eight months that I was at Yale University, I published two papers which are often cited to this day.

At Yale, I was already receiving a special fellowship from NIH, so our lifestyle and living standard improved greatly. That was the first time we had money to buy a new car. I still remember that it was a grass-green Chevrolet station wagon. When we took long trips, the children would take turns to sleep in the backseat. We lived in an apartment building close to the campus and hired an Italian nanny to take care of Faith and help Felicia with the household chores. Our plans for the imminent future were already on track — that gave both of us time and space to appreciate and savor the joys of research and family life. We were at Yale only for a brief span of eight months. During that period, we often drove to the Albert Einstein College of Medicine to take care of matters relating to our set-up of the new laboratory. The excitement at the prospect of having our own laboratory gave us an inexplicable sense of euphoria.

Albert was at Yale University for four years. It proved to be a time of discovery in his young life during which he was able to test waters and take on new challenges. He told me how Felicia had taken him to see the campus, how she arranged for a senior student to meet him, and how she had taken him to see the old laboratories and told him all about our daily life at Yale. The three children were closer to Felicia, because she single-handedly managed their academic pursuits, leisure activities, and extracurricular involvements like sports and music. Of course, I too am close to my children; however, their mother's influence and attention have always been greater. Felicia was undoubtedly a capable wife and good mother. She never came up short with regard to my life or the children's lives, and what I have been able to achieve today is largely attributed to Felicia.

The sands of time continue to flow. Though one can visit, at some time one must also inevitably leave. Every person who enters the world must also leave; such is life. Does time drive us or do we drive time? Regardless of the answer or whether we are talking about the past or the present, we must conclude our Yale segment on this family tour of rediscovery.

The three children and I went for a short visit to Yale University in March 2000. That single day alone held all our sweet memories. Felicia and I left Yale University in 1972. We took David and Faith, packed up all our research expectations, and relocated to New York, where I took up my post at the Albert Einstein College of Medicine.

It was early spring then and still snowing in New York.

6

Our Research and Life Together

In January 1972, I received a research grant from the NIH and was also conferred the "Career Development Award." That gave me the means to conduct my laboratory research as well as provided me with a salary. As far as the Albert Einstein College of Medicine was concerned, with us becoming their faculty heralded an infusion of new blood into the biophysics department as well as the beginning of a new era at the medical school.

The Albert Einstein College of Medicine is a part of Yeshiva University, an educational institution established by the Jewish community after World War II. At the time of the university's founding, Albert Einstein was consulted for permission to have the medical college named in his honor and he accepted. Although Yeshiva University is not as well-known, its medical school is ranked among the top ten in the United States.

Felicia and I chose to join the Albert Einstein College of Medicine for two reasons. First, Bernard Horecker, then associate dean of the medical school, hoped I would set up a laboratory for the school's newly created biophysics department. That certainly presented an exciting opportunity. Second, I was enticed by the possibility of studying and discussing ideas with Jerard Hurwitz, a renowned scientist in the department of developmental biology and cancer. I believed his knowledge and experience would be of invaluable help to me in my endeavor to utilize biophysics techniques, such as fast reaction techniques and fluorescence spectroscopy, in studying the molecular mechanisms of gene transcription.

Those two factors aside, there remained the question of whether a faculty position at Einstein would be available to Felicia. We brought up the subject with Horecker. He was well aware of the fact that Yale had offered Felicia good opportunities in its effort to retain her and in appreciation for her invaluable contribution to the university. He explained that there was no opening for an assistant professorship at that time, but in half a year's time the university would certainly be able to offer Felicia a position. Upon receiving this assurance, we relocated ourselves to the greater metropolitan area of New York.

Taking the First Step in Our Scientific Careers

New York became the place where Felicia and I would establish our footing in the academic world. When we first arrived in the United States, all we brought with us were our dreams; all we knew we had to accomplish were to study hard, conduct research, and publish our research results. Being just thirty years old, we confronted the boundless academic world with a fearlessness of which only the young and inexperienced are capable. Little did we know that our naiveté coupled with our untiring perseverance in the beginning propeled our first stride to establishing a place for ourselves in the scientific world, a step at a time.

At the Albert Einstein College of Medicine, I was an assistant professor of biophysics and was eligible to have my own laboratory. As Felicia was to take up her faculty position half a year later, she spent the first six months conducting postdoctoral research in my laboratory. My research required advanced equipment of high precision to measure the extremely rapid reactions involved in gene transcription. However, such cutting-edge precision instruments were not yet available at the time, I was therefore left to my own devices to not only develop, but also build these instruments. As I dedicated my time to create new instruments, Felicia helped me in the day-to-day essentials of running the laboratory, including conducting biochemical experiments. As research collaborator, she was the most important member of my laboratory.

That was our first time working together in the same laboratory. Our achievements at the time were monumental; the papers we published a year later captured international attention of the academic arena. Albert Einstein

College of Medicine was where our budding career in the scientific world bloomed and we had fond memories of our time there. However, those seven years at Einstein were also the most unstable, rocky period of our careers.

The Origin of the Names

Albert was born at the Albert Einstein College of Medicine Hospital. Of course, the hospital was a mandatory stop in our itinerary of rediscovery. As I stood with Albert in front of Albert Einstein's commemorative bronze statue, I told him the reasons we gave him the name Albert — he was born in this hospital, and the hospital was named in the honor of Albert Einstein.

The origin of each of our children's names is unique. The eldest child, David, was born in Cleveland. Our time in Cleveland was the toughest phase in our lifetime, but the mentorship and nurture from my advisor, Professor David Goldthwait, guided us through. His kindness was deeply etched in my heart, and so I named our eldest child, David, after him. The second reason we named him David is that, in English, David means "one who is being loved." After the complicated childbirth and premature death of our first son, Felicia suffered emotionally. The birth of David eased the pain of her loss, so we named him David to express our love for him.

Faith is our only daughter. She was, at the same time, born into a free and liberal America, and also to parents who were overseas students, and still held on to the Chinese traditional values. The relationship between Chinese parents and their daughters was a dichotomy of heart pain and anticipation. Chinese parents are torn apart with a sense of loss that the daughter they love so much will someday be married off, while on the other hand, they wish their daughter will find her final refuge of everlasting happiness. But we understood that unlike in Taiwan, American women are expected to be more independent. So we named our daughter Faith, hoping that she would grow up with self-confidence and courage to confront discrimination that women sometimes face in the society. Furthermore, the meaning of her Chinese name, Fei-Su (a phonetic equivalent of her English name), harbors our hope that she would be eloquent, intelligent, and able to take on the world as a modern woman in every other way.

When Albert was born, we were in the process of building our careers at Einstein. Albert's Chinese name, Ya-Po, reflected our hope that he would excel in academic pursuits, make a significant contribution to society, and find enjoyment in books and learning. Indeed, during his childhood we ourselves were fully engaged in the pursuit of knowledge, and immersed in a scientific world that seemed as vast as the sea.

This is the passage of time and the journey of life, one generation after another. Cao Cao from the ancient Chinese epic, *Three Kingdoms*, once remarked that in battle, he gives everything he has into each thrust of his weapon, and the very act wakes him to the "reality" of his existence — but at other moments in life, everything seems like a transient dream. I have none of his heroic flair, but I have savored the happy and sad moments of life, the euphoria of union and the sorrow of separation. Every day, especially when I say my prayers for Felicia, I have the feeling that time is in a race with me, chasing after me; before I know it, in a flash, it has been ten, twenty, and then thirty years.

As I visited the Albert Einstein College of Medicine with my children, my former colleagues of thirty years ago came together and gathered with us, and as we reminisced, waves of fond memories of the days when Felicia conducted her research at Einstein inundated us. At that time, she, in fact, suffered hardships and unjust treatment at Einstein due to the uncertainty of her appointment status.

The Elusive Teaching Appointment

Felicia worked in my laboratory as a postdoctoral fellow, and our joint research at Einstein went very smoothly. In addition to conducting research on the molecular mechanism of RNA polymerase, she was also responsible for all the routine tasks that are essential to maintaining a laboratory. We had joined the Albert Einstein College of Medicine at a time when their staffing situation was extremely unstable. Felicia and I were unsure of the details; all we knew was that Yeshiva University itself had operational difficulties, and every year the medical school was forced to turn over a million dollars in order to offset the university's deficit.

The medical school considered the policy extremely unfair, and they had made plans to split away from the university and become an independent institution. However, the news of breakaway autonomy leaked, the university president and the board increased their vigilance and responded in a lightning speed with an action plan up their sleeves. One weekend when the dean of the medical school was away campaigning for more funds, the university president sent notification letters to every faculty member informing them of the dean's dismissal. Associate Dean Horecker was, at the same time, affected by the incident and he was, thus, forced to leave the school.

Half a year came and gone. I had no alternative but to seek out interim Associate Dean Arthur Grollman to explain to him and inquire about Felicia's promised position. When asked whether there was any supporting documentation to certify this promise, I was speechless. At the time, Felicia and I had complete trust in Associate Dean Horecker because he was a respected and well-known scientist. It also never crossed our minds that we might need a proof of the promise. Moreover, how were we to know that the Albert Einstein College of Medicine would undergo such a dramatic administrative upheaval within half a year? In the end, Felicia had to continue conducting research in my laboratory. Two years later I was promoted to associate professor, and Felicia was appointed to a post as a lecturer, but she continued to commit her time working in my laboratory.

Documenting Allosterism

Felicia focused on her biochemical research and I, on biophysical research, side by side in the same laboratory. I had set up my instruments, and we worked relentlessly day after day, publishing numerous important papers under the names "Wu & Wu." At this juncture we already had a firm standing in the academic community, and my laboratory gradually became the largest laboratory in the Einstein's biophysics department. Our application of fast reaction techniques and fluorescence spectroscopy in the study of gene transcription mechanisms was considered the most advanced one, but that was also the first spark that ignited the scientific community's interest in our research.

In the 1960s, two Nobel Prize-winning scientists from the Pasteur Institute in France, Jacques Monod and Francois Jacob, discovered that proteins have two different forms or conformations, and that proteins are able to switch interchangeably between these two conformations. Switching between the R and T conformations is a phenomenon of biological regulation. Suppose an enzyme usually exists in the R conformation. The binding of various biological substances to it causes it to change into the T form; this transformation is called allosterism or allosteric transition.

For example, some people suffer from diarrhea when they drink milk because the lactase synthesis mechanism in their genes cannot be activated. Since lactase is the enzyme in the body responsible for breaking down lactose, these patients are thus unable to break down the lactose in milk. Usually, these genes are inactive due to a protein, called a lac repressor, residing on the promoter region of genes encoding for lactase. If a lactose molecule binds to a lac repressor, it causes the lac repressor to change from one conformation to the other. After the transformation, the lac repressor separates from the promoter region and allows the genes to be activated and used for lactase synthesis. Once this process occurs, one can drink milk without any risk of suffering from diarrhea.

This chemical process was first described by Monod and Jacob in the 1960s. They predicted that the lac repressor was an allosteric protein. When lactose was present, it would bind to lac repressors in the R conformation. The lac repressors would then change from the R conformation to the T conformation and separate from DNA, leaving RNA polymerase free to bind to DNA, carry out transcription, and start the synthesis of lactase. But despite Monod and Jacob's continued efforts to prove their theory, they were unable to do so.

In the 1970s when Felicia and I were setting up our laboratory, we were highly interested in the binding mechanisms between enzymes and other molecules, leading to observations of the conformational changes that take place. We were initially unaware that Monod and Jacob had been searching for scientific proof of their theory since the 1960s. By using the fast reaction instrument I developed, Felicia and I were able to observe conformational changes. When the lac repressor binds with lactose, it assumes one conformation. When it binds with genes, it assumes another. Because the speed at which it changes conformations is extremely rapid (about 1/100,000 sec), it is impossible to observe without specialized instruments. It is no wonder that Monod and Jacob were unable to prove the theory that they had proposed.

We published that paper in the *Journal of Biological Chemistry*, not long after the set-up of our laboratory. It attracted international attention, including that of the Pasteur Institute in France. They invited Felicia and me to speak at a NATO summer school held in Greece as well as at the Pasteur Institute in Paris. These sowed the seeds of doing research at the Pasteur Institute for a year during our sabbatical. Of course, the turn of events were unforeseen and unexpected.

The Storms at Albert Einstein College of Medicine

We have fond memories of our time at the Albert Einstein College of Medicine. I remember that day when I was teaching a class and midway through Felicia stopped in front of the window and announced, "I'm going to the hospital to give birth." Amidst cheers, she smiled and waved goodbye to the class and went to the hospital by herself. By the time I finished the class and rushed to the hospital, Albert was already born.

As a baby, Albert was not as good-looking as his older brother and sister. Felicia even jokingly commented why this child we produced was such an ugly baby. On the contrary, Albert grew up relatively handsome, and he was even a part-time model. We often recounted to Albert the story of his birth, which always led us to break out in uncontrollable laughter.

Five years at Einstein, our laboratory became the largest in the biophysics department. Our funding came from the National Institutes of Health, the National Science Foundation, and the American Cancer Society. With ample research funds, we were able to publish numerous high quality papers, thus elevating our standing in the scientific community.

However, the biophysics department, since the eventful incident of autonomy, was still unable to recover from its unstable staffing situation. For the last eight years we were led by an acting department head. One day the acting department head told me he had raised a proposition that the biophysics department be dissolved, and that he himself planned to take up a position as a professor of internal medicine through internal transfer. His words left me completely dumbfounded, and I blurted out, "What would happen to us and the other professors?" The head responded indifferently, "You'd do best to fend for yourselves."

The research Felicia and I conducted at Einstein was extremely successful, and our papers were well received and critically acclaimed, our chances of securing new employment opportunities were fairly high. With the help of my former mentors, Professors Hammes and Stryer, in less than a month, I had two excellent offers: the first was a section head position in the laboratory of molecular biology at the National Cancer Institute; the other was a full professorship in the department of biological chemistry at Washington University, St. Louis.

The Albert Einstein College of Medicine realized our intentions of leaving, the dean quickly appointed a committee headed by Hurwitz to review the situation. After the meeting, the committee recommended that Felicia and I stay on, and furthermore, they proposed to me to assume the position of head of the biophysics department. Felicia and I had extensive discussions, we shared our thoughts that the establishment of our laboratory had not been a simple task, and that to give it up would be regrettable. We therefore decided to stay on at the Albert Einstein College of Medicine. However, I was ambivalent about taking up the department head appointment. I was still young then, and taking on administrative duties too early in my career would impede progress and deprive my time to do research, which I dearly loved.

The dean had officially offered me the position of biophysics department head, but I was still deliberating on whether to accept it. The appointment decision was, however, pending approval by the faculty search committee which was a bureaucratic formality of the university. It was at this point when things took an unexpected turn. News of the appointment reached the ears of the acting head who had originally planned to transfer to the department of internal medicine, and he voiced extreme displeasure over the lack of recognition for his eight years of service as the acting head of the department. He groused that though there was no achievement he could claim credit during his tenure, he did dedicate his time and effort to run the department.

Once I heard the news, I reacted immediately by approaching the dean of the medical school and told him that I was in fact not interested in serving as head of the biophysics department, and that I would rather spend more time doing research. I added that if my presence in the department would affect the employment or advancement opportunities of other professors, then Felicia and I would rather change departments. The dean was apologetic for the way the situation had developed, he could do nothing but respect my decision. Thus, Felicia and I transferred from the biophysics department to the biochemistry department. I was promoted to full professor as recommended by the committee a year ago, and Felicia assumed the position as assistant professor, which eventually enabled her to have her own laboratory. With this tenure came the independence and challenges to apply for grants to fund her research as well as draw up her own research proposals, but she was full of confidence and enthusiasm to take her research to another level.

In 1969, while doing research for my doctoral dissertation, I discovered that there were two zinc ions in *E. coli* RNA polymerase, but I was unsure of their function. This was the first time that a link had been found between metal ions and gene expression. To put it another way, two zinc ions had been found in an enzyme involved in gene transcription, but no one understood their function. This was an extremely important lead for inorganic biochemistry, and I was regretful that after all these years we had not investigated further.

In 1978 when Felicia began the process of forming her own laboratory, we thought this would be an ideal focus for her research. On one hand, this was one of my doctoral research discoveries, on the other hand, Felicia's background in chemistry made her an ideal successor to carry on this research. Thus, Felicia started to write her research plans, focusing on the role of zinc ions in gene transcription. Her research proposal was impressively written, and she was awarded a three-year grant by NIH. Felicia was well on her way to becoming fully funded in her research endeavors, and she was gradually gaining recognition from the scientific community.

Over the years, our colleagues at the Albert Einstein College of Medicine have stood by us. We met up with Dr. Susan Horwitz, a world-renowned researcher of the anti-cancer drug, Taxol. Felicia became the only patient to complete the twelve-session Taxol treatment when her cancer recurred.

My heart ached when I recounted to Dr. Horwitz the Taxol treatment Felicia had undergone and the excruciating pain she had to endure from the side effects of chemotherapy. Dr. Horwitz reiterated that she was still trying her best to do clinical studies on Taxol in the hope of being able to offer patients an effective drug with minimal side effects. Was this all predestined or was it a cruel joke played on us by Heaven — we both tearfully lamented that her research had to be used on Felicia.

That day as my children and I strode down the familiar old corridor, my children conjured up fuzzy recollections of our old colleagues. Felicia, known for her warmth and hospitality, never failed to organize annual medical school get-togethers for her colleagues and students from her laboratory. So during this reunion, my children were able to revisit their childhood memories as well as meet their mother's former colleagues and friends who held fond thoughts of her.

Ah! Before I knew it, it had already been thirty years, and these dear friends were as warm-hearted as ever. That day, the gathering was not organized by Felicia. The luncheon prepared by the former colleagues was their expression of love and fond memories for Felicia. Reminiscing her, Felicia's name was constantly on our lips. That day we met Jack Peisach, Fred Brewer, Philip Aisen, Olga Blumenfeld, Irving Listowsky, Sam Seifter and other old pals. It was a simple lunchtime gathering with an air of nostalgia. The confluence that brought old friends together did not come by chance. It was specially arranged to share our memories of Felicia — her life, her passion and her remarkable scientific achievement. Those three decades were memories that would never fade.

Obstacles to Settling Down

The Albert Einstein College of Medicine is located in the northern part of Bronx in New York City. The southern part of Bronx is known as the most dangerous neighborhood in New York. It is a paradox that the public order in this part of New York City is deemed relatively safe because it was reputed to be near the homes of many mafia leaders — an affluent neighborhood of high security and high-class residences.

When Faith was very young we rented a house in the nearby town of Larchmont in the Westchester County. Our landlord was an unemployed American who gave us many bothersome rules such as keeping windows closed at all times so that heat from radiator would not "escape," and minimizing the usage of hot water during showers because these utilities would lead to energy wastage and high energy bills. There was once while Felicia was giving Faith a bath, the landlord suddenly cut off the hot water supply. Poor little Faith was shivering in the cold. This incident convinced us that we had to move out of the house.

We relocated to New Rochelle. Not long after we moved, Albert was born. With three children, Felicia's dual responsibilities at work and at home increased dramatically. Although we employed a nanny, Felicia was still frantically busy tending the family, so not long after Albert was born, I decided that for the good of Felicia and the young children, I ought to find a full-time caregiver.

Luck was with us, and we found a kind-hearted African American woman named Margie Pea. Perpetually bright and cheerful, she had a round face that was always smiling, just like the faithful servant of Vivien Leigh's character, Mammy, in *Gone with the Wind*. When Margie joined our household, Albert was just born, Faith was only two, and David was seven. Our three children were raised by her practically throughout their growing-up years. Margie was like our family member and she remained with us for sixteen years, until we left the United States so that I could work in Taiwan. Margie and the children shared a deep emotional bond. When Faith and Albert graduated, they both asked Margie to come to their university graduation ceremonies many years later. Margie died a few years after Albert's graduation. All our children went to attend the funeral at her hometown in South Carolina.

My parents believed that if we were to settle down in the United States, we definitely needed to buy a house. My father had always wanted to help us pay for our place in the United States because he believed that owning a home helps the family to settle in. Although I was appreciative of my father's offer, Felicia and I decided to wait until our financial condition stabilized before deciding to buy our first house in Scarsdale, a town that is half an hour's drive from the Albert Einstein College of Medicine.

Our first residential property was an elegant little house with a luxuriant green lawn; our neighbors were all professors and academics. The backyard, overlooking a little woods, is an open space with a basketball goal post, swings and a barbecue grill. Looking beyond from our backyard, we could see the elementary school which our children attended.

My children and I reluctantly parted with these old friends at the Albert Einstein College of Medicine. We continued our journey down the memory lane — making visits, reminiscing and putting details of the past in context. We returned to Scarsdale. The sun started to wane and the sky deepened into a riot of vibrant colors. I thought of an old saying familiar to every Chinese: *the evening sun is beautiful; how regrettable that the day is almost over ...*

7

A Sabbatical Year in France

I remember the school field trips I went when I was young and everyone was singing together, "In front of my house there's a small river, behind it there's a hill, on the hill blooms of wildflowers drape the slope, and the wildflowers red as fire…" That evening, with the waning sun behind us, the children and I returned to our former home in Scarsdale. On each of our children's faces was a sweet, innocent smile. I knew that our hearts were stirred up and each of us was full of thoughts and emotion. To the children, this place held their childhood memories, and to me, this was the home that Felicia and I had built with our own efforts.

There was a gentle slope in front of our house, and a bed of flowers lined the path connecting the garage and the front door. My parents used to plant tiger lily, loofah, and other vegetables in the wide open space between the back of our house and the hills flanking on both sides. The harvest from their efforts satiated our voracious craving for Chinese food. There was no river stream next to the house and the hill beyond the backyard stood sparse and barren, but still, this was our home. Our shared memories and strong family ties forged the connecting bond to this house.

The brown tiles, white wall, thick forest, and barbecue grill at the backyard presented the happy setting for countless family gatherings filled with chatter and laughter. Faith still remembers waking up every morning to watch Grandfather and Grandmother practice *tai chi*. David spent his elementary school and junior high school years here. Albert recalls fondly the walks to school he took with his older sister, holding her hands, and the big welcome smile of Margie upon their return from school. I could still remember after dinner Felicia would always sit with the children at the big dining table, guide them one by one in their schoolwork, and then teach them to play the piano. In autumn, Father and Mother would rake up the fallen leaves, three to four times a day, keeping the backyard immaculate.

Vacation days were the most enjoyable. The autumn sun shone warm and bright and the maple leaves turned fiery red. During autumn vacation, the city would close the Bronx River Parkway to car traffic so that residents could ride their bicycles out on the road. On our bikes, basking in the warmth of the clear, blue sky and the balmy breeze, we sped through against a beautiful backdrop of rich autumn foliage made up of red canopies of maple leaves, and the gently undulating wavelets of the clear lake. The picturesque sight already etched an indelible imprint in our shared memory as a family.

The waning sun slowly sank until it disappeared behind the clouds. We lingered along the path around our former home, rounds after rounds, but in the end we had to say goodbye to the bygone days and conclude our walk down this memory lane. We turned our heads and looked behind us one last time. The glow of the day was gradually diminished by the fall of the night sky.

The Unique American Education

Even when David was little, he was a pensive, serious child. When he was five, maybe six years old, he would play with a watch or a camera, take it apart and put it back together again. When he played the Chinese chess or the *Go* chess with me, he had to win no matter what; if he lost, he would definitely cry. As for me, I thought this child had to learn to deal with failure, so sometimes I would purposely refuse to let him win. The chessboard, where we sparred our chess skills, thus became a platform for learning, for mentoring my son, and most importantly, for bridging close bonding between father and son.

David not only matured at an early age, he was also quite gifted intellectually. Even in preschool, he displayed an aptitude for mathematics. As I recall, the summer after his fifth grade, his superlative performance in mathematics and science had led his teachers and even the principal to suggest that he skip a grade. At first, I did not allow him to jump grade, since I had always believed that children should progress through school grade by grade, step by step. However, in the end, his teachers and the principal prevailed upon Felicia and me to allow him to take mathematics classes at high school level, and after careful deliberation and extensive consideration of his gift, we finally relented and allowed him to try attending lessons at a higher grade.

From then on, it became the principal's and the teachers' responsibility to see and drive David to and fro the local high school for mathematics class. The dedication and concern demonstrated by these educators gave us a good impression of the American educational system. As parents with school-going kids, the experience was indeed eye-opening.

I remember that when David was in fourth grade, the school conducted political science class as the curriculum. In one of the terms, the focus of their class was on the United Nations. The class was divided into "countries" represented by two to three students each. David became the representative for Cuba. The teacher taught the students how to use library resources to conduct research of their respective countries, and then took the students down to the United Nations Building in New York City to interview officers of the respective countries they were "representing." The teacher requested the students to understand the cultures, political situations, and the international roles of the countries they represented. At the end of the school term once they completed their research, it would be their turn to take the stage, submit proposals, debate, and campaign to win votes for the country they represented.

That day was the big moment for the students of the political science class to demonstrate what they had learned in class. The school held a mock United Nations assembly for the students, and the parents were invited to attend too. On that day, David dressed up as Fidel Castro and spoke eloquently on stage. He criticized America's superpower dominance of the world, he argued that the current state of international politics was unfair to Cuba, and he spoke emotionally of Cuban citizens' hopes for the future. He made his passionate speech, at the same time campaigning for Cuba to swing the opinion of other "member nations" to vote for Cuba.

Felicia and I were full of praises of the uniqueness of the American educational system which is designed to foster students' independent thinking, and the focus is in sharp contrast to the traditional Chinese educational system, which emphasizes "teaching" and "learning." The difference between the two is enormous. The interactive approach, openness, and spontaneity advocated in the pedagogy guide students to form political viewpoint as well as develop their critical thinking on other fronts and fields, and that truly are the hallmarks of education. David's political science class in that semester opened our eyes to the discovery of the unique spirit of the American education.

Parting with My Parents

The two years that my parents lived with us in Scarsdale was the last time they were ever in the United States, and also the last time that we lived together as a three-generation family under the same roof. Those two years, Felicia and I were very focused and busy with our research. Margie helped with the household chores, but Felicia still managed the children's education single-handedly. I was extremely busy too. When weekend came, I set aside time so that the whole family could take a day trip or venture into New York City to enjoy Chinese cuisines in restaurants, but on other weekdays my parents could only sit at home and wait for the plan and arrangement made by us. On the other hand, the children were growing up and they had to attend school every day, hence my parents gradually began to feel lonely staying in the house. So they eventually decided to return to Taiwan.

Felicia and I felt a sense of reluctance. Especially I did not want to see them leave. Since young, my parents loved me most, and they always hoped that I would be able to continue to live with them forever. When we left Taiwan, my parents would continue to set places for us at the dining table. Seeing the empty seats, the thought of us being far away and the uncertainty of when they would be able to see us again moved them to tears.

Every little concern and affection of my parents were deeply engraved in my heart, and I always hoped my parents would come and live with us permanently in the United States. When they decided to return to Taiwan, I knew that in the future, chances were slim for them to come back and see us in the United States.

No matter how my heart was unwilling, how I could not bear and how I did not want to see them leave, I knew that I had to let them go. Before parting with them, I took them on a trip to Hawaii. That week, I was down with a cold and fever. The thought of the imminent separation from my parents brought sorrow and pain in my heart, and for a long time, I did not recover fully from my cold, from the heartache. I saw them off at the airport. As I watched my parents' silhouettes disappear in the crowd, their wrinkled hands locked into each other, I was unable to stop the flood of tears from my eyes. That afternoon at the Hawaii International Airport, I stood lingering for a long, long while, reluctant to depart…

The European Experience

Felicia and I published papers on the studies of gene transcription under the names "Wu & Wu." These papers were well received all over the world, especially at the Pasteur Institute in Paris. In 1976, we received an invitation to attend a life sciences summer school, sponsored by NATO, at the Spetsai Island in Greece; we were also given an opportunity to speak. The summer school was two weeks long and attended by well-known scientists from all over the world. Both of us felt extremely honored to be invited to present our lectures at such an established conference.

It was a five to six-hour boat ride from Athens to Spetsai. This was our first trip to Europe, and the sight of Athens — the cradle of the ancient Greek civilization and Greek mythology — gave us the feel of exhilaration and excitement. As soon as we disembarked at Spetsai, sprawled before our eyes were the white-washed houses, the little elegant lanes lined with flowers, and the vast expanse of sea. Joyous and uplifting — that were the exact words to describe our first trip to Europe.

Among the speakers invited to the two-week summer school, many were Nobel Laureates. Felicia and I were the youngest of the guest speakers, but our lectures won acclaims and were well received. The person who invited us to attend and participate the summer school was none other than François Gros, who was then the director of the molecular biology department at the Pasteur Institute in Paris. After the conference, he initiated to invite us to present a lecture on the same topic to members of the Pasteur Institute. He said our research induced high level of interest from Pasteur Institute.

Setting foot in Europe for the first time, we were drawn by its unique and long history. As we had never been to Paris before, we accepted his invitation eagerly. After the conference at Spetsai, the two of us immediately presented our lecture at the Pasteur Institute on the allosteric mechanism of the lac repressor. What we had not expected, though, was that this trip would ultimately create an enormous impact on the future of our entire family.

That summer in 1976 was our first time in Paris. The whole audience of scientists listened raptly to our lecture. Among them, a female scientist by the name of Agnes Ullmann shed tears as she listened. After the lecture, she told us, eyes still red and watery, "I wish that Dr. Monod were here to hear you speak." We later found out that she had worked with Dr. Jacques Monod, a Nobel laureate at Pasteur, for many years, and that he had passed away just recently. He had spent more than ten years attempting to obtain experimental evidence to support his theory but had not been successful. It was beyond anyone's expectation, our experimental results actually proved Dr. Monod's theory. But, it was a pity that he did not live to see it.

That evening, Dr. Gros treated us to a dinner. We were completely intoxicated by the beautiful Parisian night. We saw sophisticated Parisians enjoying fine cuisine and the medieval architecture sparkling and glittering under the illumination of modern urban lightings. It all looked so spectacular. We could only use words such as, "absolutely beautiful," to describe the scene.

That night Dr. Gros told us that he hoped in the future we would consider taking a sabbatical year to do research at the Pasteur Institute.

We had since been working at the Albert Einstein College of Medicine in 1972. In the United States, it is possible to request for a year of sabbatical after teaching seven years at a university. Felicia and I both thought Dr. Gros' invitation was a valuable opportunity to immerse in the various different academic environments, learn advanced research techniques, and enhance our knowledge. Three years later, after the summer school at Spetsai, Felicia and I applied for a year of sabbatical from Einstein to do research at the Pasteur Institute. At the same time, I was successful in my application for a research scholarship to serve as visiting professor at the French National Health Research Institute (INSERM). So in 1979, the whole family's move to France was finally realized.

Our trip to Paris in 1979 was a life-changing experience to everyone of us in the family. Other than our research career, the shared memories and enriching lives of our family in that one year were to become our favorite fodder for conversations for years to come. The year in Paris was just a milestone in our lives, but it was a fulfilling, enriching and stimulating year for our entire family.

Our Research Results in France

I spent seven years at the Albert Einstein College of Medicine. I used biophysical techniques to study the molecular mechanisms of gene transcription. It required large amounts of purified genes and proteins, which at that time were only available from bacteria. However, as a medical graduate, I naturally wished to conduct my research using human or animal cells. The late 1970s was the period when genetic engineering first took off, so it was an opportune time to extend my research to mammalian or human cells.

Before Felicia and I went to the Pasteur Institute, a professor of molecular biology at the institute, Dr. Henri Buc, came to the United States to discuss with us the possibility of doing research at his laboratory in France. He hoped to venture into the field of molecular biology in order to conduct research on gene transcription.

Dr. Buc is an eminent scientist who later became our good friend. However, at that time when he visited the United States to invite us to France, I had already committed to do research with a well-known scientist at the Pasteur Institute, Dr. Moshe Yaniv, who studied gene expression in animal cells. But the tremendous heartfelt sincerity that Dr. Buc showed in his invitation by traveling personally from France impressed Felicia to the extent that she decided to join his laboratory. This marked the beginning of our separate paths in scientific research.

That year in France, the research that Felicia and I engaged in progressed relatively smooth. On our first day at the Pasteur Institute, Dr. Paul Berg, an internationally renowned scientist who later received the 1980 Nobel Prize in Chemistry, came to speak. His research involved inserting human genes into animal viruses and expressing these genes in mammalian cells. That day, he mentioned that since animal viruses have finite structures, the number of genes that can be expressed in this manner is invariably limited.

After listening to the talk, Dr. Berg and I went to Dr. Yaniv's laboratory to continue the discussion. I suggested to him to insert the genes of animal cells into bacterial plasmids and then transfer the plasmids to bacteria — in other words, to use bacterial phages as vectors and simultaneously add promoters of SV40 genes to the vectors. A bacterial phage is like a virus, except for the difference that its host is not an animal cell but a bacterium. This procedure could be used to produce a significant amount of animal genes. The bacterial phages or plasmids used in this process are called "shuttle vectors."

Both Dr. Berg and Dr. Yaniv thought this idea was worth a try, so my main research topic at the Pasteur Institute in that year was to develop a type of shuttle vector to express genes in bacterial or animal cells. The research results produced that year at the Pasteur Institute had a far-reaching influence and impact on the future development of genetic engineering and biotechnology.

Meanwhile at Dr. Buc's laboratory, Felicia was conducting the bacterial gene transcription research. They were investigating the mechanism of transcription initiation. When Felicia joined this research team, the researchers in Dr. Buc's laboratory had already extracted a substance similar to SV40, a simian virus mini-chromosome, from the nucleus. But the amount of chromosome-like substance that they were able to obtain was quite small, too little even to support the meager needs of their own research laboratory. Fortunately, Felicia came up with an idea to utilize the plasmids found in *E. coli*, an intestinal bacterium, and these types of plasmids naturally contain large amounts of complex nucleo-proteins. Felicia and her co-researcher were thus able to confirm their composition and structure, and elucidate their function in gene transcription.

In the short span of four months, Felicia's plasmid idea had enabled other research teams to expand their research capabilities. However, Felicia had always thought she should take advantage of the opportunity in France to explore a new field, so after accomplishing the research goal in that four months, she concluded her research at Dr. Buc's laboratory. Through Dr. Buc's and Dr. Yaniv's recommendations, she proceeded to the largest cancer research center in France, the Institut Gustave-Roussy, to study anti-cancer drugs.

Felicia developed an interest in anti-cancer drugs when she was doing her postdoctoral research at Yale University. She thought that with her organic chemistry background, she could accomplish more by doing research in anti-cancer drug discovery. After arriving at the Institut Gustav-Roussy, she started working with a well-known scientist, Jean-Bernard Le Pecq, on experiments relating to anti-cancer drugs. They synthesized new anti-cancer drugs and studied their mechanisms of action. Felicia published a paper that detailed the results of the experiments. Though the effectiveness of the drug at clinical trial stage did not turn out as expected, the fact that she could produce results in as brief a period as six months already demonstrated her capability and great potential as a researcher.

That year in France, besides making great strides in scientific research, we also made great friends. Even after we returned to the States, we still maintained frequent contacts with Drs. Buc, Yaniv, and Le Pecq.

France, however, was not the only exciting experience happening to us that year. That year we also decided to leave the Albert Einstein College of Medicine and relocate to the State University of New York, Stony Brook.

Adjusting to Life in France

When we first arrived in France, David was in the eighth grade, Faith, third grade, and Albert, first grade. Felicia and I could not speak a word of French, so we had to rely on our family translator, David, who had studied three years of French in junior high. With Dr. Buc's help, we rented an apartment in southern Paris. It was a modern Western-style apartment with an elegant garden. We lived on the second floor, and every morning when we woke up, we would look out to admire the beautiful blooms of the garden below us. The refined lifestyle and the appealing environment — we had completely settled in our new home in Paris. The subway was our mode of commutation to the Pasteur Institute.

Our first primary agenda was to make arrangements for our children's schooling in Paris. Dr. Buc helped us to settle the arrangements. First, we enrolled Faith and Albert in a French elementary school which was near our home and a mere five to six-minute walk for the kids. Whereas David would be attending a bilingual school where classes were conducted in both English and French. He commuted by subway to get to school which was located near the Eiffel Tower.

That one year in Paris was pivotal to David's choice of academic pursuit when he returned to the United States. When David started his lessons in school, the teachers realized that he was exceptionally intelligent and they suggested a "floating" approach for David, which means he should select classes according to his level of ability in each subject. Back in the United States, we were opposed to David skipping grades, but after arriving in France, we contemplated the factors that since the American and French educational systems were completely different, and David would only be in France for a year, we decided to take the teachers' suggestion.

We never expected that after one month, David would float from the eighth grade to the twelfth grade in several subjects. In other words, in France, David immediately became a high school senior. Well, come to think about it, David's unusual educational experience would became a special imprint of memory of his time abroad thus Felicia and I did not worry too much and allowed David to study whatever that made him happy.

In the French educational system, students take a nationwide examination called the baccalaureate after high school graduation; this examination determines their eligibility for college. Though David was only fourteen years old and had only attended the final year of high school, the teachers made arrangement for him to sit for examination along with the rest of the students. Surprisingly, he passed.

We were thus reassured about David's educational progress, but Faith and Albert were still young and did not understand French. On their first day of school, we accompanied them to school and found out there was only one teacher who could speak English, but that teacher taught neither Faith's nor Albert's grade levels. At that moment, we were certainly a little concerned.

The next day, Felicia and I had a discussion. We decided we needed to know how our kids adapt to the school, so after they had gone to the class, we went over to the school to take a look. We arrived during the recess, and immediately saw Albert sitting on a bench in the schoolyard playing with a seven or eight-year-old French girl, they were both pulling and pinching each other's nose. After looking a little longer, we spotted our energetic little Faith happily playing tag with a little French boy. We heaved a sigh of relief and laughed. Children have their own ways of developing personal relationships. It looked like Faith and Albert would have no problems adjusting their lives in France.

Having seen that our three children had all adjusted well in their new environments, we felt reassured and were able to dedicate our energies into our work.

I remember the discussion meeting at noon on our first day of work at the Pasteur Institute. Dr. Yaniv faced the members of the laboratory and said, "We have Professor Wu joining us from the United States today; please speak and discuss in English." A female researcher responded, "Why is it then when we go to the United States, the Americans do not speak French?" I replied confidently, "You don't have to worry; since we are in France, we plan to learn French." Thus, starting the next day, Felicia and I attended French classes at the Alliance Française, an institution that provided French language instruction. However, Felicia and I were intensively involved in our research. We had to publish our results in papers, and at night, we had to spend some quality time with the children. We had our hands full, and after three months, we gave up the French lessons. Looking back, we admitted that our language aptitude was not as strong as our kids but nevertheless those three months of French lessons were enough to make our everyday communication significantly easier.

Margie, our housekeeper in the United States, did not come along with us to France, so Felicia was obviously much busier. In addition to her full dedication to her research in laboratory, Felicia had to take care of the grocery marketing and also cook for the family after work. Because of the language barrier, she and the vendors communicated with hand gestures. Next, she would be in her kitchen apron to prepare dinner. After dinner, she would coach the children in their homework, help look up words in the dictionary, and at the same time, study French. Her life was always hectic and busy.

That was Felicia — once she was committed to do something, she always saw it through to the end with meticulous attention. Where parenting and children's education were concerned, she was strict and was never slack. Since young, there was nothing that the children did not discuss or share with Felicia. This was the lifetime harvest she reaped from her motherly devotion. Her dedication was her expression of selfless sacrifice and passion. Needless to say, the love and care Felicia gave me were beyond measure. On this journey of life, the mutual affection and trust we shared were unimaginably strong.

Touring Europe

Europe is a continent where many countries are geographically close by. Since we were already in Europe, we felt that we should take advantage of this opportunity to visit each country. Felicia was an energetic, outgoing and outdoorsy person. On weekends and holidays when she was free, she would take the children out for a gastronomic experience to enjoy world-renowned French cuisine, pastries and coffee, or a historical tour of the Parisian sites, such as the Louvre, the Palais de Versailles, the Eiffel Tower, and the Arc de Triomphe, where we left our footprints together as a family. Our sightseeing excursions were learning trips too. With complete information and guide on hand, we explained to the kids the background of the places of interest as we traveled. Thus, holidays enriched the knowledge and experiences of our children as they learned more about the world.

We later bought a small red Renault 5, the most popular car in France. With a car, we were able to take road trips outside of Paris. That year, we visited more than ten European countries; it was certainly an enjoyable time for our family. Once, we drove down to Cannes in southern France. We had no fixed destination; so it came as a serendipity that it happened to be the Cannes Film Festival on that day. The city was all lit up and illuminated. Throngs of people, streams of cars, bevies of glamorous women and dashing men who were waiting to be talent-scouted, and the motorcades of international stars whom we did not know or recognize — shrouded Cannes in a frenzied mood of merry-making. This was the first time our family had witnessed such a spectacle. Though we had ended up there by chance, we too became caught up in the excitement, and joined the starstruck crowd in laughter and anticipation, especially Felicia.

On another occasion, we spent two weeks touring Spain which is the second largest country in Western Europe after France. Spain's language, culture and customs are unique and notably different from the rest of Europe. Ninety-five percent of the population are Roman Catholic, and because of the vivacity and liveliness of the Spanish people and culture, religious rites and ceremonies are joyous occasions celebrated like festivals. Spain is also the cradle of the art and the birthplace of many world's famous painters such as Picasso and Dali. We immersed ourselves in the diverse cultures of Spain on an enjoyable journey of fun and laughter. We traveled all the way to the

Straits of Gibraltar, stood a long time gazing at the African wilderness on the opposite coast. Reluctantly we left and drove away. The two continents are separated only by a thin strip of water, and yet the people, culture, and the way of life are so vastly different. It is through the travels of our vast earth that culminated the feeling the greatness and cultural diversity of our planet.

Every time we went on a trip, we tried to make do with modest simple accommodations, but we did not skimp on food. Felicia loved cooking and picking up recipes, and the children and I love to eat too, so we took every opportunity to try the local cuisines and specialties. Of course, we did our homework before each trip, that is, reading up the countries' geographical and historical background. Before setting off, we would always prepare relevant reference and guide books. While I drove, Felicia and the children would read and discuss about what they had seen and experienced. Travel and learn, that was how we enjoyed and gained a deep appreciation of the unique culture of each country and region we visited. A Chinese saying goes: Reading thousands of books is not as useful as traveling for a thousand miles, and this means experience is still the best teacher. However, it brings greater pleasure to our lives to combine and blend reading and traveling together, like what we were doing.

Constructing a Cosmopolitan View

Indelible in our memory cache were the beautiful recollections of our extensive travel in Europe. But perhaps the most memorable of all was our journey to East Germany from West Germany when East Berlin and West Berlin were still divided.

The wall that divided them was like a sword thrust into the stomach; it sliced the city in two and created two radically different identities. West Berlin was prosperous, dynamic, and full of life; the people's faces were in smiles. But on the other side of the wall, stern and cold faces filled the quiet and still streets of East Berlin. That wall even divided a house in two. Under the same roof, by the mere separation of the wall, two completely different worlds existed, beyond one face of the wall, it was West Berlin and beyond the other face, it was East Berlin.

We brought the kids to visit the East Berlin railway station. Nervousness pervaded in the air and the sardine-packed human congestion brought the train station to a standstill, we could barely move, and we were forced to simply shuffle along with the crowd. Waves of people surged past us. On every anxious face was the frozen expression of tenseness and impassion. Even the young people's faces portrayed the emotionless frigidity. We wanted our children to learn about different societies, cultures, and political systems as well as how these factors cause deep rifts of difference in people's lives and the environment they live in. Felicia and I wanted to nurture our children to develop a perspective and fundamental view about the whole world, so that they would not be entrapped into their own tunnel vision. An exposure to the world not only expanded their horizon but also strengthened their ability to adapt to today's constantly changing world. That year, our travels in Europe added the most colorful brushstrokes in the memory canvas of our entire family.

Our year in Paris is a memory that will never fade. As the years go by, we inevitably create footprints in our minds telling tales of the past, some of which were deeply and indelibly imprinted in our lives. They are the detailed footnotes in our life until the moment we take our last breath and are reunited with our beloved ones in the Heaven above.

Half a year after Felicia passed away, I visited Paris to attend an academic conference. Recollections of what happened twenty years earlier when I took my family to Paris during my sabbatical year came back. Our life was filled with both sweet memories and bitter disappointments. The only way of reliving that fleeting moment is through the memories in our hearts. Time passes and there is no turning back. We are unable to chase the past, we can only stride forward, and no one can predict what lies ahead. There is always a past, a present, and a future at various stages of our lives — together they form a trilogy. As I walk on the giant wheel of time, the past catches up on me. I will always have Felicia to rely on, so I will never feel that this life has been without meaning. That year in Paris was a truly special year in our lives as a family.

Contemplating the past brings back a flood of memories. Inevitably.

8

The Long Island Days

The time spent in Europe gave our three children a new perspective on life. Upon return to the United States, Faith continued to study French through junior high school, high school, and college. In college, as a student majoring in political science, she participated in an overseas study program and studied in France for a year. After graduation, she secured an internship in Paris with an assemblyman from the Champagne region of France and later worked with a political party headed by a former Minister of Environment. She did research and submitted two Master's theses written in the French language.

David received his doctorate in chemistry from the University of California, Berkeley. He went on to do his postdoctoral research in Cambridge, England. There he met our future daughter-in-law, a ravishing Parisian mademoiselle by the name of Christelle Bousquet. At that time, she had already completed her law degree in France, but she furthered her study at Cambridge to obtain a Master of Law.

My youngest son Albert did not choose to continue studying French; rather, he chose to study Spanish. Albert, among the three children, is the most friendly and warm-hearted, he also has the passion and congeniality of a Spaniard; perhaps that is why he chose to study the language.

Taking up Our New Positions at Stony Brook

While we were in France, our former colleague at the Albert Einstein College of Medicine, Arthur Grollman, was at the State University of New York (SUNY) at Stony Brook, serving as chairman of the pharmacology department. The Governor of New York then was J.D. Rockefeller; he had invested a great deal of money in the school, hoping that the State University of New York at Stony Brook would become the East Coast equivalent of the University of California, Berkeley. At that time, the Stony Brook campus was in aggressive stage of development. Physics Nobel Laureate, Frank Yang, had even been invited and attracted there to take on a teaching position.

The first time Dr. Grollman came to visit us, I had no intention of giving up my laboratory at the Albert Einstein College of Medicine. Furthermore, Felicia and I were both busy with the preparations for our sabbatical in France, so nothing conclusive resulted from the meeting. Grollman's persistence did not wear off even we were already at the Pasteur Institute. He told us that he hoped Felicia and I would visit Stony Brook, where he would arrange for me to give a special lecture. I finally accepted his invitation to return to the United States to deliver the lecture and visit the Stony Brook campus.

At that time, Stony Brook was in the midst of an extensive development teeming with dynamic energy. The university was outfitted with the latest cutting-edge equipment. The offer of appointment was extremely attractive; besides offering me a three thousand square feet laboratory and a chair professorship, they offered Felicia an associate professorship. The university also raised a one million dollar endowment fund for me to maintain and develop the laboratory. And what was even more tempting was that Stony Brook is located in the picturesque, upscale residential neighborhood of Long Island.

The second time I returned to the United States from France, Felicia and I went together to visit Long Island. At the time, the school arranged for me to meet Frank Yang. This gesture manifested to me just how much the school had valued Felicia and me. I had given the proposition much thought, my research had been successfully applied in biophysics and biochemistry to study gene transcription, my next step then in the future research was to study mammalian and human gene expression. In order to break new grounds in my research, I would require new advanced equipment, and upgrading equipment in an existing old laboratory would certainly be more difficult and challenging.

The prospect of venturing into a novel research arena was one of the leveraging factors. Stony Brook, being a comprehensive university, offers multidisciplinary academic programs such as the engineering and humanities faculties which a medical school lacks. The interdisciplinary structure of the university fosters a much vibrant research culture than a medical school. Thus, the comprehensive breadth in the academic disciplines was also an important criterion.

Of course, our foremost concern was the children's education. We both knew that Long Island is one of the most prestigious residential addresses in the United States; many lawyers, doctors, and business honchos working in the New York City choose to live on Long Island. Some of the best public schools in the country are located on the Long Island, hence we felt reassured that our children would receive quality education.

Felicia and I talked over it for a long time after we returned to France. Although we found the terms and option quite attractive, we still felt we should seek the advice of our fellow senior scientists. So when we returned to the United States again, we talked with Dr. Jerard Hurwitz. He told us that the terms Stony Brook offered us were excellent, and moreover, the Albert Einstein College of Medicine would never be able to match Stony Brook's offer. However, he suggested that we go and speak to one of his old friends, Dr. Seymour Cohen, who was a member of the National Academy of Sciences and had been on the faculty of the pharmacology department at the State University of New York at Stony Brook for a year.

So off we went to visit the affable and warm-hearted Dr. Cohen. The knowledgeable scientist welcomed us to the Stony Brook campus. He said he had a fulfilling experience there thus far. He added that the school had made preparations to support us in any essential way, and they were only awaiting our affirmative answer. Dr. Cohen was the last person we consulted. We decided that if an academician as well-respected as Dr. Cohen recommended Stony Brook with such high regard, then we should take up the positions offered to us after our sabbatical.

A Tranquil Life on Long Island

We returned to the United States and relocated to the Stony Brook campus. Before assuming our new positions, the school and the pharmacology department organized a welcome party for us and invited William and Florence Catacosinos, who had donated one million dollar to the endowment fund that was to be designated as the Catacosinos Cancer Research Professorship. The president of the Stony Brook campus attended our welcome party and presented us the professorship award.

Felicia and I were excited and elated to have a laboratory that was comprehensively equipped with up-to-date instruments and facilities. Apart from the three thousand square foot laboratory and nice offices, we also had our own cold room, instrument room, cell culture room, and library. Occupying nearly one-quarter of the floor area of the building where it was housed, it was the largest laboratory in the medical school.

Felicia and I remained at Stony Brook from 1980 until our return to Taiwan in 1988, so Long Island was where Faith and Albert spent their growing-up years. Geographically, Long Island is shaped like a fish. The fish's head faces Manhattan, and the northern part, which is shaped like the fish trunk, faces the Long Island Bay. Connecticut is on the other side of the bay. The northern shore of Long Island is where the rich and famous live, in their stylish residences and mansions; the southern side with long stretches of pristine white sandy beach, is a haven for water sports. When we first arrived in Long Island, we lived by the waterfront on the north end. We had our own private beach. Swimming, frolicking in the water and catching mussels became our family's favorite activities.

Although beachfront living was enriching and alluring, we thought the beach might be a little dangerous for the children, so we moved out after just three months, and a year later, we bought a house in Setauket. The house had six bedrooms and a wooded backyard; it was just the kind of house that Felicia and I had dreamed of to raise our children. The woods covered a land area of more than three thousand square meters, and the built-up area added to another one thousand and seven hundred square meters. The open and expansive space was what appealed to us as the conducive environment for quality living.

When we first arrived in Long Island, the children thought that it was like a large, wild forest, as all the houses were well hidden in the dense forest. Our three children, who had grown accustomed to city life, were at first unused to the peace and quietness of Long Island, but after a period of time, they came to enjoy the forest, beaches, library, and the pond in deep aquamarine color, which were all only a stone's throw away. Wild dabbling ducks and geese swam languidly in the ponds, and the slender branches of the willow trees swayed in the breeze and dangled into the water. Sauntering on the little path by the edge of the pond, the mirror-like stillness of the pond surface, with occasional rings of ripples, and the dense canopy in different shades of green set a picturesque scenery before our eyes. The changing color of the autumn leaves was particularly spectacular, turning Long Island into a glorious blazing red that resembled a phoenix being consumed in the flames of fire and reborn in eternity.

The children, especially Albert, enjoyed taking walks to the pond and feeding the ducks which became close to him like his friends. The familiarity was so intense that Albert could even tell every duck apart. Felicia and I enjoyed running by the pond in the midst of the beautiful surroundings. On weekends, we would change into our swimsuits, and then the whole family would cycle to the seaside for a dip. Life on Long Island was peaceful and comfortable, and it was a lifestyle that anyone would loathe to give up, so I am eternally moved by the sacrifice Felicia and the children had to make — for giving up residency in America and for giving up a research career at its peak — in order to support my decision to return to Taiwan.

At that time, when we chose our place of residence, another important consideration was its vicinity to our children's schools. When our family returned to the United States, Faith was about to enter the fifth grade, and Albert, second grade. Attending school was very convenient for them as the schools were in close proximity to our home. However, after less than one term, the two children were placed in a high achievement educational program and had to attend schools in a different neighborhood, so the school bus became their mode of transport to school.

David Enters Harvard

Matters concerning David's schooling took a startling turn — which unfolded like a dramatic opera, leaving us at a loss as to how to react — when we returned to the United States. Originally, David was to start his tenth grade study when we returned. However, when we took David to enroll and gave the school a copy of his transcript, the school told us that the high school curriculum would be too elementary for David, and the school advisory board suggested that he enter university instead.

In the United States, when a child enters university, it means he can fly the coop and leave his home. As soon as Felicia heard what the school said, she became extremely worried. She told the teacher that David was only fourteen years old, and we did not want to lose him. I was, on the other hand, not as worried as Felicia because I rationalized that firstly, David had not attended any American high school, and secondly, he had yet to pass the college entrance requirements on the SAT and PSAT. He might not pass, and even if he did, the colleges might not accept him. So I posed the teacher a question, if David did not score high enough in these examinations to be accepted by the universities he applied, could he come back and study at the high school?

The teacher said that it would be possible to appeal to the school board. With this understanding, David took the SAT and PSAT. To our surprise, David passed with flying colors with nearly perfect scores in both exams. Never in our wildest imaginations would we have thought that would happen. Finally the notion sunk down on Felicia and me that perhaps David should attend university.

We sent in David's application for university admission to the best colleges in America which included Harvard, the Massachusetts Institute of Technology, Yale, Princeton, Stanford, and the California Institute of Technology. We originally thought that given David's brief stints in American schools, these crème de la crème colleges might not accept him, but two months later, all the colleges we applied to, except Harvard University, offered David a place. I took David to visit each of the universities that accepted him. Then one Friday evening in early April, I received a telephone call from a lady from the admissions office of the Harvard University.

She told me that the school was reviewing David's application. His young, tender age was a great concern. Harvard was concerned if David was mentally prepared for and was able to adapt to the liberal culture of Harvard where male and female students live in co-ed dormitories. I told her that we would not know either; we did not know what David's reaction would be. Then I told her that Felicia and I were from Taiwan. We were thinking that perhaps we could send David to Taiwan for a year and let him understand more about his roots and cultural background. We proposed to Harvard to admit David a year later when he would undoubtedly be more mature.

She hesitated a moment, then said decisively, "We must see the boy." The call came on a Friday evening; the following Monday we immediately drove David to Harvard University. On the way there, I related to David the story why his mother and I came to the United States. I explained to him the characteristics of Taiwanese culture, and the reason why we remained in the United States. After about six hours, we finally reached Harvard.

The director of the admissions office was already waiting for us in the office. As she and David exchanged words, I was stopped at the door. She told me, "Professor Wu, please wait outside. Today, the person being interviewed is David." She and David went into a different room, but not long after in less than five minutes, they came out again. Stepping out of the room, she said David was extremely mature, and his matriculation would not be a problem; in fact, he would become an asset to the academic world. Less than a month after that interview, Harvard University mailed us David's entrance form, indicating that he had been admitted for that academic year. The meticulous process and great interest that Harvard University took in considering David's admissions application was a strong factor in his decision later to attend that university.

The Struggle Over Staying in Taiwan

Felicia and I discussed the issue of David starting college at age fifteen several times and finally decided that he really was too young, so we persuaded David to defer his admission for one year. That summer I planned to take the whole family to Taiwan for vacation and let David settle down there.

This was the second time Felicia and I returned to Taiwan after we left for the United States. The first time we returned was 1974, when Faith and Albert were still very young. Though Felicia and I were preoccupied with running around looking after our two toddlers on the flight home, our hearts were a head-spinning mix of emotions, that of the yearning for home and the unknown feeling of trepidation and fear. Because we were gone for nine years, home felt at once close and yet seemed so far away. This time, in the blink of an eye, it had been six years later. Other than making arrangement for David to settle into Taiwan, Felicia and I hoped to bring the children back home so that they could learn and know where their parents came from, as well as to get to know our relatives and friends in Taiwan.

During that month, I explained to David the reasons why we hoped he should remain in Taiwan. I reasoned it out with him that though he was born in the United States, by blood and birth, he is still a Taiwanese. I also told him the story of the Japanese American professor, Sakami, who fought against Germany for the United States in Europe during the Second World War, but when the United States declared war on Japan, he was imprisoned in an internment camp because he was a Japanese. Although he was an American citizen, he was still essentially an Asian with yellow skin. I told David that the future world is going to be a very complicated place. If he returned to Taiwan and learned a little more about the East and Asian values, he would benefit when he grew up, and by then, he would have many more avenues open to him.

Although it was my wish that David would stay in Taiwan, I hoped and expected that the decision to come from him. Three days before our return to the United States, I asked David if he had already made up his mind. If he had not, what were the issues that he was considering? David answered that he was afraid that if he stayed, he would have no one to communicate with on an intellectual level. But he was still willing to consider the idea. After that, he shut himself up in his room, thought for an hour, came out and said to me affirmatively that he had decided to stay.

The second day, I was still uneasy. I asked again, "David, are you sure you want to stay?" David said, "I'll think about it over again." He locked himself in the room once more, came out an hour later, and told me that he had decided to stay. But I felt David was already struggling a little inside him. Finally, on the day before departure, I asked David again, "David, are you really sure you want to stay?" David went to his room and pondered over the question one last time. After an hour, he came to me face-to-face and said yes, he had decided to stay.

That night, I tossed and turned, unable to sleep. I started to reflect on my past — the pressure and expectation that my father had placed upon me to study medicine, and the compromises I had to make in order not to disappoint him. However, I later went against my father's wish, I did not practise as a doctor. Instead, I focused myself on a research career which was fulfilling and gave me a sense of satisfaction. David should have the right to choose. But that night I realized in my heart, I had already decided to take the entire family back home to the United States the next day.

The next day, I told David, "You don't have to stay in Taiwan. Come home with us." That day, David vehemently refused to go home with us, because to him, he had put his mind and heart together to derive this difficult decision, and I had just simply refuted and negated it. That day I asked Felicia to pack his bags. At the airport, David was still unwilling to get on the plane, but we forced him. On the flight, David's tears flowed profusely. He refused to speak a word to me until several days later.

From my involvement in handling David's "to-stay-or-not-to-stay-in Taiwan" dilemma, I learned one important lesson, that is, in the interaction between parent and child, the role of a parent, at some point, is to be someone to whom our children could turn to for guidance and advice. Each individual's life is in the control of one's own hands, hence, even though our intention is in the best interest of our children, that should not be the basis to hold them down in making their own decision. Through David's incident, I learnt a few things and reviewed my perspective about being a father.

When we returned to the United States, the academic term at Harvard had not begun, so David passed his time by going to the library and attending university classes at Stony Brook. Felicia and I knew in the heart that our young David was about to leave home and off to college. Finally, it dawned upon us that our first child was like a fledgling bird, with plumes of feathers on its wings, ready for its first flight out of the nest.

Suffering from Unfair Treatment

The research that I conducted at the Stony Brook campus utilized a combination of biophysics, biochemistry, molecular biology and genetic engineering techniques. It consisted of research on gene transcription mechanisms, exploration into new research areas, and most importantly, the use of human cells to study cancer genes. At Stony Brook, Felicia was already an associate professor; she studied the role of metallic ions in the regulation of gene expression as well as anti-cancer drugs. In the research field that investigates the function of metallic ions in genetic expression, Felicia was a pioneer; thus, due to her achievement, she was able to obtain a five-year research grant from NIH and was often invited to speak and present lectures around the world.

Because of our outstanding achievement in scientific research, Felicia and I were jointly-appointed professors at the biochemistry, chemistry, pharmacology and other departments at Stony Brook. Ironically, Felicia also faced discrimination in getting a promotion and thus, she became the subject of unfair treatment there.

When we arrived at the Stony Brook campus in 1980, Felicia was given the appointment as an associate professor due to the procrastinating delay on the part of the Albert Einstein College of Medicine in giving her entitlement for a full appointment. So when Felicia came to Stony Brook, she worked extra hard, hoping that through her achievements in research, she could become a full-fledged professor in two or three years.

After three years, Felicia applied for a full professorship. At the time, Felicia was already a leading researcher and authority in the research of metal ions in gene expression. After the application was submitted, the department head said Felicia's research achievements were certainly exceptionally outstanding but the Stony Brook pharmacology department set high bar for full professorship, hence, Felicia had to first receive international recognition in order to attain the rank of full professor. The department head had made the stance clear, and Felicia was confident that her achievement in research was widely recognized and known in the acadamia, she gladly accepted the challenge. Half a year later, Felicia was invited to give a plenary lecture in Prague, the capital of Czechoslovakia, at an international conference organized by the World Biochemistry Congress which was held every four years. This was a special honor, and certainly a strong, concrete proof that she had received worldwide recognition and affirmation as a leading researcher in her field. Therefore, the next year she again applied for promotion to the rank of full professor.

However, the department head still insisted on setting up a committee to review Felicia's credentials for advancement. The members of the committee were all nominated by the department head; nevertheless, the evaluations of the committee were extremely positive. What was incomprehensible was that the department head still would not approve Felicia's promotion. He rationalized that although the review committee's assessments were positive, they were for reference only, and the committee within the faculty did not approve the review. Usually, I was a member of the departmental faculty promotion committee, but because Felicia is my wife, I was abstained from the review to rule out any possibility of nepotism. Though I felt that Felicia had received unjust treatment in promotion, I had very little say in the matter.

What angered Felicia most was that there was a Caucasian male associate professor in the same department whose research achievements were far less stellar than hers, was actually promoted to the rank of full professor that year. Felicia realized that the department head was discriminated against Asian women. She could no longer tolerate the injustice.

Fighting Back Furiously

An earnest attitude, and a forthright, honest personality. That described Felicia's character. When confronted with inequality or injustice, she would challenge it to the end. She was intolerant of the department head's act of discrimination and was even prepared to hire a lawyer to file a lawsuit.

At that time it was already 1986. I was busy recruiting scientists for Academia Sinica's Institute of Molecular Biology and Institute of Biomedical Sciences. Felicia was by my side offering her encouragement and helping hand. Meanwhile, she was actively pursuing the issue of promotion. I urged her not to waste her energy to fight for her promotion in Stony Brook where there was a lack of transparency and equality. I knew that we both had received recognition and acclaim in the American academic world; if we made a transfer to join another university, Felicia would no doubt be offered a full professorship.

Thus, I let out news to the academic community that Felicia and I were considering to leave Stony Brook. At that time, New York University and Cornell University approached us. Both universities were in constant contact with us, and Cornell University, in particular, offered me a position as head of the biochemistry and pharmacology departments and Felicia a full professorship.

Cornell University's medical school is located in the northern part of Manhattan. Cornell University offered us a posh penthouse apartment on the east side of Central Park. Felicia loved New York, especially Manhattan. An art and cultural metropolis that has a lively vibe pulsating with a flourishing arts, music and theatre scene, and a bustling urbanite lifestyle, this is the confluence where the famous, the talented and celebrities converge. When we saw the living accommodation that Cornell University was offering us, Felicia almost felt an impulse to accept.

That was 1987. I had already agreed to return to Taiwan for a year in 1988 to establish the Institute of Biomedical Sciences at Academia Sinica and serve as director for one year. Therefore, if I were to accept the post at Cornell University, it would have to be after 1989. When we told the university that we first had to return to Taiwan for a year, they readily agreed.

Although Felicia had decided that leaving Stony Brook was a possibility, she continued to challenge the department head to voice her protest. Before we returned to Taiwan, Felicia engaged her lawyer to write a letter to the university in protest of the unfair manner and lack of transparency in which the department head had dealt with her promotion. Felicia refused to yield and back down because she felt strongly that she deserved the promotion which she worked hard for. Not someone to give up easily, she saw a cause to put right this injustice, so that in the future, Asian females would not have to suffer any form of discrimination at Stony Brook.

That was Felicia. She would not succumb to any compromise, if her conscience tells her to fight for a moral cause, she would be willing to sacrifice herself and give her all to accomplish it. I believe that her spirit of perseverance, strength, and fearlessness in the face of adversity were the reasons why she was able to fight cancer for thirteen years. Felicia — she was such a unique person with true feelings and great passion for life.

The Belated Justice

In the year 1988, I returned to Taiwan to establish the Institute of Biomedical Sciences and serve as director. The president of Stony Brook at the time, John Marburger, went to Hong Kong for a visit, so he made a detour to Taiwan on his way back. He was deeply impressed by the infrastructural groundwork we had done to establish the institute. He was superfluous with his praises on our work, saying that building a research team in the East that met international standards was a stupendous achievement. That evening, we organized a dinner for him. The conversation at the dinner table drifted to the issue of Felicia's promotion. The school president was astounded to learn Felicia's plight and stated that upon his return to the United States, he would look further into the matter.

Upon his return to the university, the president specifically asked the Provost to assemble a special committee with internationally renowned academics sitting on the panel. Two weeks later, the special committee passed the motion and review. They voted unanimously for Felicia to be promoted to full professor and overturned the department's ruling that rejected Felicia's promotion. The university president himself even wrote a letter to the department head to inform him of the special committee's decision, and he requested the department to honor it. So Felicia finally received her due justice and was promoted to the rank of full professor.

This is the anecdote of Felicia's promotion at the State University of New York at Stony Brook and the journey in her academic career. She endured the unfair treatment of gender discrimination, but remained determined in the face of every disappointment and obstacle; she never flinched and wavered. The greatest moment of anguish, and the greatest trial that Felicia faced in her life, was, however, the moment when she discovered she had cancer. I walked with her on this journey, and being the dearest person in her life, the poignancy and heartrending experience were beyond mere words.

SECTION III

TRANSITION PERIOD

9

Discovering Breast Cancer

After Felicia and I received the offers of faculty positions from the State University of New York at Stony Brook, we gave careful consideration before accepting. We even sought the opinion of Professor Seymour Cohen, a highly respected academic in the Stony Brook pharmacology department. At that time, he reassured us that there would not be any personnel problem at Stony Brook. However, we later discovered that there were intradepartmental issues, and Felicia also encountered numerous setbacks in seeking a promotion. I spoke to Professor Cohen about these issues. By then, Professor Cohen became our very close family friend, and the children all called him Uncle Seymour. He said, "You had just come, and the school had given you excellent terms which do not come by easily. I did not want you to change your mind about the school's offer simply because of something what I said. And besides, I sincerely hoped that you would come to Stony Brook."

The old professor's words expressed his concern for us. Felicia's and my research at Stony Brook were smooth-sailing. We might encounter some unpleasant situations, but they did not adversely affect our scientific careers. I was elected to member of Academia Sinica in 1984, but I was already busy laying the foundations for the establishment of its Institute of Molecular Biology in 1983. Felicia was assisting me with the planning: making contacts to organize conferences, staff recruitment, and other related tasks. Though the planning and preparation work for the institution kept us extremely busy, we were nevertheless happy and contented to be given the opportunity to do our part to contribute to our country.

Chinese American scientists and a number of members of Academia Sinica residing in the United States all participated enthusiastically in the development of science in Taiwan. At that time, the members who played active role in the development of the Institute of Molecular Biology included Paul Ts'o, James Wang, Ru-Chih Chou Huang, Ray Wu, and others. James Wang, Ru-Chih Chow Huang, Ray Wu, and I took turns to return to Taiwan to serve and act as director of the Institute of Molecular Biology during sabbatical leaves to see through its preliminary stage of development.

Academia Sinica's Institute of Molecular Biology and Institute of Biomedical Sciences jointly placed advertisements to recruit scientists. The planning for the Institute of Molecular Biology was in the works for some time, and the process of recruitment went fairly smoothly. Plans for the Institute of Biomedical Sciences, however, progressed much slower. So I told Shu Chien, a key member of the advisory committee for the Institute of Biomedical Sciences, about the Institute of Molecular Biology's plan for four rotating directors.

Shu Chien was quite impressed with the plan. He suggested to Dr. Paul Yu, chairman of the Institute of Biomedical Sciences advisory committee to invite me to join the committee to assist with the establishment of their institute. I was thus involved in two committees and actively engaged in the scientist recruitment for both institutes. Starting from 1985, I returned to Taiwan more frequently for work related to the two institutes.

While I devoted my time to do my part for Taiwan, Felicia was busy doing her part: planning conferences, writing abstracts and synopses, sending meeting notifications, and making food and accommodations arrangement. Although she was not a committee member, she devoted herself whole-heartedly in helping the establishment of the two institutes. If Felicia had not shared my responsibilities, I think my recruitment trips back to Taiwan those couple of years would not have been so fruitful and smooth-sailing.

In 1986 on the eve of Thanksgiving, I had a trip to Taiwan as planned. At that time, David had already graduated from Harvard University and was studying for a Ph.D. degree at the University of California, Berkeley. Even though he was already a graduate student, he was still young at the threshold of his twenty years of age, and Felicia was worried about him living away from home by himself. So I always stopped by to see him on my way to Taiwan.

The plan to spend Thanksgiving in Berkeley with David never materialized. David was planning a duck feast for me. He started preparing this meal a week earlier, and had even called Felicia to ask for recipes and special cooking tips. However, I never had the opportunity to enjoy the feast he prepared, because on the eve of Thanksgiving in 1986, Felicia discovered that she had breast cancer.

Discovering Breast Cancer

It was on the eve of Thanksgiving, two days before I was scheduled to attend a meeting in Taiwan, Felicia was busy packing my luggage. That night before she went to sleep, she unexpectedly felt a hard lump on her left breast. She told me immediately. I could also feel a two-, perhaps three-centimeter lump on the outer part of her left breast.

Felicia had always been in the pink of health. She had been a sportsperson since young. In college she was a member of the school's volleyball, track and field and archery teams. And we led an active lifestyle when we entered adulthood, our vacations were lined up with activities like mountain climbing, trekking and camping. In the United States, regardless of how busy our work was, we would still jog and swim on a regular basis. In everyday life, Felicia took special care to maintain a well-balanced and nutritious diet. On top of that, she even had regular health examinations. For her, even catching a cold was a rare event.

The other reason why Felicia placed such high priority about her health was that her mother was diagnosed with breast cancer when she was sixty years old. The cancer later spread to the liver and took her life. Felicia was clearly aware of her mother's medical condition. Her mother underwent surgery for a benign breast tumor in Taiwan, but the wound never healed. Her mother later went to the United States, and stayed at her son's house (Felicia's brother). Felicia's mother underwent a more extensive examination. At this point she discovered what she had was breast cancer.

Though she endured a series of painful treatments, in the end, the cancer still spread to the liver.

We were at the Albert Einstein College of Medicine at that time when my mother-in-law came to stay at our house for about three months and received medical treatment at the Albert Einstein College of Medicine Hospital. Felicia felt for her mother's pain and suffering. This had a particularly deep effect on Felicia because she was very close to her mother. My mother-in-law suffered the agony of cancer for ten years before she passed away at the age of seventy.

Because of her mother's medical history, Felicia paid special attention to have regular medical examinations. She would have a mammogram almost every six months. In fact, at the time when she discovered the lump in her breast, she had a mammogram just four months earlier. So at first we did not think anything could be seriously wrong.

Nonetheless, the next day we immediately telephoned a few physicians at various cancer research institutions including Dr. Paul Carbone, director of the cancer center at University of Wisconsin-Madison and one of the world's pioneer oncologists. These physicians all recommended Dr. Frank E. Gump, a surgeon at Columbia University who had operated on over a thousand breast cancer patients. I consulted Dr. Shu Chien, then at Columbia University. He also concurred that Dr. Gump was the most respected authority in his field. I then contacted Dr. Gump and took Felicia to the Columbia University Hospital to have an examination on that same day.

Dr. Gump was an amiable and warm-hearted gentleman. He immediately performed a biopsy of the lump in her breast; by that afternoon we had the results. He confirmed that it was breast cancer and suggested that she undergo mastectomy as soon as possible.

To us, the revelation came like a bolt of lightning that suddenly struck on a clear blue day. Felicia, especially, found it hard to believe the fact. She said that she just had a mammogram four months ago and was given a clean bill of health; how could that be breast cancer? Moreover, how could that happen to Felicia, who had always led a healthy lifestyle and made conscious effort to have regular medical examinations?

But these were, after all, doctor's diagnosis, and we had no choice but to accept the cruel reality. So after returning to Stony Brook, I immediately canceled the trip to Taiwan, informed David of his mother's condition, made arrangements for Felicia's surgery, and admitted Felicia to the hospital to do further tests.

Everything occurred too suddenly. During this period of time, Felicia was at an emotional low. She constantly asked herself disbelievingly, "Why me?" She even blamed the doctor who conducted her mammography for not being thorough enough in the examination. But the bout of depression was transitional and did not last very long. I believe Felicia's positive and optimistic nature stand her in good stead to confront the unexpected — once she decided to face it, she would no longer be depressed and would fight the battle head-on. Of course, the main reason that made Felicia get up on her feet was her young children who still needed the love and nurture of a mother. Felicia had to be strong, she did not want to be a cause of worry, and wanted her picture-perfect family to be intact.

Receiving Treatment

Two weeks later, Felicia entered the operating theater and had her left breast removed. That day, both Shu Chien and Ming-Neng Yeh, my former classmate in medical school and a member of the faculty of the Columbia University Medical School's obstetrics department, came to observe and offer their assistance. After the surgery, the doctor immediately conducted tests on the tissues and confirmed that it was breast cancer. Dr. Gump also discovered that the lymph nodes showed signs of swelling and removed them as well. He told me later that out of Felicia's nine lymph nodes, seven already contained tumor cells.

When Felicia was diagnosed with breast cancer, it had already reached the second stage. As the semi-radical mastectomy (partial breast removal surgery) revealed that the cancerous cells had spread to her lymph nodes, the doctor recommended Felicia to undergo adjuvant chemotherapy as soon as possible after she recovered from the surgery. Adjuvant chemotherapy is a treatment that patients receive after a surgery to remove tumors; it eliminates any cancer cells that may be left in the body and prevents cancer from recurring.

In 1986, mankind's knowledge about cancer was not as comprehensive as today, the same could be said of anti-cancer therapeutics. Nevertheless, we found the best doctors and scientists working on the most advanced research in cancer to give their opinion on Felicia's condition. Felicia and I wanted to know what type of drugs should be used for chemotherapy.

As Felicia was involved in the research of anti-cancer drugs, she was knowledgeable about their use, side effects, and success rates. So before the chemotherapy process, she participated in all discussions as a patient and as a researcher. At that time, the drug treatment most commonly used was a three-drug combination: cyclophosphamide, methotrexate, and fluorouracil (CMF). Based on the past statistics, the five-year survival rate of patients in the second stage using CMF was approximately twenty percent. Felicia was unwilling to accept this kind of odds.

After Felicia had her left breast removed, she was determined to win the battle against cancer for the sake of her family and her loved ones. Under no condition would she allow the cancer cells in her body to survive. We hence sought consultations with various oncologists, hoping to find a more effective anti-cancer drug.

At that time, there was a potent new drug called adriamycin that was also quite toxic and had detrimental effect on the heart, but was very effective against cancer cells. Felicia and I knew about this novel drug treatment. We consulted our doctor and scientist friends about the possibility of using this new drug.

It is not hard to imagine Felicia's state of mind. She wanted earnestly to use the most effective drug to treat her illness. After several rounds of intensive discussions with the doctor, we decided to use AMF; in other words, the cyclophosphamide in the CMF combination is replaced with adriamycin, in order to increase the chances of a complete cure.

After the drugs for chemotherapy had been determined, it was further decided that Felicia's chemotherapy would be conducted at the affiliated hospital of the State University of New York at Stony Brook. She had to undergo eight sessions of chemotherapy and after which the hormone therapy. Felicia deeply felt the agony of chemotherapy that her mother went through — now she, too, had fallen ill and experienced the suffering. The pain that she had to undergo would be greater than what her mother had endured because she had chosen the strongest possible drug treatment. Felicia was not one to resign herself to fate. Cancer had taken away her mother's life but she refused to allow cancer to triumph over her. The belief and the determination became the constant motivating force to live.

A Portrait of Struggle

It was an afternoon in early spring. The sunlight penetrated the dense foliage of Long Island like streaks of thin golden thread, and the wind blew softly through the woods. The children and I arrived in Long Island and returned to the house and garden that Felicia and I had tended with so much loving care.

That day was bitterly cold. We drove the car up to the doorstep of the house, or perhaps I should say, to what used to be our home. In front of us was a vast and open expanse of green grass. It seemed the present tenants preferred having an open and unobstructed view. The densely forested woods that used to be there were now gone. I said to myself, "This is the house in my memory — that holds important milestones in Felicia's and my life, and marks the growing up years of our children's lives. Time flies; things have changed."

We looked around the house at the entrance, and that sparked the curiosity of the house owner. He opened the door; the children and I explained why we were there. The resident cordially invited us in to let us walk in the garden. Albert strode to the window of his old bedroom and said the first thing he would do in the morning was to walk to the window to watch the swaying shadows of the trees in the wind and listen to the chirping of the birds. David walked to the rear of the house where a tree nearly twenty-five meters tall stood. It was he who first discovered that the tree was sick with bug-infested branches. Faith celebrated her sixteenth birthday here in this garden. Beaming in her sweetest smile, Faith was as ravishing as a princess. Like a bright moon accompanied by myriads of stars, she was basked in the warmth of the well-wishes of her classmates and family.

Felicia would always enter the house through the kitchen's door to discuss about dinner preparations with Margie when she came home in the evening. Margie's round face and warm-hearted smile was just like a ray of sunlight that brightened our dining mood and atmosphere.

Walking past the garden, I could not bring myself to recapture the memories of the Thanksgiving eve when Felicia discovered she had breast cancer and I could not retrace those moments of tenacity and courage as she underwent chemotherapy treatment. Instead, images of her frail silhouette and her bouts of nausea recurred in my flashbacks.

Back to Stony Brook, Felicia underwent chemotherapy treatment. The first time, I accompanied Felicia to the affiliated hospital and stayed with her for the procedure. Dr. Madagenicz, the doctor-in-charge, explained in detail the side effects of chemotherapy which include nausea, vomiting, physical weakness, heart palpitations, and loss of hair. In reality, Felicia was already quite clear about the success rate, survival rate, risks, and side effects of the therapeutics. She was determined to fight for the chance to live. She had prepared herself mentally for the side effects of the chemotherapy and was ready to confront them.

In my recollection, I only accompanied Felicia for the first chemotherapy. And that was the first and only time she rested at home after the chemotherapy. For the subsequent sessions, she would always return to the laboratory immediately to continue working.

The first time she received AMF, the adriamycin's toxicity to the heart rendered her nauseous, weak, and short of breath with breathing difficulty as soon as she reached home. Felicia's countenance was a sickly pallor, and she felt weak to the point that I had to support her as she walked. The first chemotherapy treatment already took a toll on her but Felicia was able to steel herself and fight through the same side effects, sessions after sessions.

Altogether, there were eight sessions of AMF chemotherapy treatment; each session would span approximately over two weeks. When the drug is administered into the body for the first time, the patient's white blood cell count decreases after the first week, which is deemed as the critical condition for the patient. It is necessary to wait until the patient's white blood cell count rises before the second chemotherapy treatment can be administered.

Felicia's chemotherapy treatment took approximately six months, during which she lost all her hair. We went to New York City together to buy wigs and breast pads; she was not daunted at all, and was not affected by the loss of her hair — considered as the crown of glory for women — because to her, these "three thousand strands of frustration" amounted to nothing compared to her precious life and her family she loved so much. Right from the beginning, Felicia fought bravely against cancer, and not once in the thirteen years in her battle had I ever seen her downcast and disheartened.

The children and I walked along the periphery of the pond. Joggers, panting and their cheeks flushed, zipped past us. Albert sat on his favorite rock. This was where he sat to feed the ducks; that was why he called it his rock. It was still early spring. There was no graceful drapes of the long, slender branches of the willow trees touching the surface of the pond. On the snarled-up, entangled branches were sprouts of green shoots that quivered in light breeze, which appeared like ripples in the reflection of the pond. I did not know for sure whether we were captivated by this picturesque sight, or because our thoughts had flown to some faraway place, but on the little path, everyone was quiet. Perhaps we were all absorbed in our recollections of the past.

It had already been more than ten years since we left the United States. At the affiliated hospital, it came as a serendipity that we ran into Dr. Madagenicz, the doctor who had conducted Felicia's chemotherapy treatment. He welcomed us heartily and said, "Every time Felicia completed her session of chemotherapy treatment, she would always leave in a rush. I advised her to take sufficient rest, but Felicia always insisted on getting back to the laboratory to work." Dr. Madagenicz recalled that Felicia came across to him as someone who did not appear as a sickly patient despite her condition, because she, for someone in scientific research, would ask medical staff very precise and detailed questions about her treatment and then, she would be seen carefully taking down notes. "Among the many cancer patients I have treated for chemotherapy, she was the toughest, the most enthusiastic and positive I have ever seen," Dr. Madagenicz said.

During those six months of chemotherapy treatment, Felicia lost substantial weight, as evident from her emaciated face, but she remained energetic and optimistic. I told Felicia that I would take her somewhere for a trip after she recouped some rest following the treatment session. Those six months, she still kept herself busy with laboratory research, household chores, and the children's activities. Whether these were music lessons, outdoor sports or school celebrations, Felicia would participate to show her support for the children. Looking back, I think perhaps these were the source of Felicia's strength, because in fulfilling these different roles, she derived renewed hope and mission to cherish life. This was the meaningful life that Felicia wanted to have, and she would not allow her sickness to have a hold on her.

The Energy of Recovery

Six months later, I took Felicia to New Orleans to attend the annual national biophysics conference. In fact, my purpose was to let Felicia have an opportunity to spend some time away from work. At that time, she had completed her eight chemotherapy sessions and was on the path of recovery to regain her strength. Eager to be up and about, Felicia could hardly wait to go with me. We did not know until we reached New Orleans that it happened to be the last day of Mardi Gras. For someone who loved festivities, Felicia would never give a major event like Mardi Gras a miss.

The ebullience on the street was contagious and Felicia stepped out too to immerse herself in the gaiety. I thought: "My God!" We had never seen such wild revelry in our life — swarms of revelers held on to their beer bottles, and drank to their hearts' content; and everyone was flamboyantly dressed. Look! There were people in Hawaiian grass skirts dancing the hula. Beautiful women danced and sang with wild abandon on the elaborately decorated parade floats, from which fountains of perfumed water were showered onto jubilant revelers flanked on both sides of the street. An intoxicated mood of mystique pervaded. The merry-making and energy of the day lifted all revelers to the zenith of euphoria.

Glittering gold coins and small, shiny mementoes cascaded from another parade float like a waterfall. The revelers thronged in for their share. Amidst the mad rush, laughter filled the air, happy emotion emanated from the crinkles of the revelers' eyes. Felicia reached for the shimmers too along with the rest of the crowd. She forgot that she was wearing a wig, so in the midst of the commotion, her wig was immediately pulled off. I thought losing the wig would definitely be a bad idea because it might not be possible to buy another one there, so in my fastest response I strode forward, snatched up the wig, and helped Felicia put it back on her head.

Felicia looked back and realized what I had done; we smiled at each other and laughed at this funny episode.

That night, we returned to the hotel, extremely exhausted. As Felicia removed the wig and was about to step into the bathroom, a hotel service staff knocked on the door. Felicia did not stop to think and opened the door. The service staff naturally did not expect a bald-headed woman, so the poor chap just stood there dumbstruck and speechless. Felicia tried very hard to stifle her giggle. After closing the door, the two of us broke out in laughter like two mischievous children who had just succeeded in playing a trick on someone.

These two incidents clearly reflected Felicia's personality — her passion and optimism for life. She did not fall into the depths of despair and frustration when faced with a life-threatening illness. On the contrary, she fervently savored every living moment of her life, and every opportunity presented to her to be a part of the world. If I were to distill the message Felicia wanted to share with us about the purpose of her existence in this world, it would be to cherish life and to value the love in one's heart.

On learning Felicia's sickness, our friends were all very concerned about her recovery and emotional state. Dr. Shu Chien and his wife were among them who showed concern. When I informed them that Felicia's recovery was progressing well, and she had an open and positive outlook as before, they were extremely happy and invited us to their thirtieth wedding anniversary celebration.

Felicia and I readily accepted the invitation. Felicia even went as far as to personally pick and buy their presents. She prepared two presents and had the couple's names engraved on them. We attended the party in happy spirits with loads of our well-wishes for the couple.

The couple had spent a great deal of time learning tango so that they could perform the dance for all of us that night.

Tango dance demands lithe and graceful movements. The ease and familiarity with which they performed the dance steps went to show how much time and energy they had dedicated in their practice. There is this particular dance step, called the "dip," in which the female partner arches her back to the floor, and the male partner supports her with his arm. While the couple was engrossed performing the "dip", Felicia picked up a stalk of rose, scurried nimbly over to Dr. Shu Chien and placed the flower between his lips. Laughter broke out in the room full of guests. Till today, Felicia's antics still warm the cockles of the couple's hearts.

Though Felicia underwent surgery and chemotherapy after being diagnosed with cancer, her energy and enthusiasm returned relatively quickly. Felicia had to be on a long-term medication of anti-cancer drug to prevent the disease from striking again.

The medication that Felicia took was a synthetically produced drug called Tamoxifen. This drug, often given to women in high doses, has a chemical structure similar to estrogen. Its main function is to cause the suppression of estrogen function, known for stimulating breast cancer development. Its estrogen suppression properties arise from its chemical structure, which enables it to competitively bind to sites that estrogen usually binds to.

Felicia took this medicine every day and went for a health examination every half year. At that time, the rule of thumb frequently cited in the medical field was that if the patient is in remission for five years, the patient is considered to have recovered and cured of cancer. In my heart, I knew Felicia lived her life by a measurement span of five years, she was waiting to see what her body condition was going to be like for the next five years.

Felicia took Tamoxifen for a period of eight years, until the cancer recurred. Today, medical researchers have discovered that if Tamoxifen is taken over a period of more than five years, it will start to lose its suppressive properties. Every time I think of this, my heart aches. If, at that time, medical research had advanced to present stage, perhaps Felicia's fight against cancer would not have been difficult and painful.

Devoting Heart and Soul for Taiwan

Towards the end of 1986, Felicia discovered she had breast cancer. In July 1988 we returned to Taiwan. During that period, we were busy with the planning work for our return to Taiwan. On top of that, we had our usual laboratory duties and submission of research proposals for the following year to work on. Before we left for Taiwan, Felicia had also successfully applied and received a five-year research grant from NIH. Of course, we were actively involved in the recruitment exercise for Academia Sinica's Institute of Molecular Biology and the Institute of Biomedical Sciences.

Though we had a busy schedule and multiple responsibilities, being able to make a small contribution to our homeland made us feel gratified.

The original plan was to return to Taiwan and serve as director of the Institute of Molecular Biology, however, I ended up succeeding Dr. Shu Chien as director of the Institute of Biomedical Sciences. The change in plans arose from a discussion I had with Shu Chien before he returned to Taiwan in 1987. He said that the Institute of Molecular Biology already had its first three or four years planned, but the Institute of Biomedical Sciences only had him returning to serve as director for its first year, and so he hoped that I could succeed him the following year.

The Institute of Biomedical Sciences was in need of a scientist with experience in both medicine and research who could steer and spearhead the planning for its establishment, and to headhunt such a person in such a short timeframe would not be easy. I told Dr. Shu Chien that I had already accepted the post at the Institute of Molecular Biology. Dr. Shu Chien and Professor Paul Yu, the chair for the Institute of Biomedical Sciences' advisory committee, made a special request to the Institute of Molecular Biology to release me so that I can be appointed as director of the Institute of Biomedical Sciences during my sabbatical year. The Institute of Molecular Biology agreed, so I returned to Taiwan in 1988 to assume the appoinment as director of the Institute of Biomedical Sciences.

When we returned to Taiwan in 1988, Felicia and I had originally planned to take just one year of sabbatical and do as much as we could for our homeland. However, life is always unpredictable. What was meant to be a trip to Taiwan turned out to be our homeward-bound journey to sink our roots permanently. The years ensued were also the time I stuck through thick and thin with Felicia in her fight against cancer. I was forty-nine years old when I came back to Taiwan. In the blink of an eye I am already over sixty. Time and tide wait for no man, and Felicia had left this world. The present and future that I embrace, I could only share with Felicia my beloved, in memory of her…

10

Imparting Our Knowledge as Our Contribution to Taiwan

Felicia and I returned to Taiwan in July 1988. More than thirty scientists returned with us, and the brain gain was considered a major groundbreaking news of the 1980s in Taiwan's scientific community. All the returning scientists shared the same dream, that is, to build a strong foundation for the medical field in Taiwan and to develop Taiwan's biomedical capabilities and technologies to achieve world-class competitiveness.

As long as you have a dream, you will have the desire to fulfill it. Shu Chien, who came back to Taiwan before me, had already laid the basic structure and set up the system for the Institute of Biomedical Sciences. This solid beginning enabled me to take over his responsibilities with ease and steer ahead confidently. Back on home soil at last, Felicia and I were filled with vigor and passion to nurture and grow our idealistic vision for our motherland. We originally planned to stay for just a year, but the degree of our commitment and fervor seemed to win us over.

Life's Little Adjustments

That summer, our whole family returned to Taiwan. David was at Berkeley doing his doctoral study; Faith had graduated from high school and had already set her mind to attend Cornell University.

Albert was just beginning his tenth grade, equivalent to the first year of high school in Taiwan. David and Faith spent their time in Taiwan only during their summer vacations and they also expected the entire family would be together again in the United States after one year, hence, they were not too greatly affected by our move to Taiwan.

Albert, on the other hand, had no alternative but to study for his tenth grade in Taiwan. Besides being separated from his friends in the States, the new school environment in Taiwan would also pose a challenge for him. We explained to Albert that this would be a precious opportunity for him to explore his own roots and gain an appreciation for Taiwan's culture, its unique society, as well as foster a bonding with his relatives. Albert is always an obedient child, so he was naturally receptive of the idea. But I knew back then, in his heart, he was telling himself to try to stick out for a year, and after which, he would be able to return to the United States.

We understood that year was going to be extremely difficult for Albert. He was at the age when interaction and communication with his peers constituted an important process of growing up. He would be relatively lonely as his friends were all in the United States and his older brother and sister were not with him; his social circle changed entirely as soon as he arrived Taiwan. And he had to attend Taipei American School (TAS) in Tianmu, which was far away from where we lived in Nankang. The TAS bus did not come as far as Nankang, so Albert had to leave the house at six-thirty every morning. When he came home after school, it was already past seven at night. Aside from the commute, the vast difference between the Taiwanese and American school systems also made Albert's adjustment more difficult.

As for Felicia and me, our lifestyle in Taiwan was also quite different from what we had enjoyed in the United States. My main responsibility — which was to steer the establishment and development of the Institute of Biomedical Sciences — was primarily an administrative position involving frequent meetings, both internal and external. These meetings took up most of my time, and the demands of my busy schedule inevitably infringed upon my family time. In the United States, Felicia and I were known as a "twenty-four hour" couple. We went to work together in the morning, ate lunch together, came home together at night, and even attended social gatherings together. In Taiwan, because the nature of my work and responsibilities were drastically different, my family time with Felicia and the children was reduced dramatically. At first, Felicia was not accustomed to these little shifts and changes in life at all.

Indeed, the adaptations that Felicia had to make that year proved challenging to her. From the time Felicia and I got to know each other, we were practically inseparable in school as we studied and attended lessons together. If there was any one time that we were not physically together, that could be the period when she left the country to do her Master's degree in the United States and the period when I served in the army at Kinmen. Otherwise, we were together from day to night. Now, at most, all we could do was to squeeze in time to have lunch together. There were several occasions when she attended meal gatherings with me, but soon she stopped doing so, partly because she felt bad about leaving Albert alone at home, and partly because she felt that these business meals and social networking in Taiwan dry and boring. Eventually, she came to understand that the scope of duties and responsibilities as expected of my administrative position were unlike my previous research work, and she reconciled herself to adapt and accommodate these changes in life.

Researching Vitamin K3

In the United States, Felicia's research focused on metal ions and their role in gene expression. Though her research had already received international recognition, this was not the critical area of focus in Taiwan's research directive. Thus, before the move back to Taiwan, Felicia had already started planning her research initiative that would bring benefit to Taiwan and propel the research and development here.

Since 1982, cancer is ranked first among the top ten causes of deaths in Taiwan, and the number of people suffering from cancer annually has surpassed thirty thousands. But at that time, Taiwan's cancer research as well as drug discovery and development lagged far behind the developed countries. The country also lacked drugs to treat cancers that are of high prevalence in Taiwan, such as liver cancer. Felicia's other primary research area was anti-cancer drugs, hence she decided that upon her return, she would focus on this area to develop new cancer therapeutics and treatments, and to enhance the basic clinical research of cancer in Taiwan.

For this reason Felicia carried out research on the anti-cancer properties and mechanisms of Vitamin K3. Vitamin K3 was originally used as a coagulant and it was by chance in 1982 that the American scientists discovered that Vitamin K3 has anti-cancer properties. However, it was not known how Vitamin K3 act to kill cancer cells, so Felicia's research team began investigating the mechanisms of action. Her laboratory in Taiwan was the most successful in the world in the investigation of the anti-cancer mechanisms of Vitamin K3 and also the first research group to conduct clinical trial of Vitamin K3.

As for my work in Taiwan, I assessed the research directives based on the illness statistics and health profile of Taiwanese people, and also the specialties of the returning scientists recruited from overseas. Thereafter, I organized the research structure of the Institute of Biomedical Sciences into six divisions: the structural biology research division, the epidemiology and public health research division, the cardiovascular diseases research division, the neuroscience research division, the infectious diseases research division, and the cancer research division. Felicia took on the responsibility of coordinator of the cancer research division. Felicia did not show a single trace that she had been afflicted with illness as evident in the dedication and long hours she put in, usually into late night, in her research work. Had it not been the relapse eight years later, her colleagues in the laboratory would never have known that she herself was a cancer survivor.

Everyone Encourages Us to Stay in Taiwan

Taiwan's medical community hoped that, given Academia Sinica's paramount status, the establishment of the Institute of Biomedical Sciences would integrate and synergize medical research and clinical practice thereby improving the quality of medical science and healthcare in Taiwan. Thus, the medical community expressed its strong support and held high expectations of the Institute's research plans and future opportunities for collaboration.

As I came onboard the Institute of Biomedical Sciences, the progress of its development was akin to the powerful energy of an arrow ejected from a bow — fast and steady, and destined to travel for a long haul. Every member of the research teams showed their commitment to work towards the same goal. And at that time, Felicia and I started to feel the pressure and obligation to stay rooted in Taiwan to continue the work.

Felicia's love for our homeland was no less than mine. She might take awhile to get used to having less time with me at work and at home, but she adapted pretty fast and integrated well into other facets of life. For instance, many of the returnees from the United States were afraid to drive on the roads of Taipei which they deemed as chaotic traffic, but Felicia was a picture of calm when she was behind the wheel. She not only drove, she also commuted by taxi and bus, did her grocery shopping in traditional markets, and immersed herself in the diverse offerings of cultural performances, and even indulged in the pleasure of local sauna. Though we returned to Taiwan under the pretext of our sabbaticals, we certainly felt deeply for our homeland, no doubt about that. However, if we were to consider living in Taiwan for long term, that would indeed be difficult and a struggle for us.

The stress I had to deal with surfaced as soon as I returned. It was around August and September, the first two months after my return, the Institute of Biomedical Sciences had to present a proposal for the following year's budget. I had already foreseen that, with the fast-paced and dynamic development of the Institute of Biomedical Sciences, the building and facilities would no longer be sufficient to sustain its growth in two years' time. So I submitted a proposal and budget for the construction of a new building. The proposal further heightened everyone's expectation of the future of the Institute, even drawing attention from the government and various sectors.

The scientists who returned with us were extremely enthusiastic and efficient — a series of collaborative medical research projects and training programs were launched. Deserving further elaboration here is the training program initiative. Taiwan was at least ten years lagging behind the United States in cancer treatment. We did not even have medical oncologists. Since cancer is Taiwan's top killer, the training of medical oncologists was imperative. So the Institute of Biomedical Sciences drafted the preliminary training proposal, put forth jointly by Paul Ts'o, Jacqueline Peng-Wang, and me. We specifically invited Paul Carbone, a leading oncologist of international renown, to Taiwan to conduct the training program. This program paved the road for the development of the subspecialty of medical oncology in the country, and at the same time, created collaboration opportunities between the Institute of Biomedical Sciences and major Taiwanese hospitals. The medical community already pinned great hopes on the institute to flex its leadership in the academia to integrate the diversity of medical fields in Taiwan.

The budget for the construction of a new building for the Institute of Biomedical Sciences was approved by Academia Sinica and submitted to the Executive Yuan. At that time, the Minister without Portfolio Jun-Shan Shen was the administrative officer responsible for the review and allocation of the Executive Yuan's science and technology budget. He stated that the government was extremely supportive of the plan. However, there was a catch. He believed that if I continued to be at the helm of Institute of Biomedical Sciences, the Executive Yuan would definitely allocate and grant the fund. But if I stepped down and left Taiwan, the Executive Yuan would regard the future development of the institute as uncertain, and this might influence their decision to approve the budget.

It happened around February or March of the following year. The group of thirty or so scientists, who joined and came back with me, met the then Academia Sinica President Ta-You Wu. They voiced out their aspiration that I would continue to stay on and work with them towards our common goal of propeling research and building a firm foundation for the biomedical sciences sector in Taiwan. If I stepped down, they too would consider leaving. Their ardent support proved a tipping point that I found myself in a dilemma, both awkward and difficult, because they were the scientists whom I personally invited to come with me to Taiwan. These scientists had left their jobs in the United States and returned to Taiwan out of love for their country and their strong faith in me. If we were to lose these scientists, the loss would not just be their jobs and careers in the United States, the greatest loss of all was, in fact, Taiwan's. Thus President Ta-You Wu also expressed his wish that I would remain in Taiwan.

Even academicians based in the United States, such as Shu Chien, Jacqueline Peng-Wang, and Ru-Chi Huang-Chou, hoped that I would continue the work in Taiwan. Jacqueline Peng-Wang said that if my decision was to stay, in two years' time she would also return to work with me. And though there were some overseas scientists who were unable to return to Taiwan in the short term, they were ready to do everything they could to offer their expertise to push Taiwan's development of medical science, so that we could all realize our mission together.

Considering the Reality

Felicia and I discussed and pondered the dilemma at great length. We had our concerns, the foremost being our children's education. As David was in the graduate school and was growing up, matured and responsible, we did not have to worry much about him. Faith just began her studies in the university; her understanding was that we would return to the United States after one year. Supposing we continued to live in Taiwan, the long distance and vast ocean that separated us would be a huge obstacle for us to render her immediate assistance and attention should anything happen. And our greatest concern was Albert actually. Having been schooled in the American system, it was impossible for Albert to enter the normal Taiwanese high school system. Even at Taipei American School, he was already facing the challenges of adjusting, as their school system was quite different from that of the American schools. Should Albert experience problems adapting to school and life in Taiwan — which could affect his studies adversely — he might not be able to return to the United States for university; the consequence could thus have a negative impact on his future.

Of course, the other problem before us was the most realistic, our financial status. The tuition fee and living expenses for our three children in the United States constituted a large part of our family expenditure. Taking into account of our remuneration in Taiwan, there was no way we could afford the high education expenditures of our children. The loan that we had taken out on our housing mortgage was another financial burden. These realistic considerations put into perspective why the question of "to remain or not to remain in Taiwan" was such a difficult decision to make.

Felicia also recognized the importance of us staying in Taiwan. She was a person with great love for her family and her homeland, so she was not at all opposed to coming home. But in her opinion, the move would be more appropriate three or four years later when all our children would be in college. By then, we would be free of financial worries and concerns, and we could focus all our attention and energy on the development of biomedical science in Taiwan.

When President Ta-You Wu asked me whether I was considering the possibility of staying on long-term, I explained to him our difficulties and suggested to him to invite overseas scholars who were about to retire to return and take on the position. Their children would have grown up, and they were less likely to be held back by the economic demands of their children's education. I also told President Wu that after our sabbatical, we had already given our in-principle confirmation to take up positions at Cornell University, I as chairman of the biochemistry and pharmacology departments, and Felicia as a full professor. Assuming we turned down the appointment in Cornell, there were lecture courses at Stony Brook that Felicia and I, as senior professors, were responsible for teaching. If we did not return to Stony Brook, the school would have scheduling problems, and that would affect the academic and leave plans of other professors.

On top of that, we had other considerations. In our laboratory back in United States, Felicia and I had over thirty students, research assistants, and postdoctoral fellows who wished we could return soon from our sabbatical to continue to supervise and mentor their research. Furthermore, before returning to Taiwan, Felicia had applied for and received a five-year research grant from NIH. I also had three ongoing research projects funded by NIH, the National Science Foundation, and the American Cancer Society. With these research commitments in tow, the management of grant, project planning and laboratory resources planning were no easy tasks. Thus, after evaluating the real situations and considering the practicalities, a plethora of difficulties was foreseeable if we remained in Taiwan.

A Turnaround Finally in the Midst of Twists and Turns

However, things took an unexpected turn. The year when I was in Taiwan, Dr. John Marburger, then president of the State University of New York at Stony Brook, had a scheduled visit to Hong Kong, so he stopped by Taiwan. I made arrangement for him to meet President Ta-You Wu. At the meeting, President Wu broached the topic on me and said how he wished I could stay in Taiwan to help the country establish the Institute of Biomedical Sciences. President Wu also explained my difficulties — which included the remuneration, research projects, and the course lecture duties — to Dr. Marburger.

To my surprise, President Marburger declared that I brought glory and great honor to the university as a professor hailing from the State University of New York at Stony Brook to establish a research institute of such prominent scale and world-class standard in Asia. He offered to help with regard to Felicia's and my salary considerations. Felicia and I could continue to receive salaries from Stony Brook as professors on secondment to Academia Sinica's Institute of Biomedical Sciences in Taiwan. He would take care of the other issues with the school to alleviate our concerns so that Felicia and I could concentrate on our work in Taiwan. In short, the president gave his words that we could continue to receive our paycheck from the university while we continued our work at the Institute of Biomedical Sciences.

In an instant, these words from the school president settled all our problems and concerns. It was as if we emerged from beneath a dark cloud, saw the silver lining, and finally the sunray.

In fact, at that time, besides the appointment offer from Cornell University to assume the chairman position of its biochemistry and pharmacology department, in January 1989 I also received an invitation from Stanford University to serve as chairman of its pharmacology department.

Actually, after President Marburger made known his well-intentioned proposition to President Wu, I had indeed made up my mind to stay in Taiwan to help my home country break new ground in biomedical science. That night Felicia and I had another round of earnest discussion about the possibility of the two of us to remain in Taiwan.

Besides the children, career was also pivotal in Felicia's consideration. Her career in the United States was at its peak, and the discrimination issue that affected her promotion had been completely resolved, and there were other top American universities offering her full professor positions. In any case, the academic research culture and environment in the United States then was much more conducive than that in Taiwan. I was embarking on a new challenging career in establishing the Institute of Biomedical Sciences, but for Felicia's case, as a research scientist, to give up what she had already achieved to start all over again was tantamount to putting a reverse gear on her career, thus dragging her down from her pinnacle. That was certainly unfair to her.

Furthermore, supposing we were back in Taiwan for good, Felicia and I would have to give up our retirement pension. In the State University of New York, the university retirement scheme stipulates that the university would contribute twelve percent of one's salary every month whereas the individual himself or herself contributes three percent to the Individual Retirement Account. At the age of sixty-five after retirement, he or she is then eligible to withdraw the money in the retirement pension. However, if Felicia and I were to return to Taiwan, then we could only withdraw the three percent that we contributed and had to relinquish the other twelve percent accumulated over the past ten years we had worked in the State University of New York. As this worked out to quite a substantial sum of money, generally anyone would have deep, serious thought about giving it up.

Family was another factor. Felicia's family had all immigrated to the United States, and she was one who strongly valued family ties. Though she and her siblings lived in different states, it would still be easier to keep in touch or meet if she were in the United States. So Felicia was naturally hesitant to remain in Taiwan and be separated from friends and family in America.

Though our financial problems could be resolved, Felicia was still concerned about the issues of children, friends and family, and her research career. I knew that these issues never left her mind. At that time, my high school classmate Shiao-Lei Yu had just returned to Taiwan from the United States, and he made a telephone call to inquire how we were doing. Felicia explained the situation to him, adding that she was giving the possibility of staying in Taiwan serious consideration. The career and achievement that she built over the years in the United States had by no means been easy, however, since the country really needed us, then she probably would really stay.

Establishing the Medical Chair Professorship System

In reality, even if the proposition of the Stony Brook president was viable, meaning that we could still receive our U.S. paycheck while in Taiwan, this would not do as a long-term plan. Ultimately, there were two key factors that reinforced my decision to stay in Taiwan and for Felicia and I, to give up our research careers in the United States.

I said to President Wu, it was true that the State University of New York granted us the permission to stay in Taiwan to advance the development of the biomedical sciences field while retaining our tenure and salaries with the university. But my belief was that since we were truly committed to returning, we should sink roots in Taiwan, resign from our academic appointments and give up the option of having a backup plan to fall back on. The future development of the Institute of Biomedical Sciences was not something that I could achieve single-handedly. Hence, the recruitment of talented scientists from overseas is a continual process, and it would be my responsibility to lead by example and be a role model — to give a sense of security to returning scientists and also the assurance that I would continue to be at the helm. This would also be an important criterion in the recruitment process of scientists. However, my resignation from the State University of New York would put me into financial difficulty, and my salary in Taiwan would not be enough to cover both household expenses and our children's education.

The other factor was the medical community's support for the Institute of Biomedical Sciences. The medical community had high expectation of me to stay on, hence, they were very supportive of the clinical research and training projects, such as the medical oncology training program I mentioned earlier. National Taiwan University, Veterans General Hospital, Tri-Service General Hospital, and the Institute of Biomedical Sciences had all invested a substantial portion of their resources in a collaboration to establish the clinical research centers. Because everyone knew and were under the impression that I was only planning to stay for a year, they looked upon me as a visiting academic. A visiting academic is usually not accountable to fulfill obligations for the institution, as such, if I did well, they would naturally be pleased, and if my performance did not achieve their objective, they would not voice any strong displeasure either. But playing the part of a visiting academic, I would never be able to integrate and become one of them. This would not only undermine the institute's intention to consolidate the medical community and provide leadership within the scientific academia, it would also hold back the mission of integrating basic medicine and clinical medicine in Taiwan.

President Wu took my words and understood the impact. He shared the same sentiment that the goverment must resolve the issues of remuneration and policies governing returning scientific talents, since I and many other distinguished scientists vouched our commitment to stay in Taiwan to make a contribution. So President Wu and Shu Chien paid a special visit to Lee Teng-Hui, the President of Taiwan at that time. As soon as President Lee understood the situation, he immediately declared his wish that I should stay and he decreed the Executive Yuan to draw up a special policy plan establishing the "Medical Chair Professorship System," which included the remuneration and welfare provisions for ten medical chair professorships matching with the benchmark set in overseas. The reward of salary and other welfare benefits would be based on the meritocratic consideration of one's achievement, and thus the institute could exercise flexibility in offering favorable terms and incentives to scientists. This policy would not only benefit me, it would also act as a stimulus to attract top researchers from around the world.

The policy was a pioneering initiative in Taiwan. In the past, the salary of civil servants in Taiwan followed strictly to a set of rigid systems and guidelines which were difficult to change. President Lee's initiative to draft new policies enabled me to recruit top scholars and this set a precedence that paved the way for other research institutes in Academia Sinica to recruit and attract outstanding researchers.

Soon after the Executive Yuan approved the "Medical Chair Professorship System," President Wu organized an exquisite dinner function and invited eminent physicians and academics from the medical profession, including my mentors Jui-Lou Song, Chen-Yuan Lee, and the presidents of the medical school and teaching hospital. They expressed their earnest hope that I would sink root in Taiwan to develop and launch initiatives that bring the integration of Taiwan's life science and medical research communities. That night, the sincerity of all these scholars and medical school presidents struck a chord in my heart.

The moment that Felicia and I had to make a decision had certainly come. President Lee had given his strong mandate to overhaul the old policies to lay the foundation for a new system, and the medical community's persistent encouragement to urge me to stay on had also attested their atmost sincerity and support. Now, Felicia was the key deciding factor whether we would or would not stay.

Felicia Consents

Like me, Felicia had a deep feeling for the homeland. Being a mother and an accomplished scientist at the peak of her career made her decision even more difficult to make. As a parent, she did not want to be separated from her children. She was also worried that Albert would not be able to adjust well in Taiwan, adversely affecting his future academic pursuit. On the career front, returning to Taiwan would mean she had to put aside and conclude, at her peak, some twenty odd years of research effort in the United States and start all over in Taiwan. Whereas for my case, I would also be giving up my academic research, but it marked a milestone in my life to embark on a new career. This would not be the case for Felicia. The sacrifices that she had to make, as well as future difficulties she would encounter, were far greater than mine. These were well-founded grounds why it was difficult for her to make a decision.

At that time, our friends in the medical community were constantly telling Felicia their wish — that she would agree to stay with me in Taiwan. Hence, in the same vein, she had to give her choice careful deliberation.

Our talk that night still remains firmly ingrained in my mind. I felt indebted and was greatly moved by Felicia's support for me. If she had not consented, then there was no way I could remain in Taiwan. Felicia shared her view, and her point of view was certainly not without reason: she believed that our return would be more appropriate and well-timed three or four years later when all our children would be older. Furthermore, the prospects and appointments from the State University of New York at Stony Brook, Cornell University or Stanford University were substantially higher and more attractive than that in Taiwan, and what's more, we were able to attain even greater heights in our research. Thus, Felicia was filled with queries in her mind and really questioned whether this was the best time to stay.

I listened and brought up issues close to my heart; the first one was the state of her health — although her recovery was progressing well, it was impossible to predict if her cancer would relapse. Her research career was at its peak, but the demands of the academic environment in America were greater. If someday her health deteriorated, she might lose the opportunity to do research. In Taiwan, although she had to start from scratch, she could control the workload at a pace that she was able to cope physically. In addition, we had a close relationship with the medical fraternity in Taiwan, and if she were to seek treatment in the future, it might be more convenient and accessible in Taiwan than in the United States. I would feel more assured and have a peace of mind.

I related to Felicia a heart-to-heart conversation we had together during our courtship days. As a youth, I worshipped the idealism of Dr. Albert Schweitzer who gave up all he had in life to practice medicine in Africa to save the people of Africa. It was my dream to give up everything, go to Africa, and make the most of my abilities as a doctor. So I once asked Felicia, if one day I really decided to go to Africa, would she come with me? Felicia said yes, she would come with me.

That night I told Felicia I was at that moment, overwhelmed by the same feeling and emotion like the time I was trying to decide whether or not to go to Africa. This time, my heart was filled with my aspiration and passion for Taiwan. I told her it would be a life-changing decision and many uncertainties would lay ahead, and I was driven by a sense of mission for Taiwan, and I needed her, and her support, to fulfill it.

Then, Felicia looked at me, serene and calm. She didn't say a word. I knew that she had already consented. At that moment, I was filled with unspeakable gratitude towards her.

It is never easy for a married couple to look in the same direction with one heart and one mind. The oneness carried special significance — Felicia's selfless love and trust in me. For my sake, Felicia gave up her career, she also did what I knew to be most difficult for her — to live with the separation from her children. Felicia was the epitome of motherhood — her children were her source of strength, her selfless devotion and deep attachment for them meant the whole world to her. Now, for my sake, she had to give up her natural calling as a mother — the maternal instinct to be close to her brood. The emotional struggle that she had to overcome as a mother was unthinkable. It was our neverending love and mutual trust that grew stronger by the years that transcended everything else for that difficult decision.

I felt indebted to Felicia's support for me; she expressed it through her action — her love for me. For my sake, she was willing to give up her longing for her children and family whom she cherished most. For my sake, she was willing to stand by me and work together with me, our hearts as one.

11

Life after Returning to Taiwan

The decision to stay in Taiwan was my choice. Because it was a calling to make a contribution to the motherland, I did not view my decision as a sacrifice, and I have never once regretted it. However, I know in my heart the sacrifice that Felicia and the children made — the sacrifice of living apart when we treasure our family togetherness most. The impact on our young Albert was, undoubtedly, particularly great.

Albert's First Year

Albert started as a first-year high school student at Taipei American School. That year, he had difficulty adjusting. About half of the student population in the school are Taiwanese. Taiwanese parents typically value the importance of education and their high expectation of their children to excel academically engender a stressful learning environment. Rivalry and competition are intensive among the students. The learning environment that Albert had been exposed to in the States was distinctively different, hence, that first year was extremely trying for him.

In addition, Albert had to deal with loneliness. Felicia and I were extremely busy at work, his older brother and sister were in graduate school and college respectively in the United States, and all his friends he grew up with were there as well. Waking up early and returning home late became his daily routine during the first year. Most of the time he came home to an empty house, as Felicia was still at the laboratory. Previously, though we were busy at work, Margie would be waiting at home to welcome him with a big smile. Now when he reached home, he had to make a telephone call to the laboratory to tell his mother that he was home, and she would then call it a day at the laboratory, come home and prepare dinner for him.

Friendship and peer support are crucial in the development and growing up years of a fifteen-year-old boy. Albert's struggle with lonesomeness during the first year struck us with a regretful conscience and deep concern. Now, it was definitely difficult to tell our three children, especially Albert, that we had decided to stay in Taiwan.

That year, Albert corresponded with his American friends by mail (the e-mail technology then was not as advanced as it is today), telling them he was sure to return after one year, and he hoped they would not forget him. It is clear from his anticipation to reaffirm and keep the bonds of his endearing friendship that Albert felt isolated and lonely during his first year in Taiwan. His transition was by no means an easy one.

However, we still had to tell Albert our final decision. Felicia knew that Albert would find it extremely hard to accept, and given how much she loved her children, she was at a loss over how to broach the subject with him. But I felt that no matter how difficult it was, we needed to have his understanding and acceptance. So I picked and found an appropriate opportunity to tell him of his parents' joint decision.

I will never forget his reaction. The first words that he shot, "How about me? If I don't go back, my friends are going to kill me." He was crestfallen.

I explained to Albert why we had to stay in Taiwan. I told him although he, David and Faith were all born and bred in the United States, Mom and Dad were both from Taiwan, and we had a deep emotional bond with our homeland that was inherently a part of us. I went on and said the opportunity to do our part for the good of our homeland brought the ultimate, the highest purpose in our life. I told Albert we should instill and value a sense of purpose and mission in life.

I told him he still had to return to the United States to attend university. I encouraged him to value the two years as an immersion experience to develop a greater understanding of Taiwan and its heritage, as well as the

Chinese culture. In time to come, he would understand why it is important to embrace one's own root and identity. Furthermore, his experience here would empower him to acquire a broad and all-encompassing global outlook, and he would also be able to develop a kaleidoscopic perspective of the ever-changing world beyond the American context.

That night Albert did not say anything. He was pensive and lost in thought. Two days later, Albert looked in my face and said that he understood our decision. During this period, he would put our interests first before his. He said, "Mom and Ba (dad), you guys do your best here; don't worry about me." Albert has always been extremely respectful towards his parents, he is also tremendously thoughtful. Felicia and I were greatly moved and comforted knowing that we had Albert's support and understanding. We were even more deeply moved that our child was such a considerate, loving person.

However, I remained concerned and worried about Albert's academic performance and his adjustments to daily life in the next two years. It would be a lifelong regret to Felicia and me if the decision to stay in Taiwan would have adverse effects on his studies, thus affecting his choice of college. Fortunately, the worry was unfounded. Albert had already identified his future goal during his high school years — he wanted to pursue a combined M.D. and Ph.D. degree. Albert knew that if he wanted to enter a well-known American medical school, his academic record had to be impeccable.

Once, Albert asked me why people have to strive and work so hard their whole life.

I explained to Albert it really depends on how one views life. It takes people of different walks of life, race, creed or color to make up the society, and each individual has a different role to play and everyone has different expectations of himself or herself. There are people who hope to be able to contribute something back to the society, like his parents. And then there are some who just hope to be able to get through life without any ups and downs, which is perfectly fine too. The important thing is what he himself wants out of his life. In the game of life, which playing piece would he choose to be?

I do not know what effect that conversation had on Albert, but I noticed that after our discussion, Albert was more studious and diligent than ever. He knew that those two years would be critical to decide his chance in getting into a top American medical school. His academic record had to be near perfect, or else he would not stand a chance.

Gradually Adjusting to Life in Taiwan

Albert opened up and he enjoyed his second and third years in Taiwan. He started to make new friends, participate in school clubs and societies, and play in the school band. Albert played the trumpet, and every year he would perform at the American Club in Taipei's Yuanshan District. The school also organized an annual dance for parents in conjunction with the band performance at the American Club. Felicia and I always looked forward to attending this dance, with the school band being its main music accompaniment, because we could then enjoy and appreciate our beloved son's trumpet-playing.

Albert gradually came to like life in Taiwan. He enjoyed Chinese cuisine and local snacks at small, roadside stands, and the local dessert served in ice shaving. I still remember his first time sampling the dessert — he bought shaved ice from the roadside stands and experienced bouts of diarrhea at home. He was undeterred by the sicked and unpleasant feeling from the diarrhea episode. The shaved ice proved much too tempting. So, he continued to love his shaved ice, and of course he has not experienced diarrhea since.

His Chinese also improved by leaps and bounds. On communication front, he was already able to fend for himself in everyday life. Like other young Taiwanese, he enjoyed hanging out at the Ximending district and he loved the youth culture of Taiwan and blended well in the unique and diverse lifestyle of Taipei youths. Also, Albert started to study the Chinese language in school; he took a keen interest in the four-character idioms originating from classical Chinese that are commonly used in daily conversation. At that time, Felicia became Albert's teacher in Chinese idioms; every day she would recite an idiom and explain the etymological orgin of the phrase so that he could understand and remember.

Albert made significant progress in his studies during his second and third year of high school and along with his gradual assimilation into the Taiwanese culture, his life certainly became enriched and varied.

There was another unexpected incident which added a positive experience to his life — he became an amateur model, beyond anyone's expectation.

On a bus ride one day, Albert was spotted by a talent scout from a modeling agency. The woman gave him a business card and asked him if he had any interest in becoming a model. She knew that Albert was young and still schooling, so she told him to discuss with his parents. She urged him to give her a call upon receiving parental consent.

My view of the situation was that as long as the modeling assignment would not affect his schoolwork, then I would have no objections to him doing it. After all, it certainly seemed a unique experience for Albert. Felicia, though, was absolutely thrilled with the idea. She took Albert to the screen test, and recounted every last detail to me when she got home. After the screen test, the modeling agency signed up Albert as their model. His first assignment was a print advertisement for IBM. Among those who appeared with Albert in the ad was Zhi-Ying Lin, who later became a popular teen idol.

And so this became Albert's unique experience in Taiwan. Even during his college days, the modeling agency always arranged him to model in advertisements and appear in commercials in print and electronic media when he returned to Taiwan during summer vacation. As I recall, he had appeared in Yamaha motorcycle and Misiguo drink television commercials, as well as on the large advertising billboard at SOGO, then the biggest department store in Taipei. And because of his modeling experience, he also undertook projects in the United States shooting commercials. Take a recent case, for instance, he appeared in a print advertisement for Boeing Corporation and this advertisement appeared in major international publications. Thus, a serendipitous bus ride certainly resulted in a valuable and significant experience for him.

Those two years, Albert became much more positive and open. He increasingly came to love Taiwan, his adjustment problems naturally dissipated, and his schoolwork likewise improved. Other than his modeling assignments, he also tutored students in mathematics and English during winter and summer vacations. Indeed, those years were an extremely enriching and rewarding experience for him.

Entering Yale University

Before Albert's graduation from high school, he took part in an entrance examination for American and European colleges. He did extremely well with near perfect scores. He submitted his application for college and was accepted into his first choice, Yale University. Albert was the first student from Taipei American School to be accepted into Yale University in many years. It was a load off our chests, and, finally Felicia and I were able to rest easy with regard to our educational responsibility towards our three children. Our Albert had realized his dream of gaining admission into one of the world's leading universities.

It was one of those casual chats after Albert got into university. Looking back, he said the three years in Taiwan were extremely stimulating. His experience in Taiwan sharpened his acumen to think far and long-term, trained him to adapt to and deal with new environment, built up his confidence to take on future challenges, and broadened his outlook to embrace non-American perspectives. It also helped that he studied at Taipei American School, where students were of different nationalities, and he had made friends from all over the world and learned to look at things from different points of view.

My heartfelt gratitude to Felicia for bringing up Albert into a fine man. Felicia accompanied Albert through three difficult years; every day, she put his interest first, lovingly taking care of him and helping him overcome his feeling of isolation — being the only child among his siblings to come and live with us in Taiwan. I am deeply ashamed to say that because I was so busy, any credit for Albert's education must go to his mother. If Albert had not had Felicia's tender loving care those three years, perhaps he would not be as mature as he is now.

Faith's New Life

That year also had a significant impact on Faith's life and future. Personality wise, Faith is similar to Felicia in many ways. She is sensitive, active, outgoing, lively and lovable. To raise a daughter in the United States is not easy. Felicia and I, on one hand, upheld our traditional Chinese values; we were undoubtedly strict in bringing up our daughter. We hoped she would have the gentle poise and refined air of a Chinese female. But on the other hand, the environment she grew up in was open and liberal — this being an American Society. Since young, Faith has to learn to adopt and adapt two different cultures which exist in dichotomy. This could not have been easy for her.

In America, girls are allowed to begin dating when they are fourteen, or sometimes fifteen years old. Felicia and I were not comfortable with Faith being alone with boys at such a young age, so we did not give her the green-light to date. Looking back, it is difficult to say whether this was good or bad. Before college, Faith indeed had no experience in dating.

Faith began her university life. Felicia accompanied her to Cornell University to help her get settled into the dormitory and then immediately returned to Taiwan. It was the first time that Faith left home to live far away from her family. In America, almost all college-going youngsters leave home — which is equivalent to abandoning the nest — to attend college. But we were in Taiwan, far away from her. The sense of forlornness being inevitably separated from her family fermented in her lonesome heart. It was much later that Faith shared her feelings with us, she said she felt very lonely and desolate that year.

Felicia maintained close relationship with the children through weekly telephone calls to them, having small talks and casual chats to find out how they were doing. However, even the comfort of the phone call every week hearing the familiar voices could not alleviate Faith's longing for her family. She returned to Taiwan for her first year's summer vacation, I noticed that she had gained weight which was a sign that she was not adjusting well. In my heart, I felt agonized and sorry.

Something happened in Faith's life during her freshman year. She had a boyfriend in college. Faith was serious about her first relationship but it seemed that her boyfriend did not reciprocate with the same intense feeling. Hence, when he initiated to break up, Faith was extremely hurt.

She called me. She poured her heart out in tearful sobs, unable to understand why her boyfriend wanted to break up with her. I told Faith that love is a two-way street, it takes two to dance the tango. No matter how much she liked someone, if he was not meant for her, he would eventually leave. If he was the one, he would never leave her. I told Faith, just because two persons show a liking toward each other does not necessarily mean that they could get along; love just does not work that way. In any relationship, it is a continual learning of understanding each other, making "give-and-take" compromises, sharing joy and woes, and — what is deemed the most difficult of all — gaining mutual trust. I told Faith, this would be her first life lesson in managing feelings, and this relationship would also be an invaluable experience which, in the future, would be her guiding beacon to help her bond with and choose her lifelong companion.

Faith's freshman year was chronicled in loneliness and disappointments but that did not put a damper on her active, effervescent personality. During the first year, she participated in various club activities and she proved her mettle. For example, she founded an a cappella choir and asked my friend, Cornell University professor Ray Wu, to be their advisor. Faith also directed and arranged all the choir's practices and performances.

During her first summer vacation in Taiwan, I told Faith our decision to stay in Taiwan. Faith reacted differently from Albert; she did not seem to be affected. It could be attributed to the first year of living by herself away from home and the disappointments and setbacks she faced that had honed her independence. Faith's cheerful personality puts her in good stead. She even took the opportunity to work at a law firm during that summer vacation in Taiwan. The new life experiences away from home as a freshman had helped her mature a great deal.

Faith majored in political science because of her interest in international relations. Felicia and I were careful not to force our children to live according to our ideals or decisions. We were well aware that as children grow up, their parents' influence on them diminishes. We believe, as parents, we can teach and influence our children by setting good examples. For each child, the steering control to chart the direction of his life is in his own hands, and thus, only his own decision is key to what he wants in life. Of course, as long as the bonding between the parents and child is close, then the personal experience of the parents could naturally serve as an exemplary reference for the child.

Albert majored in biochemistry at Yale University. His ambition was to graduate with an M.D. and a Ph.D. This was his own decision; both Felicia and I were happy that he was able to achieve his goal. Faith wanted to become a legal counsel specializing in international relations; this was also her own decision. David became a scientist specializing in theoretical chemistry; we had similarly hoped for his success. Our three children each have their own hopes and dreams in life; nevertheless, Felicia and I have always respected their decisions and we tried our best as parents to support their ideals.

Faith's Experience in France

During Faith's third year in college, she learned of an interesting one-year overseas study program which was conducted in France. The study program was granted accreditation by Cornell University and course credit could be earned. Faith always has a deep affinity for France. She has fond memories of her elementary school days there. When we returned to the States, she continued to take French courses; her sixth grade had a weekly program to learn French and she continued studying the language through junior high to high school. She always hoped that she would have the opportunity to return to France someday, and the overseas study program seemed like the perfect chance. Faith desperately wanted to participate in the program.

Felicia and I, of course, supported her decision to study in France. We felt her trip to France would enhance her global exposure, and what's more, the long distance already separating us would not make any difference or have any bearing on her decision. That summer before her studies, Faith worked full-time as a waitress in a restaurant in France. She became fluent in the French language and close to its people.

That Christmas, Faith arranged for the whole family to travel to Corsica. Our whole family always made an effort to get together at least twice a year during summer vacation and the Christmas season. We had two objectives to visit France that Christmas: first, to get together as a family and second, to better understand Faith's life in France.

After the overseas study program ended, Faith returned to the United States. We knew that she missed her life in France and hoped to return there to do an internship after graduation. As expected, upon graduation, she applied for and was granted a research internship position; the project was commissioned by France's former Foreign Minister Bernard Stasi. Faith carried out international relations research under his guidance. A year later, Faith produced a thesis written in French, "Referendum of the Treaty of Maastricht: An Analysis of the Marne Region Constituency." Her work was to provide a geopolitical, sociological and economic analysis of the Marne electorate, both historically and of the Referendum, to help Mr. Stasi strategize for the upcoming legislative elections in March 1993.

That year Faith was happy and enjoyed her life in France. She told us that she hoped to stay for another year. At first, I did not give her an affirmative consent, but then my mind told me perhaps it was Faith's aspiration to build a life and career in France. Felicia and I knew the goal Faith had set for herself would not be easy, we thought we should at least give her a chance to try.

Faith stayed in France for another year and wrote a second thesis, "The Identity of Generation Ecology: A Sociological and Ideological Study of the Activists of an Ecologist Political Party" with the support of the ecologically oriented "Generation Ecology" political party. During those two years in France, Faith became well-versed not only in French politics, she also became a connoisseur of French culture, haute cuisine, and fine wine.

Felicia and I both knew that Faith really loved France. She hoped to live there, but I urged her to return to Asia. I told her the present era is predominantly Asia's, known as the "Asian Century." All over the world, large multinational corporations are competing to establish themselves in the Asian market. Furthermore, Asia has become a pivotal focus in the political agenda of many developed countries in the Western hemisphere. With her interest in international relations, Faith should return to Taiwan and concentrate on establishing her career in this respect.

Working at The Ministry of Foreign Affairs

Half a year later, Faith returned to Taiwan. She had tried for half a year to make a life for herself in France, but was unable to find a suitable employment, and so she finally decided to return to Taiwan. But upon her return, we realized that she was unable to work in Taiwan because she held a U.S. passport and was on a tourist visa. That she was unable to legally work in this country was a situation that Felicia and I had never foreseen.

After much twists and turns, I finally thought of Shu Chien's younger brother Fu Chien, then Minister of Foreign Affairs in Taiwan. I asked him what could be done about Faith's visa problem. Fu Chien especially arranged a meeting with Faith. He had a very good impression of Faith and offered her a job appointment at the Ministry of Foreign Affairs. Her main responsibility would be to edit outgoing correspondences that the Ministry wrote to other countries.

That began Faith's career at the Ministry of Foreign Affairs. Because she had a keen awareness of the international political situation and was adept at identifying the key points of each document that she edited, Fu Chien held high regard for her abilities. Ultimately, even the important letters that Fu Chien wrote to the United Nations went through her hands and were drafted by her. After a period of time, Faith was transferred to the Department of International Organizations and worked mostly on matters relating to Asia-Pacific Economic Cooperation (APEC). Fu Chien had come to regard Faith as an important aide.

Faith's work in the Department of International Organizations was extremely demanding, but she enjoyed it because she had finally launched a successful career in the arena of international politics. At that time, Taiwan had just joined APEC and there was some tension in the cross-strait relations; thus it was crucial to maintain careful and open communications. Faith participated in the APEC meetings as a member of the staff and shouldered the responsibility of assessing and evaluating the state of affairs from outside the meeting. At any point of time when there was a new turn of events, she immediately had to write a memo of discussion points, bring these memos to the officials at the table, giving them sufficient and relevant information to field the challenges of China and other countries. The representatives who attended the APEC meetings, including Chi Hsue, Bing-Kun Chiang, Rong-Yi Wu, Paul Hsu, and Foreign Minister Chien, all held the highest opinion of Faith's work.

One of the most memorable assignments in Faith's career was her trip to Saudi Arabia and Jordan with the entourage of President Lee Teng-Hui in 1995. The Ministry of Foreign Affairs assigned Faith to be the interpreter for President Lee's wife, First Lady Wen-Hui Tseng. Faith was extremely nervous at the time, thinking that her Chinese was not good enough to fulfill her duties satisfactorily as an interpreter. Fortunately,

Faith's performance on this trip was stellar, and she lived up to everybody's expectation for the great responsibility tasked to her.

Felicia and I knew that Faith felt deeply disappointed when she returned to Taiwan because her dream to work in France did not materialize. Three years with the Ministry of Foreign Affairs, Faith had the opportunity to become familiar with the communication and negotiation strategies on the international political stage, learn new exciting things, and do her part for Taiwan tapping on her strengths. Other than regaining her self-confidence, she finally realized that she had to make a thrust to climb the corporate ladder to advance her career. Three years later, Faith shared with me her hope to return to school to obtain a law degree. Felicia and I naturally applauded her decision.

When we returned to Taiwan, David was already doing his doctoral studies at the University of California, Berkeley. He studied with a determined mindset for six years, obtained his Ph.D. in chemistry, and went to Cambridge University to do postdoctoral research. As for our decision to sink roots in Taiwan, David did not have a hard time coming to terms with us because he had already been living by himself away from home for a long time, and had taken his own initiative to learn and discover his culture, his root and identity. Felicia and I were both very happy about it.

When I decided to return to Taiwan in the long term, I had the unanimous and unconditional support of Felicia and our three children. Their selfless actions touched me. Towards them, it is a sense of deep gratitude that remains forever in my heart. Had it not been their understanding and acceptance, how could I continue to move forward and pour all my heart and soul into biomedical science in Taiwan?

In order for me to return to Taiwan, Felicia and the children had to make difficult adjustments in life. Today when I look back, I am extremely thankful that the academic pursuit and the career of our children were not affected in any way; otherwise, I do not believe I would be able to forgive myself.

Adjustment and Recovery

Since settling down in Taiwan, Felicia focused to sow the seeds for her research. Her work was demanding, but she indeed paid more attention to her health than before, aspiring that the cancer was completely under control. She drew up detailed plans on her dietary regimen, excercise timetable and schedule for recreational activities. Her sole objective — to keep cancer at bay.

As one of her regimens, Felicia and her colleagues at the Institute of Biomedical Sciences formed a volleyball team. They practiced on a regular basis, and played matches against other institutes. As for a facility to play and practice, Felicia requested Academia Sinica to build a volleyball court on the lawn in front of the Institute of Biomedical Sciences. She even organized weekend treks and holiday hikes with her colleagues. As Felicia always thought that I did not exercise enough, I was also one of the reasons why she instituted the hiking regimen, and I naturally accompanied her every weekend. Felicia even participated in aerobic dance classes sponsored by the institute. Felicia's health improved and recovered steadily, and she was teeming with inexhaustible dynamic energy.

The first year after our return, Felicia traveled back to the United States for periodic physical examinations, and as her doctor recommended, she could also have her condition monitored in Taiwan at the same time. However, since we had decided to stay in Taiwan for good, it was necessary and logical that future examinations to be conducted in Taiwan. It was also an opportune time since the Institute of Biomedical Sciences had already begun a program to train medical oncologists. Many cancer specialists such as Dr. Jacqueline Peng-Wang, who moved back to Taiwan two years later, were devoting the greater portion of their time in Taiwan. By then, the quality of cancer treatment on home ground had already gradually improved, and I felt reassured about Felicia having her follow-up examinations in Taiwan.

The doctors who were in charge of Felicia's follow-up examinations in the United States and the physicians who monitored her condition in Taiwan all believed that she had an excellent prognosis. She was even stronger than any normal healthy individuals. Felicia herself was perfectly confident about her recovery. As before, she enjoyed all sorts of outdoor activities, especially swimming. As soon as she hit the water, she was like a fish, swimming about leisurely without a care for the world.

Breast removal surgery had made putting on a swimsuit extremely inconvenient, so three years after her mastectomy, Felicia told me she wanted to have breast reconstruction surgery. Her doctors determined that her strength had completely returned, and she personally felt her health had recovered to a fitness level before cancer struck.

During the first two years of her illness, she used breast pads. My main concern was Felicia's health, as I believe health takes top priority and everything else is secondary. Thus, not in the slightest degree was our relationship as man and wife affected at all as a result of Felicia's breast removal. But I could understand Felicia's desire to live like a normal person, so I respected and supported her decision.

Felicia's determination to go for breast reconstruction surgery was what differentiated her from most people. During her recovery period, her spirits were consistently high. Felicia's fearless confrontation of reality, indomitable human spirit and optimistic outlook are all qualities that made her unforgettable and forged her ahead to try new things and take on new challenges, and in her fight against cancer, she was able to stand resolutely for thirteen years.

When I reach this point in the story, my heart breaks, because the pain that Felicia was to endure in the years thereafter is a story that can hardly be told through words.

12

Cancer Recurs

Felicia's breast reconstruction surgery was performed by Dr. Norman Hugo at the Columbia University Hospital in New York. When Felicia decided to have the surgery, she went back to the United States and consulted Dr. Gump. He was very confident about her recovery and was impressed by Felicia's determination to battle cancer and return to a normal life. Dr. Gump gave his support and referred her to an excellent surgeon, Dr. Hugo.

Felicia returned to Taiwan to discuss with me once again. She said that she would go back to the United States for the surgery after she had attended to work and duty arrangements in the laboratory. She would put up at the house of my medical school classmate, Dr. Ming-Neng Yeh, a professor of obstetrics at Columbia University. The entire reconstruction process — painstaking and tedious — would take almost two to three months. But because of my heavy work commitment, and Albert had to be looked after in Taiwan, I was unable to accompany her.

A Paragon of Bravery

As we travel the journey of life, each chronological date on our timelines represents a past event. Sadly, returning to these events — being physically there and reliving them — evoke tears, grief and wistful emotions again. Our family has come to terms with Felicia's passing. Walking the paths, the roads we once trod as a family, coming face-to-face with every encounter and every acquaintance in her life, memories came back to us but they were not merely passing scenes of the past that bore no trace, no impression, and no scar, instead they really were tangible proof of a life that has lived out to the fullest.

The children and I went to New Jersey to visit Dr. Gump and my old classmate, Dr. Ming-Neng Yeh. That was a precious piece of memory in our family's journey of recollection. The trip enabled the children and me to better understand Felicia's feelings and thoughts, and her aspirations when she was alone making plans to rebuild her future, her life. Felicia was like a larva that, at the very last drop of its precious life-sustaining moisture in her protective cocoon, broke free of its confinement, emerged as a butterfly and took off in flight, without a trace of self-pity. That day, our meeting with Dr. Gump and Dr. Yeh enabled us to develop an even greater admiration for Felicia and induce a deeper yearning to hold on to her in memory.

Dr. Yeh said during Felicia's recuperation at his house, she was in her bright and cheerful self every day. Back then, all Dr. Yeh knew was that Felicia underwent a breast reconstruction surgery at the Columbia University Hospital. After her surgery, everything about her seemed normal. She loved communicating and interacting with people, sharing news snippets about our children, me and her ultimate "infatuation" — scientific research. She was even open to talk about her medical condition. The Felicia he knew was like the sunshine, warming everyone who came close to her.

An incident happened that unveiled the reality behind the cheerfulness. Mrs. Yeh and Felicia were chatting, Mrs. Yeh unintentionally patted Felicia's left shoulder lightly. Felicia suddenly cried out, "Oh! It hurts!" Mrs. Yeh was completely startled by her exclamation.

"I'm sorry. What's wrong?" Mrs. Yeh asked. Felicia replied, "I'm sorry to alarm you. I didn't cry out on purpose, but that is really painful." It soon dawned on Mrs. Yeh that Felicia put up a brave front — the sunshine smile on Felicia's face was a shield to hide the unbearably excruciating pain she had endured from the surgery. She never cried out or even expressed it. If Mrs. Yeh had not accidentally touched Felicia, she and Dr. Yeh would never have realized the severity of pain Felicia had to endure on a daily basis.

Dr. Gump said, from diagnosis to mastectomy, Felicia requested for an honest and open communication with doctors, she wanted the doctors to advise her before the mastectomy of all the possible outcomes that might occur. He also explained to her the recovery process following surgery and the side effects of chemotherapy. Felicia would jot down the details one by one as he explained them. In his recollection, Felicia was the most special, unique and exceptional of all his patients in that she was the only one who did not repel against finding out more and gaining full details of one's medical progress. Dr. Gump saw in her a living example of courage and a fiery will to live and fight.

"I have too many patients; there's no way for me to remember all of them, but I remember Felicia. I even remember what Felicia told me before she was discharged from the hospital. She said, 'I hope I never see you again.' How strong and resolute her words were! As a doctor, I could understand her thoughts and feelings, and I couldn't help but marvel at her unique character."

It was an early morning in spring. The children and I sped through in the car towards Dr. Gump's house in New Jersey. He greeted us warmly, and before long, Dr. and Mrs. Yeh also joined us. We chatted and reminisced at length everything about Felicia. The spring breeze, still bitingly cold, blew gently, but the sun cast its golden glow that felt like the warm caress of a mother's love. Spring is the season when Mother Earth reawakens. That brought an alternating intermittence of bitterly cold and warmth in the air, and we felt the two sensations of spring — sometimes it was a bone-tingling chill, and sometimes, it was the soft caress of the golden sun. The sensation exactly fleshed out how the children and I felt at the time: painful thoughts, but sweet memories.

Exceptional Scientific Achievements in Taiwan

We came back to Taiwan in 1988. In 1994, eight years after Felicia was diagnosed, her cancer spread to the liver. Before the relapse, she was in excellent health, and I would even think her physical stamina was even better than a normal healthy person. She was a member of the volleyball team at the Institute of Biomedical Sciences, and when the team played friendly matches against other institutes in Academia Sinica, she could play four matches a day without feeling tired. During that five years, no abnormalities prevailed in Felicia's physical condition. Based on the medical care yardstick at that time, Felicia was considered completely cured, however, she continued to take her medicine on schedule and visited the National Taiwan University Hospital for regular examinations. Back then, it really seemed cancer would not threaten her again.

Felicia had an extremely successful research career. She was the coordinator of the cancer research division at the Institute of Biomedical Sciences, and she was obtaining good results with her research on the anti-cancer properties and mechanisms of Vitamin K3. Using cancerous liver cells as specimens, her research group found that cells treated with Vitamin K3 would stop their cancerous activity, wither and die (which is known as apoptosis). After conducting experiments with animals, they entered the first phase of clinical trials for Vitamin K3. This research result excited her colleagues in the cancer research division, and I was gratified to see that despite switching research fields, her performance was just as exceptionally outstanding.

The other research topic that Felicia investigated was the anti-cancer properties and mechanisms of the adeno-associated virus (AAV). Though there exists in the world all sorts of viruses that are potentially harmful to humans, AAV is benign to humans. Studies conducted twenty or thirty years ago found that patients suffering from cervical cancer and prostate cancer possessed fewer antibodies against AAV than healthy individuals.

Realizing this, Felicia developed another research plan: to explore the mechanism and anti-cancer activity of AAV in human cancer cells. Using cancer cells and mice as specimens, she discovered that there is a DNA segment in AAV that has anti-cancer properties. In humans, AAV does not cause disease; rather, it binds itself to a specific site between the No. 17 and No. 19 chromosomes and performs its anti-cancer function. The knowledge that the DNA of AAV possesses anti-cancer properties, and that it could itself act as a gene carrier, made it an excellent candidate for use in the development of gene therapies for cancer.

Thus, Felicia immersed herself in her work to begin her breakthrough in another field of research. Ever since our son Albert left home to attend college in the United States, she would pour all her energy into research. At times I would remind her not to work too hard and to have balanced rest. I was still worried about Felicia's health, but eight years had already passed and Felicia remained completely healthy. Going by her well-disciplined lifestyle and great physical endurance and stamina, no one would ever think that she was a cancer patient. So I was hopeful that the cancer nightmare would finally be over, and Felicia could commit herself in the research she enjoyed so much in her tip-top condition.

The Significance of the Asian Conference on Transcription

Felicia channeled her full-throttle energy to her research in the laboratory, but she did not overlook the big picture. She was extremely concerned about the entire ecosystem of research and development (R&D) in Taiwan. Upon our return to Taiwan, we always felt that though Asia had its share of large-scale scientific conferences, there were no small-scale conferences that focused on specific research fields, such as the Gordon Conferences in the United States. Although such small-scale conferences accommodate fewer participants, the conference topic and discussions are more focused. Participants can then exchange opinions on topics that are directly related to their own research and this would encourage research and academic collaborations. Thus, such conferences elevate the research profile of the scientists.

In 1990, Felicia and I went to Seoul to attend the inaugural annual Conference of the Asian Pacific Organization of Biochemistry. Among the scientists who attended were Koreans, Japanese, Indians, and Chinese. All agreed that there was a need to hold small-scale scientific conferences in Asia. After the conference in Seoul, Felicia and I proposed the "Asian Conference on Transcription" (ACT) to be established and held by rotation in a different country every two years. Scientists from various Asian countries who attended the Seoul conference supported our suggestion at once, and it was decided that the inaugural "Asian Conference on Transcription" (ACT I) would be held in Taipei the following year.

In 1991, ACT I was held at the activities center in Academia Sinica. It was modeled after the Gordon Conferences. I served as chairman of the international organizing committee of ACT I, and Felicia the co-chair. In fact, Felicia took care of all the logistics of organizing the conference, such as contacting people, planning the conference schedule and making arrangements for accommodations and transportation.

There is a Chinese proverb that goes, "Getting started is always the difficult part." Our Asian scientists were deeply impressed by the careful and detailed planning of the ACT I. Many of the scientists who attended ACT I, including Akira Ishihama and Nobuo Shimamoto from Japan, Dipankar Chatterji from India, and Changwon Kang from South Korea, were our previous colleagues or students who had worked with Felicia and me in our laboratories. This time, everyone worked together to ensure that every aspect of ACT I was smooth and successful.

The pre-conference preparation was a flurry of activities which saw Felicia busy with the collation and publication of research papers as well as making arrangements for meals and accommodations. After finalizing the conference program, she also arranged sightseeing trips for scientists to visit Taroko Gorge in Hualien, one of Taiwan's most scenic spots, and to tour the world-renowned National Palace Museum in Taipei. The participants gained much knowledge from the conference and all became eminent scientists in their own countries. Felicia's meticulous planning in putting together a well-thought and compact conference made a strong impression on all the scientists. Thus, ACT I became a model for all the subsequent planning of the ACT conferences.

From then on, Felicia enthusiastically participated in every ACT session. In fact, it was during the ACT III held in Bangalore, India, that she felt physically unwell and realized that her cancer had recurred. In 1999 when Felicia passed away, all the scientists who had participated in ACT were saddened by the loss. At the ACT VI held in Beijing in October 2000, a poster exhibition honoring Felicia's scientific achievements and her life was organized and put up. I was asked to give the "Felicia Chen-Wu Memorial Lecture" to honor her. A documentary entitled *A Passion for Life*, featuring Felicia's struggle against cancer was screened at the conference.

The scientists participating in ACT VI had grown substantially in number beyond those from Asia to include leading experts on gene transcription from Australia, the United States, and Europe. The scientists had great respect for Felicia's willpower and perseverance, and they were awe-inspired by Felicia's highly esteemed contribution to the founding of the ACT. If there had been no ACT I as the precedent, then the subsequent ACT meetings would not be of such high caliber and great success. Thus,

Felicia's tremendous contribution in laying the foundations of the Asian scientific world was indisputable and well-acknowledged.

At this point, I would like to specifically mention Taiwan's Biophysical Society. This society was founded in 1999, and I was the founding president of the society. I was the founder of this society in name, but much of the groundwork was carried out by Felicia, similar to the level of involvement she had put in for ACT. After Felicia passed away, my former mentor, Professor Hammes, was invited to Taiwan to speak at the sixth annual conference of the Biophysical Society held at National Tsing Hua University in Hsinchu in May 2000. He traveled thousands of miles with a chief objective to give a eulogy in Felicia's honor at the "Felicia Chen-Wu Memorial Lecture." In his speech, he especially praised Felicia's early scientific research in the United States. She pioneered in a research which had a key role in shaping the present-day scientific knowledge on the structure and function of metal ions involved in gene transcription. In May 2001, the seventh annual conference of the Biophysical Society was held at National Yang-Ming University in Taipei. The society invited world-renowned scientist Charles R. Cantor to deliver a speech in memory of Felicia. It is evident that Felicia's research received critical acclaims from both domestic and international scientists, and I felt a deep appreciation for the discerning effort of the Biophysical Society.

Cancer Recurs and Migrates to the Liver

Felicia found it hard to believe that God would once again allow cancer to plague her. Eight years after she underwent surgery to remove the breast cancer, the tentacles of cancer wrapped around her. Again.

In September 1994, ACT III was scheduled to take place in Bangalore, India. That summer, Albert returned to Taiwan. He had successfully applied for and received a research stipend from the Yale University, enabling him to travel to northeastern China to research on Kaschin-Beck Disease, which is caused by fungal toxins and a dietary deficiency of the antioxidant, selenium. Albert was planning to go to Harbin and other parts of northeastern China to conduct interviews and do research.

Felicia was also making a trip to China at the invitation of the Natural Science Foundation. At the same time, she was planning to pay a visit to

Professor Bing-Gen Ru at Peking University to discuss the possibility of establishing an academic exchange. In the past, Professor Ru was a postdoctoral researcher in Felicia's laboratory at SUNY Stony Brook. Since Albert would be in northeastern China and she in Beijing, they decided to travel together. She and I decided that she would first go to China with Albert, come back to Taiwan and then travel with me to India. That year, there were two conferences in India in which we had to attend; one was the "International Congress of Biochemistry" held in New Delhi, and the other was ACT III.

Thus, Felicia and Albert went to northeastern China to conduct research on the current state and the prevalence of Kaschin-Beck Disease. Albert finally understood his Mom's conscientiousness in her research and her no-nonsense attitude towards everything. In all the field interviews that they did, Felicia took down notes all the time. When she came across something that she did not quite understand, she would always ask a string of questions until she got to the bottom of the problem, which is analogous to peeling off the threads of a cocoon one at a time to make silk. She taught Albert to analyze, make judgments and know what details to pay attention to while doing research. This trip enabled Albert to learn a great deal from his mother about being firm and determined, and the principles a scientist should uphold in pursuit of scientific research, a lesson which he found by no means trivial.

After arriving in Beijing, Felicia saw her old friend Bing-Gen Ru. He had not only become a distinguished professor at Peking University, but had also made incredible strides in scientific research. Felicia was extremely happy. After the Natural Science Foundation conference, the scientists were arranged to meet Chinese President, Ze-Min Jiang. When it was Felicia's turn, she said with a bright, cheery but nevertheless firm tone, "I am from Taiwan; I hope (one day) you will be able to understand Taiwan better." That indeed was Felicia's true spirit; when she felt that she ought to say something, she had no inhibition about making her stand known. Not many people on this earth possessed Felicia's personality traits — warm, sincere, gutsy and courageous — because she was such a unique and special person.

We immediately set off to New Delhi to participate in the International Congress of Biochemistry after Felicia returned from her China trip. Faith accompanied us. Felicia and I both delivered our speeches at the congress. I had to return to Taiwan immediately after the congress because the extramural research programs of the National Health Research Institutes would be reviewed by a panel of over sixty experts from all over the world. And my presence was necessary at the review. So I was to return home first and reunite with Felicia and Faith later at ACT III.

Upon my arrival in Taiwan, I started experiencing diarrhea. I decided that it was probably something unclean that I ate while in India. After taking some medicine, I recovered completely, and I did not give the matter a second thought. But after concluding the extramural research program review, there were reports of a plague breakout in Bombay, India. I was extremely worried because Felicia and Faith were still there. So I hurried back to India, taking with me medicine that was used to treat plague. I met Felicia and Faith in Bangalore. As soon as Felicia saw me, she told me that her stomach hurt terribly.

I asked her how did the pain happen. She said her abdomen had been hurting for several days, and she could barely tolerate the pain. I remembered the incessant diarrhea I experienced when I returned to Taiwan, and speculated that Felicia also probably got it due to unclean food. I gave her some medicine. She felt much better after taking the medicine, and I was reassured. The two of us continued to attend the entire ACT III as planned.

After the conference, we made a trip to Bombay for some work-related business. At that time, the plague was confined to one area in the suburbs of Bombay, so when we first arrived, we were not too worried. It was not until we had settled our business, and Felicia, Faith, and I were back in New Delhi preparing to fly back to Taiwan, that the plague suddenly exploded to reach epidemic proportions. The World Health Organization (WHO) was about to declare India an epidemic-striken zone, and an order was issued to stop all international flights.

I started to worry that there would be no flights for us to return to Taiwan. All international flights seemed to be postponed indefinitely. At that moment, Felicia worked up her wit and recalled suddenly that in the past she had a postdoctoral researcher who had become a professor at New Delhi University. She immediately called up her student to ask for his help. This professor was extremely well-connected in India; he personally escorted the three of us to the airport, made sure we cleared the customs, and then got us on board the last flight to Hong Kong. Thus Felicia, Faith, and I were able to board the last outgoing international flight and leave India.

In Hong Kong, we transferred to a plane bound for Taiwan's Chiang Kai-Shek Airport. Because we had come from an epidemic zone, there were already officials from the Department of Health waiting for us. But as soon as the inspection officials saw Felicia and me, they let us pass with only a brief set of questions. What worried me most when we were in India was not being able to leave. Even though I had sufficient medicine with me as a precaution, we might meet with grave consequences if we were not able to exit the country for some time. We left India and were home, I could finally let out a sigh of relief.

I recall clearly that we arrived home on a Saturday. The next morning Felicia started coughing. The plague breakout in India alerted me immediately as the disease would affect the lungs and patients would develop a cough. The consequence would be inconceivable if Felicia contracted the plague. I immediately contacted a thoracic expert at the National Taiwan University and scheduled Felicia for an examination with Dr. Pan-Chyr Yang, one of my first M.D.-Ph.D. students whom I taught after returning to Taiwan. On Monday morning Felicia had her X-ray taken at the hospital. Dr. Yang examined the X-ray and concluded that Felicia did not have the plague. But as he noticed that Felicia was still coughing, he probed in greater detail about Felicia's condition in India.

Felicia told Dr. Yang that her stomach hurt terribly while in India. Even at that point of time, the pain still persisted. Dr. Yang examined her distended stomach and was shocked that he could feel her liver, indicating that the liver was extremely enlarged. In normal cases, the liver is not easily located by feeling with fingers. Furthermore, each time he pressed her abdomen gently with his hand, she would wince in pain. Dr. Yang immediately arranged for an ultrasound examination on Felicia. The scan showed up over forty dark spots, among which were about four to five centimeters and were even as big as five to six centimeters. Dr. Yang was worried that they were tumors, so he performed a liver biopsy. The results confirmed that it was indeed glandular cancer. Felicia's breast cancer had returned and spread to her liver!

The Situation Becomes Extremely Dangerous

To all of us, especially Felicia, this piece of news came like a bolt from the blue out of nowhere. For the second time, she was afflicted with great disappointment and despair. She had done everything she could to take care of her body — but all her effort went down to the drain with the recurrence of her cancer. Going through the liver biopsy was extremely painful; furthermore, at that time Felicia was already quite weak. After all the tests, Dr. Yang arranged for Felicia to be admitted to the hospital.

The severity of her condition became apparent as soon as she was hospitalized. Her liver grew larger by the day, and the pain in her internal organs was so intense that it had to be suppressed by morphine. Felicia's liver became so large because there were over forty tumors growing inside, and they were all growing unceasingly, pushing outward against the outer wall of the liver and forcing it to swell. There is a thin membranous capsule on the outside of the liver; when the liver swelled, the membrane swelled with it, almost to the point of bursting. Such visceral pain is extremely difficult to endure, and this was the kind of pain that Felicia experienced. During her hospitalization, Felicia's liver continued to grow incessantly and her pain, sharper and more intense. The pain finally reached to a point where it hurt so much that she was virtually in a dazed, half-conscious condition the whole time. Her condition became extremely perilous.

The National Taiwan University Hospital immediately assembled a small medical team, with the deputy director-general of the hospital, Dr. Che-Yan Chuang, acting as convenor. The team included Jacqueline Peng-Wang, Pan-Chyr Yang, An-Li Cheng, Chiu-Hua Wang, X-ray specialist Shi-Jie Chen, and liver specialist Guan-Tang Huang. The deputy director-general was my older brother Cheng-Chang Wu's elementary school classmate and a very good friend of the family. Jacqueline Peng-Wang was head of the cancer research division of the National Health Research Institutes. Dr. Yang was the doctor who discovered that Felicia's cancer had migrated to the liver. Dr. Chiu-Hua Wang was the specialist who performed Felicia's routine examinations at National Taiwan University Hospital. As a student of the first graduating batch of oncologists trained by the Institute of Biomedical Sciences, Dr. An-Li Cheng was acquainted with Felicia and knew her very well. Following some discussions, the team decided to ask Dr. Cheng to serve as the physician in charge of Felicia's case.

At that time, Felicia had already entered a semi-comatose state. The medical team needed to find the effective medicine for Felicia as soon as possible; otherwise her life would be in extreme danger. The team consulted famous oncologists and cancer research scientists at medical institutions all over the world. I also contacted my university classmate Dr. Andrew Huang; he was then president of the Sun Yat-Sen Cancer Center. A cancer specialist with extensive experience, Dr. Andrew Huang had served as professor of oncology at world-renowned Duke University for many years. He came to review Felicia's condition. After studying Felicia's medical record, he shared his thoughts with me in a very serious tone.

Because the tumors in her liver were already the size of three fingers wide, the situation was extremely urgent. Furthermore, the spread of the breast cancer to the liver points to an aggravating condition. As the organ in the body responsible for the disposal of harmful materials, all medicine must pass through the liver to have its harmful properties neutralized. Thus, medication is not very effective against cancer in the liver.

In addition, Felicia's cancer was already in the final stage. The various stages of cancer can be classified as follows. In the first stage, tumors are still confined within the organ in the body. In the second stage, cancer cells have spread to the surrounding tissues. When Felicia was diagnosed with breast cancer, it had already spread to the nearby lymph nodes; thus the cancer had already reached the second stage. In the final and most dangerous stage of cancer, tumors have spread to organs farther away from their origin. In Felicia's case, the metastasis of breast cancer to the liver was an example.

My old classmate Dr. Andrew Huang told me that the spread of breast cancer to the liver was one of the most dangerous types of metastasis. According to his prediction, regardless of the treatment we used, Felicia would have at most one to two years to live. At that critical moment, the medical team was looking into every possible treatment, and it was a race against time. Felicia was already virtually unconscious. If they continued to allow the tumors to grow unchecked, once the tumors occupied more than seventy-five percent of the liver, she would experience liver failure and her life would immediately be at risk.

Selecting Chemotherapy Medicine

The tumors already posed an immediate threat to her life, something had to be done to stop the growth. Thus, Dr. Huang proposed using the strongest possible medicine to suppress tumor growth.

He suggested that we use taxol and adriamycin together; at the time, they were the strongest medicines available for breast cancer. After Dr. Huang offered his opinion, the team immediately held a meeting. The medical team thought there must be scientific justification to use the two medicines together, they ought to have some published papers or research supporting this course of action. Dr. Chi-Hsin Yang, a medical oncologist at the National Taiwan University, happened to be at the National Cancer Institute in the United States doing his further studies, so Dr. Peng-Wang called and asked him to search for related information and papers. As a result, they discovered that when the two medicines were used together, they might actually partially cancel each other out.

As there was research suggesting that these two medicines should not be used together, what could be used then for Felicia's treatment? I could understand the pressure that the medical team faced, especially Dr. An-Li Cheng. His responsibility as chief physician in that situation could not have been easy. At last, upon the recommendation of various experts, including the specialists at NIH and renowned oncologist Dr. Paul Carbone, we decided to use a combination of cyclophosphamide, adriamycin, and 5-FU (CAF), together with leucovorin (L) for Felicia's treatment. Eight years earlier when Felicia's breast cancer first appeared, the CAF combination had suppressed cancer growth. This time the research team chose to use the same combination plus leucovorin, hoping that it would also be effective against the metastasized breast cancer cells.

This complex decision-making process took place within a breathlessly short span of one week. Because Felicia was in so much pain, the doctors prescribed a large dosage of morphine to suppress it; this left her in a constant state of semi-consciousness.

Given her situation, using medicine involved taking risky gambles. There is a protocol for using medicine in chemotherapy. The first time the medicine is taken, it is necessary to wait two, maybe three weeks before taking more. Because the medicine used in chemotherapy is so lethal, it kills normal healthy cells along with cancer cells. After each dose of medicine, the patient's white blood cell count drops for approximately one week. It is thus necessary to wait one more week for the white blood cell count to return to a normal level before another dosage can be administered. If the medicine has no effect during that period, the tumors may continue to grow and pose an immediate threat to one's life.

Hence, the extreme care taken by the medical team in selecting the combination of medicine was understandable. After Felicia took the medicine, there was no real significant difference for the first session that spanned over a period of about three weeks. That is to say, the tumors did not shrink, but at the same time, they did not grow larger. That gave us some hope, but Felicia was in as much pain as before. The medical team had a meeting and decided to give her a second dosage at the third week after the first session. The second time she took the medicine the tumors showed signs of shrinking, and Felicia felt her pain subside. The medical team finally concluded that the combined CAF and leucovorin treatment was effective in the suppression of Felicia's tumors. Everyone heaved a sigh of relief, albeit only slightly.

The Relentless Onslaught of Chemotherapy

During the hospitalization, Felicia was constantly in a dazed state, she suffered from pain and the medicines' side effects. Before undergoing chemotherapy, she endured visceral pain unimaginable by others. Even after using morphine, the pain was so excruciating that she experienced vivid nightmares, one after another.

The second time she took the medicine, her pain lessened, but Felicia still had to endure a barrage of side effects that struck her body like lightning storms and torrential rains signifying the end of the world.

Generally speaking, anti-cancer drugs achieve their purpose by killing the dividing cells. But since the medicine is unable to effectively distinguish between cancer cells and normal dividing cells, they perform the task indiscriminately, killing both kinds of cells. Although the vast majority of anti-cancer drugs are most harmful against cancer cells, their effects on normal cells can be relatively quite severe. The normal dividing cells most affected are bone marrow cells that produce red and white blood cells, skin cells, hair follicle cells, and membrane cells lining the digestive tract and mouth. Hence, the anti-cancer medicine will cause patients to suffer from anemia, a lowered white blood cell count making them more susceptible to infection, hair loss and ulceration around the mouth and digestive tract that makes swallowing food difficult. Even if they are able to eat, they throw up constantly. These are the side effects of chemotherapy. Most patients are unable to withstand these effects and give up after only one or two treatments.

Thereafter, Felicia underwent ten chemotherapy sessions. She never bowed to the treatment sessions which were increasingly even more grueling and torturous. She faced every treatment with a resolve so strong that was beyond words. During the second session of the combined CAF and leucovorin treatment, Felicia's tumors gradually shrank in size, but the side effects from the drugs still left her in terrible pain. Her hair fell out and her mouth became ulcerated, causing her tormenting pain. Before every meal, Felicia would have to spray morphine in her mouth and then take slow, careful bites one at a time; every bite was a new source of agony. She knew she needed food and nourishment in order to battle against cancer, and she was determined to keep on eating no matter how difficult it was.

However, the side effects proved to be a much stronger contender, each time Felicia made such a valiant effort to eat, she would immediately succumb and throw up everything. It was heartbreaking for me to witness what she went through. Before she gradually saw the glimmer of hope and life, she had to endure tremendous pain from the treatment. If she did not have that unwavering desire to live and the constant longing and concern for her loved ones, could she have endured such hardship?

At that time when Felicia's cancer recurred, the eldest of her younger sisters, Wan-Chan, came back from the United States to take care of her. She set up a cot next to Felicia's hospital bed and remained by her side every day, watching over her elder sister every single second during this critical stage. That was a great comfort to me. Without Wan-Chan's loving care, Felicia's recovery would have undoubtedly been more painful.

I went to see Felicia every day and attended every meeting held by the medical team regarding Felicia's treatment. I knew that Felicia's cancer had recurred and migrated to her liver. I knew the struggle ahead of her would be longer and more arduous than the first one. But I had kept this promise in my heart — like the wedding vows we made to each other — to spend my lifetime by her side looking after her till the end of our lives.

SECTION IV

FIGHTING CANCER

13

Beginning a Long-Term Resistance

I read once in the introductory remarks of Aldous Huxley's *Brave New World*: "Determination is the essence of a life molded through great struggle. In the low points of one's life, strength of mind is the only way to overcome the strength of the oppressive forces around us." I saw proof of this statement in Felicia.

Mutual Encouragement from Fellow Patients

About the same time when Felicia's cancer recurred, Dr. Huai-Yao Chang at the molecular neurosciences research division of the Institute of Biomedical Sciences also found out that his nasopharyngeal cancer had migrated to his neck. Dr. Chang was an expert in signal transduction and one of the discoverers of calmodulin. Before returning to Taiwan, he discovered that he had nasopharyngeal cancer and had undergone two years of treatment. He recovered and returned to Taiwan in 1994 to take up a post at the Institute of Biomedical Sciences. During that year, he had done well in the planning and establishment of his division. The energy and commitment he channeled into his work brought him assurance and belief that he was on the road to recovery.

One day when he was playing tennis his neck felt a little sore. He thought he might have sprained his neck and went to the hospital for a checkup. But instead, he was told that his nasopharyngeal cancer had spread to his cervical spine. Dr. Chang could not believe that the cancer had not let him off. He immediately fell into the depths of depression.

Dr. Chang and Felicia were hospitalized at around the same time, and he also went through a dangerous life-threatening period. But under the attentive care of his doctors and Mrs. Chang, his condition began to show some promising progress. After the second chemotherapy treatment, Felicia felt slightly more conscious and alert, so sometimes she was able to get out of bed and walk around. She knew Dr. Chang was also hospitalized due to a cancer recurrence. She visited him and the two hospital mates gave each other mutual support and encouragement. Sometimes, when I went to the hospital to visit Felicia, I would see Felicia hook Dr. Chang's arm into hers and the two of them would walk slowly down the hall. It was a touching, heartwrenching scene of two illness-stricken lives soldiering on with a determination to live and help each other out to go through the thick and thin of their battles.

During her hospitalization, Felicia constantly encouraged Dr. Chang, "We can't be beaten. We absolutely have to recover together." Felicia stayed at the hospital for three months; her largest tumor shrank down to 1.5 centimeters. But she still had over forty tumors. However, as long as the treatment was able to suppress tumor growth and cause shrinkage, we considered that as good news.

Incredible Fighting Spirit

After Felicia's strength improved and returned to a slight degree of her normal state of health, her enthusiasm for work resurfaced. While she was still in the hospital, she made calls to the laboratory, kept up with the research team's progress, edited their papers from her hospital bed to fax back to the laboratory almost every day, and gave them detailed advice about things that they needed to watch out for. Felicia communicated with her laboratory by proxy; as a regular daily visitor at Felicia's ward, I naturally became the messenger link between her and the laboratory. A stack of reports came from the laboratory each day; she finished them and sent them back the next day without fail. Of course, at the time, Felicia's body had to endure the same side effects of oral ulceration, nausea, and vomiting as in previous chemotherapy treatments, but she approached her work with the same effervescent spirit as always.

The amount of work she took on dismayed even the doctors, who were incessantly scolding her and cautioning her to get some rest. But Felicia would simply reply, "My illness shouldn't slow down the laboratory's progress. Besides, working is a part of me. It enables me to forget my pain, forget my exhaustion, and forget that I'm ill. Working stimulates me. It's a kind of overflowing life energy that I find difficult to describe, but I know that it helps me to fight cancer."

Hearing this, the doctors would think that this was a source of Felicia's unyielding strength in her fight against the fierce disease and they gave up insisting that she rest. I recall that Dr. Pan-Chyr Yang, now chairman of internal medicine at National Taiwan University, once said that the hospital was like Felicia's office, the bed and tables all piled high with research reports and papers. To prevent Felicia from working was impossible. And while at work, she was full of energy, and she did not seem at all like a person stricken with cancer.

Throughout the treatment, incredible life strength and determination enabled Felicia to maintain her resolve in the fight against cancer. She enjoyed nature and being cooped up in a hospital room would certainly drive her to boredom. So although she was still extremely weak, as soon as her body started to show some signs of improvement, I would take her out for walks.

That was during the second month of her hospital stay. I took Felicia to Dajianshan near Nankang to admire the luxuriant greenery of the mountains in the distance and the lush green turf of the rolling slopes. At that time, Felicia could only take five or six steps while climbing the tracks of Dajianshan before having to stop and catch her breath. I supported Felicia throughout, up and down the steps, the two of us stopping often to talk so that she could have a chance to take a breather and rest. Every time we sat down, a half-hour would pass before she regained enough strength to get up again and continue walking.

Although setting out on a short journey for fresh air was difficult, Felicia still hoped that I could accompany her to the countryside at least once a week to smell the freshness of the forests and the grassland. The serious disease did not dampen her love of nature.

After three months, both Felicia's and Dr. Huai-Yao Chang's medical conditions improved dramatically. Fortunately, the two were able to overcome the odds in the face of great difficulty. When they were discharged from the hospital, they congratulated and encouraged each other, though they both knew that the path ahead would be long and difficult. But to Felicia, whatever situations or external factors that might come her way, her determination to fight on — already deeply ingrained in her heart and mind — would never waver. I knew that the metastasis of the cancer had caused her to experience a brief period of frustration and momentary sense of defeat. But once she resolved that she would not give up that easily, her tenacity naturally gave her the strength to wage another battle against cancer. She was fully aware that the road ahead would be full of brambles.

In spite of her physical weakness and exhaustion, she returned to the office immediately and sprang into action drafting new research plans. She regarded her own medical condition as a case study, she released the full details of her medical file, and held discussion meetings with postdoctoral fellows, research assistants, and students.

The laboratory research team was shocked by the extent to which Felicia made known to the public about her own condition. Her senior research assistant, Nian-Tsu Chang, said that although everyone worked round the clock in the laboratory researching on cancer, she personally had never come in such close contact with a cancer patient. At that instant, the individual standing before her and working alongside with her was not only a cancer patient, she was also a cancer researcher, and moreover, her mentoring professor. Being in such close contact with a cancer patient and upon understanding what Felicia went through in order to fight her disease, Nian-Tsu Chang was shaken and felt her heart throbbing in silent pain for what Felicia had undergone. For a long while, Nian-Tsu Chang was deeply affected. She said that it was then that she came into real contact with cancer, finally understood what the disease was, and realized the terrible damage it inflicted in people's lives.

Although Felicia recuperated well enough to be discharged from the hospital, she was still extremely weak. The doctors, the research team, our colleagues at the research institute, the children and I were all worried about her health and hoped that she would not over-exert herself with work. But Felicia simply regarded cancer as a passer-by, a temporary unwelcome guest that had come to visit. She was not willing to let any facet of her life be hindered by cancer. This included not just the quality of her personal life, but her demands and expectations as a researcher too. Thus, despite her weak physical condition, Felicia never displayed any sign of fatigue or distress of a body ravaged by disease.

Forcing Herself to Make a Speech

The following month after Felicia left the hospital, the American Association for Cancer Research (AACR) and the Institute of Biomedical Sciences jointly organized the International Symposium on Cancer in Taipei. This was an extremely important scientific conference since it was the first AACR symposium ever to take place in Asia. The planning began a year earlier. Originally, Felicia had been scheduled to deliver the first lecture at the symposium. But then, she did not expect her cancer to recur. Her physical condition was not as strong as before, so I advised Felicia that if she felt weak physically, perhaps she should cancel the lecture. Felicia was silent and did not respond to my suggestion. I knew what she was thinking then: the conference agenda had already been decided and finalized, so to ask someone to take her place then would not really seem appropriate.

It was the day before the conference, past nine in the evening, and I was still working in the laboratory when I received a call from Felicia. At that time, she was already at home. Felicia told me this conference was important to her, she should not be absent for the delivery of her lecture. She wanted to return to the laboratory to prepare. Felicia was scheduled to give the first lecture at nine the next morning. Eventually, she was standing on her feet at the podium for exactly an hour. She was energetic, her voice was loud and her performance, unparalleled. At the end of her speech, she received a standing ovation from the audience that went on and on. Following her speech, the AACR honored Felicia with an award in recognition of her scientific achievements and her unique spirit and determination in the face of adversity.

As I sat listening to Felicia's lecture, my mind and heart were a jumble of thoughts and emotions. Thinking of how bravely Felicia had fought, how strong and independent she was, and how the true essence of her character had remained unchanged despite the gravity of her condition, I could only feel appreciative and thankful beyond any words. She fought not only for herself, but also for the liberation of emotional trauma inside me and the children. Had it not been Felicia's willpower of steel and endurance, our whole family would have been enshrouded in a lifeless gloom and depression. And because of Felicia's strength and optimism, she continued to fill us with beautiful, endearing memories as a family.

There was another aspect of Felicia that had my admiration. She was given morphine to stop the unbearable pain of her swelling liver until the tumors had shrunk. The doctors decided to stop the morphine dosage once the swelling in the liver had subsided. As Felicia was prescribed morphine in high dosage for a prolonged period, the doctors and I were concerned if she would grow dependent on it, thus resulting in addiction.

What surprised all of us was that when Felicia stopped taking morphine, she simply stopped, and there were no signs of addiction or withdrawal symptoms. This exemplified Felicia's iron will. I often say that Felicia is the most unique individual I have been blessed to know in this lifetime. She had such great determination which is extremely rare in human traits.

Completely Different Outlook on Life

Dr. Huai-Yao Chang fell ill, and was admitted to and discharged from the hospital around almost the same time as Felicia. However, his situation differed a great deal from that of Felicia after his discharge.

Dr. Huai-Yao Chang came over to my office once to look for me. He said that his neck still hurt a lot. He was in so much pain that he suffered deeply, and consequently he felt he had brought burden and stress to his family. He lamented that life had lost its meaning to be alive in this state. Dr. Chang said he was extremely worried about the future development of the molecular neurosciences research division as well as his colleagues. I could sense from his tone his world-weariness tinged with harbored thoughts of suicide. Besides giving him encouragement, I told him I would take care of his research-related duties, and that he should just concentrate on getting better.

I could tell Dr. Chang was still feeling low and dejected, so I referred him to a psychiatrist who prescribed an effective drug for his condition. After the consultation and treatment, Dr. Chang's family observed that he seemed a lot better; I too noticed that his workload in the laboratory gradually returned to normal and that he would even go out occasionally with friends from the Institute of Biomedical Sciences. I was somewhat relieved.

Half a year after Felicia left the hospital, her strength gradually returned to normal. She was a person who wanted to stay active whenever given the chance. The Institute of Biomedical Sciences organized a trip to Lalashan, a mountain in the Taoyuan Prefecture known for its peaches and majestic cypresses. Felicia participated and looked forward to the trip. The whole group was making the ascent up the mountain in high spirits, and as we passed the halfway point to the summit, an urgent message was received from the Institute of Biomedical Sciences: Dr. Chang had committed suicide.

At that time, it was already evening. It was impossible to make the descent down the mountain, so Felicia and I, together with the group, stayed overnight at a guesthouse. The next morning, Felicia remained at Lalashan; I began my descent as soon as the day started to break at around five and I rushed to Dr. Chang's house.

Mrs. Chang recounted the events of the day before. She said that she left home early in the morning to buy groceries. She came home and cooked lunch; it was at the moment when she called out for Dr. Chang to have lunch and she could not find him. At first, she thought he had perhaps gone to visit a neighbor so she went and knocked on every door, but was still not able to locate him. So she telephoned his office, but he was not there either. By then, she became extremely worried. She thought of going to the neighbors again to ask if they had seen him. When she walked up to the fifth floor, she noticed a pair of sandals on the balcony outside the window. At a closer look, she realized they were Dr. Chang's sandals. Her heart was racing. Mrs. Chang quickly dashed to the balcony, looked down, and saw Dr. Chang's limpless body lying lifelessly on the pavement below… At that instant, she knew her husband had committed suicide.

The tragic death of Dr. Chang brought deep grief to the Chang family. The colleagues at the Institute of Biomedical Sciences mourned for his passing. I arranged a farewell ceremony as a final send-off for Dr. Chang. After the send-off, I finally had time to ask his psychiatrist why Dr. Chang had committed suicide when he seemed to have stabilized emotionally after taking the medicine.

The doctor remarked that Dr. Chang's physical and emotional condition were indeed more stable after the prescribed medication, but medication, no matter how effective, cannot change a person's outlook about the world. So when Dr. Chang's medical condition improved, he had gained enough physical strength to do the things that he wanted to do, including terminating his own life.

Drugs can improve one's mental state, but that cannot alter the way one thinks and views things. The doctor's words gave me much food for thought from the conversation I had with him. Like Dr. Chang, Felicia had a cancer recurrence, but she was never frustrated or depressed, and the thought of retreat never crossed her mind. Her immediate instinct was to find ways to challenge cancer, fight it, and empower herself to live every minute of her life to the fullest. Every second of her life was a beautiful moment.

A strong determination and subconscious beliefs play pivotal role in motivating a person's will to live and survive. I saw two very different forms of life expression in Felicia and Dr. Chang. I can only say Felicia's iron will and optimism saved her as well as our entire family. Felicia did not believe that leaving this earth was an avenue to resolve problems; she did not avoid her problems or hide her own medical condition, and she was unwilling to let her family members suffer because she did. Had it not been for her unique character and strength that saw her through the thirteen difficult years of journey battling cancer, would I have Felicia by my side to give me such beautiful memories?

Playing Tug-of-War with Life

During the hospitalization period when her cancer recurred, I noticed a special characteristic of Felicia that left me with feelings of awe, admiration, and a tinge of empathy for her at the same time.

She was in a semi-conscious state and was unable to leave her bed for an entire month. As she gradually regained her strength and consciousness, she showed her true colors as a scientist by recording every detail of her medical treatment. Furthermore, she personally attended every meeting held by the medical team. From a scientist's perspective, Felicia's action was seen as one guided by the principle to seek truth from facts; however, take her as a sicked patient, her courage was inconceivable because not even a normal person could demonstrate such fearlessness.

The chief physician of the medical team, Dr. An-Li Cheng, who accompanied Felicia through her struggle for life, described this period as a "spirited and courageous battle."

This time when Felicia was admitted to the National Taiwan University Hospital, her liver was full of tumors, and she also had a pleural effusion in her left lung, which meant water had accumulated within the lining of the lung. After the water was pumped out, cancer cells were discovered in it, indicating that the cancer cells had already traveled to the pleural cavity. Felicia's situation was not only urgent, but potentially life-threatening.

At the instant, her stomach hurt a great deal, to the point that she had to use morphine to stop the pain, and even then, the residual pain was still unbearable, bringing tears to her eyes. Dr. Cheng said Felicia requested him to treat her as he saw fit and not to worry that she would be unable to take the pain. No matter what, she wanted to live. She saw the meaning and mission in her life which she absolutely refused to give up.

Dr. Cheng was from the first batch of oncologists trained by Academia Sinica's Institute of Biomedical Sciences. He had previously worked in Felicia's laboratory and regarded her as both his mentor and senior. As the chief physician responsible for Felicia's treatment, he had, in the years to come, become both her doctor and her friend. Dr. Cheng spoke of the difficult challenges faced in Felicia's battle against cancer as a physician, he had to deal with the dilemma of administrating a higher drug dosage or stronger medicine on her, however, she would always tell him, "Don't worry; I can take it. Relax and treat me; I'm determined to keep on living."

"Among all my patients, she was the only patient who demonstrated such strong willpower and courage to live," Dr. Cheng said of Felicia. Dr. Cheng had a comprehensive knowledge of Felicia's treatment history and background, he knew she received eight chemotherapy treatments after her mastectomy. Adriamycin proved to be the most effective of the medicines she took then. Adriamycin is extremely potent against cancer cells, but it is just as toxic and harmful to the rest of the body, especially the heart. The lifetime limit for adriamycin use is thus five hundred and fifty milligrams (per square foot of body surface area). When Felicia underwent treatment in the United States, she had already been treated with nearly the maximum allowable dose of adriamycin.

At first, the medical doctors were reluctant to use adriamycin, or "small red berry," as it is commonly called in Chinese. But after considering its effectiveness they finally decided to continue administrating it, albeit in smaller doses. Then they added leucovorin to increase the effectiveness of 5-FU. After three sessions, this chemotherapy treatment was producing results. Felicia's tumors shrank in size, but she had also reached her limit in terms of the amount of adriamycin she could take; her heart could not take any more. She was experiencing severe heart palpitations, nausea, and difficulty in breathing.

The accumulation of adriamycin in Felicia's body threatened her health, so the medical team decided to switch medications. Dr. Cheng replaced adriamycin with methotrexate. The treatment immediately produced results. CMFL treatment was used seven more times in the seven months after Felicia's cancer resurfaced. Felicia's liver tumors shrank, and only four or five dark spots remained, of which, the largest one was reduced to approximately one and a half centimeters in diameter. The fluid accumulation in the pleural cavity completely disappeared, and no new cancer cells were detected in subsequent examinations. Felicia's cancer recurrence had been controlled. But there was still no way to completely eliminate all the cancer cells.

The War That Could Not Be Finished

The medical team had pooled the best of their expertise and resources to offer the most ideal treatment for Felicia's breast cancer that spread to the liver. Felicia was a scientist and she reviewed all the medical documentations and records on the subject. According to a documented source, in cases where breast cancer spread to the liver, the longest a patient could hope to live and survive was two years.

Through chemotherapy, Felicia's cancer was controlled, but why could it not be completely cured? Why was it that in cases of breast cancer metastasis to the liver, patients live for at most two years? There seemed to be common related factors to these two questions.

At the time when Felicia's cancer recurred, my university classmate and the president of Sun Yat-Sen Cancer Center, Dr. Andrew Huang, told me that the effectiveness of any medicine diminishes after it reaches the liver — liver being the vital organ for removing harmful materials from the body. Thus, from the outset, removing cancer cells in the liver is difficult. Furthermore, treating cancer cells in the liver that had been exposed to chemotherapy drugs was challenging and that explained the short survival time for patients suffering from breast cancer metastasis to liver.

The other important reason is that medicines administered in chemotherapy are very toxic drugs that not only kill cancer cells effectively but also bring severe stress to our body systems. There is a limit to the amount of any anti-cancer medicine that the body can take, in fact, patients would not be able to withstand the long-term damage caused by prolonged treatment of chemotherapy.

The treatment of cancer is determined by the stage of its detection and diagnosis, and the course of its progression. Treatment can include operations, radiation therapy, and chemotherapy. Ordinarily, surgeries are performed while the cancer is still in its early stages, but only under the condition that the cancer is discovered before it has a chance to spread to other parts of the body.

Radiation therapy with Cobalt-60 can also be used before the onset of cancer metastasis. Radiation therapy can kill cancer cells effectively, but it can also damage the neighboring normal healthy cells.

Chemotherapy is used on patients in which cancer has migrated and progressed to the last advanced stage, and the treatment is the most difficult to endure. In chemotherapy, usually one or several types of "medicine" are administered. These medicines are really poisonous drugs that kill and target fast-dividing and multiplying cancer cells, but also do damage to normal cells. Thus, the hidden danger of this treatment is that sometimes it is as harmful as it is beneficial to patients. The strategy of this treatment regimen is you "kill five thousand enemies, but lose three thousand of your own soldiers."

It is extremely difficult to find a perfect solution. Because chemotherapy also does harm to normal cells, the dosage of medicine administered is extremely important. If too little a dose is used, then the medicine becomes ineffective. But on the other hand, if the dosage is too heavy, it results in the death of normal dividing cells, especially blood-producing bone marrow cells. After each chemotherapy session, the patient's white cell count drops; this reduces the body's immunity to fight disease and infections. Under this circumstance, it then becomes necessary for the white blood cell count to rise before conducting further chemotherapy treatments.

After chemotherapy, patients' tumors might be destroyed or at least effectively controlled, thanks to the drug administered. However, once the treatment regimen is stopped, there is great possibility that tumors may return. However, the reality of the situation is that patients' bodies are incapable of withstanding wave after wave of chemotherapy. There are limitations to what the human body can tolerate. In the long run, even if one is not beaten by cancer, one will be destroyed by the treatment.

Cancer cells also possess their own drug-resistance mechanisms. Thus, even if a patient's body could endure an indefinite amount of chemotherapy, drugs usually become less effective after a period of time. Once the tumor starts growing again, it means that cancer cells have already become resistant to the drug. Then the doctor must switch drugs and administer a new type of chemotherapy. The sad plight of patients in the terminal stage of cancer is the emotional trauma of fear, terror, anxiety and dejectedness they have to go through in keeping up with the regimens of switching drugs and enduring their alternating side effects. It is like fighting a battle that has no end in sight, that is virtually on the defeated side.

Felicia was a scientist whose research focus was on anti-cancer drugs; she, of course, knew all the phases and cycles of chemotherapy. Felicia had controlled her cancer, but she was fully aware that the risk and probability of a relapse in the future was extremely high.

Choices and decisions are actions based on life experience and accumulated wisdom. In the face of difficult challenges or a turning point in life, how one should choose and make a decision is a grueling test of life. In her fight against cancer, Felicia overcame obstacle after obstacle and won battle after battle by trying new treatments with the latest anti-cancer drugs. She fought the battle of life and was driven by her dogged determination to survive. My grief, my respect for Felicia's long, arduous hardship — which culminated from the difficult decision she made and the high price she paid to fight for her survival — were simply beyond words. I was her closest companion. I walked her through every step of her chemotherapy regimen. The journey was my greatest pain; regardless of the efforts I made, I could not alleviate her pain. But this was also my greatest source of gratitude, because I witnessed the indomitable spirit and the noble character of the person I loved most.

14

Offering Oneself as a Lab Specimen

Felicia received CMFL treatment for eight consecutive months, from October 1994 until July 1995, and the growth of the tumors in her liver was brought under control. During that period, her strength also gradually returned, and she started to exercise and work again. Things were looking up. However, Felicia's determination to find a cure for cancer never waned.

During the life-threatening stage of Felicia's hospitalization, Ms. Shu-Fang Tsai, a colleague at the National Health Research Institutes' extramural research department, was also at National Taiwan University Hospital to keep her daughter company. She called from her daughter's hospital room to inquire after Felicia. At that time Felicia's condition was extremely critical, and she was in a ward that isolated patient from visitors. But their phone conversation left a strong impression on Shu-Fang.

Felicia told her, "It's really not fair. I was so careful about my health, why is it that cancer still wouldn't give up on me?" Every time Shu-Fang thought of these words, her heart ached. She could feel Felicia's pain, and she could understand Felicia's resolute determination to fight against cancer and find a remedy. Felicia knew and perceived that she was engaged in a battle that had no end.

And how would the medical team not feel the same sentiments and anguish? From the time when Felicia was first hospitalized, all the members of the medical team, including Dr. An-Li Cheng, Dr. Pan-Chyr Yang, Dr. Jacqueline Peng-Wang, the nurses from the oncology department, and all the other hospital employees, became Felicia's comrades in battle. The medical team contacted almost every major cancer center in the world in search of information to help them better understand the effects each drug would have on Felicia. Felicia's strong instinct to survive sent a message to the medical team, that is, to update her on any findings that had the potential to cure her. The medical team fulfilled the responsibility with resolution because their patient, Felicia, was a warrior who was determined to challenge her disease.

Discovering a New Treatment

After eight months of treatment, Felicia felt her strength returning to normal. She was anxious to know what the next treatment step was.

At that time, a foreign scientist happened to come to speak at the National Health Research Institutes. He was an oncologist who was researching on a new treatment method. During the lecture, he mentioned that NIH and other medical centers were undertaking a new clinical trial for cancer patients; this new treatment integrated high dose chemotherapy and autologous bone marrow transplantation (BMT).

As mentioned previously, the amount of drug used in cancer treatment is extremely important. If the dosage is too minuscule then the treatment is not effective, but on the other hand, an extremely heavy dosage does too much damage to normal cells, especially bone marrow cells. In high dose chemotherapy, a dosage of ten to twenty times the normal dosage is used in order to ensure that all cancer cells in the body are destroyed at one time. However, high dose chemotherapy naturally also destroys the body's bone marrow cells.

Humans cannot survive without bone marrow cells. The idea behind the autologous BMT was to do a thorough examination, administer pre-treatment medication, remove bone marrow cells unaffected by cancer, freeze and save these cells, and then administer an extremely large dosage of anti-tumor drugs to kill off all the cancer cells within the body. The last step is to re-insert the healthy bone marrow cells back into the body and let them grow. It was hypothesized that the treatment would completely cure the patient because the newly grown bone marrow cells in his or her body would also be entirely free of cancer.

In the scientist's lecture, he mentioned that the success rate of high dose chemotherapy in conjunction with autologous BMT was seventy percent. The lecture and the high success rate of this new treatment inspired Felicia. She aggressively looked for more information to fully understand the actual procedures and outcomes of this clinical research.

Assessing Feasibility

At that time, Dr. Jacqueline Peng-Wang was serving as director of the cancer research division of Taiwan's National Health Research Institutes. She had just come back from a visit to NIH and told Felicia about the clinical research NIH was conducting.

The same information coming from two different sources simultaneously made a huge impact on Felicia. I knew that in her heart, her greatest desire was to completely rid herself of cancer so that she could grow old with me, see her children raise their own families, and continue her research. She was in the prime of her life and was not at all ready to leave the world. She wanted to live on because she valued life and she loved me, our children, her family, and her laboratory colleagues. Felicia's desire was to fight cancer — to live on bravely, resolutely and happily.

In April 1995, Felicia, Faith, and I decided to make a trip to NIH in order to understand the research behind high dose chemotherapy and autologous BMT. Would this be the last glimmer of hope for Felicia to defeat cancer? Before the trip, I kept thinking: I knew Felicia dearly wanted to live on, and she saw this treatment at the experimental stage as her last hope, but I was still not convinced by the statistics produced by this clinical trial. I did not tell Felicia my doubt and concern though. In any case, she probably was thinking the same thing as me. She was a scientist herself — a very meticulous and critical-minded scientist indeed; she was undoubtedly aware of what the chances were. But because she had an optimistic outlook, she moved forward as always with a positive attitude.

Embraced with a hopeful mindset and an inquisitive spirit, we arrived at the NIH. Through Dr. Jacqueline Peng-Wang's introduction, we began our discussions with the doctors and scientists who had conducted the research. As a result, we found out that the seventy percent success rate was obtained based on a sample population that had already undergone a strict selection process.

The patients who participated in the trials had all been preselected by the researchers. Basically, those patients who were selected did not have any trace of cancer cells found in them after chemotherapy. They underwent high dose chemotherapy and subsequently bone marrow transplantation; this would ensure that the cancer cells were even more completely and thoroughly eradicated from their bodies. Of those who went through the process, the five-year survival rate was seventy percent; most of them were colon cancer patients. The result of this clinical trial did not include any patients with cases of breast cancer metastasis to the liver.

There were sixteen patients whose breast cancer had migrated to other organs. Among them, only four were breast cancer patients with liver metastases: two of them died during chemotherapy because they were unable to take the severity of the treatment, one died a year after the treatment and the only one still surviving had received the treatment only a year and a half ago, and was still under strict observation. This demonstrated that the success rate of cases similar to Felicia's was very low.

When we discussed further with the doctor at NIH, the doctor said that he would not recommend Felicia to undergo this type of treatment because it was still at the trial stage, but he would respect Felicia's decision. He was encouraged by Felicia's strong instinct to live, so he was willing to do whatever he could to help.

Resolutely Trying New Treatments

Upon our return to Taiwan, Felicia's medical team began their rounds of discussion on high dose chemotherapy and autologous BMT. The doctors could not reach a consensus and were evenly split on the treatment — half were for it and half were against it.

Those against the treatment were of the opinion that in clinical cases of breast cancer metastasis to the liver, the success rate of the treatment was practically zero. The risk was too great for Felicia to undergo the tough treatment. If complications were to arise during the treatment and caused her to lose her life, it would be too late for regrets.

Then, there were doctors who agreed that Felicia should give it a try. They knew very well that the survival rate for breast cancer metastasis to the liver using traditional treatment methods was just as infinitesimally low. The longest surviving patient documented was two years. At that time, since no viable treatment was available to completely cure Felicia's cancer, there was no absolute reason not to try a new treatment, especially since this might be the only chance she had left for a complete remedy.

Each member of the medical team had their own thoughts and reservations. I knew that the final decision rested with Felicia, because only she could decide what to do with her life. But I also knew my wife, and I could more or less predict what her decision would be.

The medical team presented to Felicia the pros and cons as derived from their discussions. The doctors knew that this would be a difficult decision; they hoped Felicia would make the final decision after deliberating all the possible scenarios.

I knew Felicia had weighed the odds and options carefully. She asked the doctor calmly, "Could you please tell me approximately how many cancer cells are there in my body right now?" He replied, "About ten million." Felicia then asked, "If I were to receive high dose chemotherapy and autologous BMT, how many cancer cells would remain?" The doctor said that if one were to estimate using pre-existing statistics, the new treatment could kill approximately ninety-nine percent of all cancer cells. In other words, after high dose chemotherapy and autologous BMT, the number of cancer cells in her body would be at most one hundred thousand.

Felicia continued the line of questioning further, "Can the body's immune system fight off ten million cancer cells by itself?" The doctor shook his head solemnly. "Then what about one hundred thousand?" Felicia probed relentlessly to the very end. The doctor replied that the immune system of a normal person might possibly be able to fight off one hundred thousand cancer cells. As soon as she heard these words, Felicia decided to undergo the new treatment.

The medical team had some reservations. Felicia explained that she was both a scientist who researched on anti-cancer drugs and a patient who experienced the painful process of cancer treatment. She committed her utmost effort in her research with an ultimate goal to find medical remedies for cancer patients. So if high dose chemotherapy and autologous BMT together could be a potential cure for cancer, she was willing to offer her body as a test case. Besides having her own cancer cured, she might be able to serve as a successful case study of this new treatment. If the treatment failed, this failure could still serve as an opportunity for doctors to study and improve future treatment methods.

After Felicia made her stance, the medical team fell into a deep silence. So did I.

The Epitome of Courage

While Felicia was away, I often thought about how she must have felt while she was contemplating whether or not to receive high dose chemotherapy and autologous BMT.

Felicia was a resolute person who did not fear difficulty or hardship. Not one who would resign herself to fate, she grasped the reins and charted her own life plan. She not only believed that she could succeed in the pursuit of knowledge, she also hoped to become a leading scientist and pioneer new fields with me. On the other hand, her family was just as important. Felicia demanded perfection in everything; her meticulous care and tender love for her family was deeply appreciated by her loved ones.

How Felicia became who she was was due to the choice she made and her persistence. She insisted on being an eminent scientist as well as a perfect wife and mother. Even while she was ill, she conducted herself in a decorum that medical caregivers gave her their greatest respect. She loved life with ardent passion and was never one who gave up. She fought courageously and embraced the scientist's attitude — of being forward-looking, and open-minded to try new approaches — in the face of challenges. Those were human qualities that the average person had difficulty attaining. But for thirteen years, Felicia fought cancer with sweat and blood, and wrote her beautiful song of life.

I could hardly bear to see her endure all the pain. But for her sake, I supported her decision. I was her closest companion; I knew the reason she wanted to keep on living. Her unshakable resolve was not for herself, but for her family and her love of life, and she also wanted to live up to her fearless determination as well as her faith for life as a researcher and a cancer patient.

Today, cancer is still an enemy to the mankind. We may one day find a cure for cancer. Over the years, we have gradually increased our knowledge of cancer and developed new drugs for treating it. But at this stage, cancer treatment still remains at a bottleneck. The pain that cancer patients face in the terminal stage and the fear that the disease cannot be overcome are the main reasons why many patients refuse further treatment. This long, slow and painful road will not be understood by those who have never experienced it, but Felicia was among those who felt this loneliness and fear most acutely.

As a scientist with a research focus on anti-cancer drugs, Felicia knew the road of research from benchside to bedside was a long and uncertain one. Besides a passion for the pursuit of knowledge, scientists who selflessly commit and dedicate their time in the laboratory need to have the faith, the belief that the research they do will later help the society, otherwise it is difficult to enjoy the solitude of being a researcher. Felicia, a cancer patient who experienced the emotional turmoil brought about by the disease was, at the same time, a researcher with compassionate love for people and strong aspiration to contribute back to the society.

I knew why Felicia eventually chose to undergo high dose chemotherapy and autologous BMT; it was her principle as a scientist to hold human life with high esteem and treat every single life as valuable. Even though success was by no means certain, Felicia was willing to try a treatment that was still in its experimental stage.

The Night Before Leaving for the United States

As soon as Felicia decided to set off to the United States to undergo high dose chemotherapy and autologous BMT, I immediately made plans for our family members to take care of her. The entire procedure was expected to take two months. Besides the children and me, Felicia's younger sister, Wan-Chan, who lived in Hawaii, would also lend her assistance. My plan was that I definitely wanted to be at Felicia's side during the most dangerous moments, the period when she would undergo the actual treatment. Thus, I scheduled David and Albert after me, and Wan-Chan before me, to accompany her through the physical examinations and to take care of her while she received the pretreatment medicines. After the timetable schedule was set, in June 1995, Felicia first went to Washington and was prepared to undergo this round of grueling and high-risk treatment.

The night before she left, Felicia and I were at home. While packing her bags, neatly and methodically, she reminded me gently what I needed to be careful about being in the house by myself. Even at this moment, she had not forgotten about me. I turned towards her. My heart went out to her. I felt sad and could not bear to see her go, but I was certain that God would give us blessing to fulfill our promise to each other. My mind was filled with a plethora of thoughts and emotions. I was unable to sleep that night.

I turned to Felicia and said, "Everyone's life is different. No one can predict what will happen in his or her life. The value of an individual's life lies not in the duration of time on this earth, but in each day how one lives, how one maintains interpersonal relationships sincerely, and how one makes the fullest use of every moment in the world."

These words later became my inspiration when I fought this battle shoulder-to-shoulder with Felicia. The same words encouraged her and reminded me that regardless of how cancer threatened her health, we had to hold on to our hope, do our best to live, and also, we must not forget the loved ones around us — all of these gave true meaning in our lives so that we were not living in vain.

The next day, I sent Felicia off at the airport. I stood watching for a long, long time as her silhouette disappeared in the crowd. Finally, with a heavy heart, I returned to Taipei. Felicia left Taipei on June 16; I planned to travel to the United States in the beginning of July. Before Felicia checked into the hospital, she stayed at the house of Dr. Jacqueline Peng-Wang. When I flew in to look after Felicia, I too stayed at Dr. Peng-Wang's place, and Dr. Peng's husband, George Peng extended his warm hospitality. Felicia and I were touched by the couple's kindness.

But we did not expect that Felicia would end up staying in the hospital for three full months for a treatment which was scheduled to take two months, and that it would become a struggle for life that was likened to torments in the midst of "raging fires and tidal waves."

This was Felicia's most painful treatment experience. Her struggle was a harrowing pace back and forth at Death's door. Those three months, thanks to her determination and endurance, she made it; she walked away from that door and came back to us. But after surviving this life-or-death trauma, even someone as strong as Felicia would describe the pain of high dose chemotherapy and autologous BMT as "living hell."

Ah! Today when I recall the days I stayed by her side and witnessed her tenacity and courage to endure the painful treatment, I still feel the surge of emotions and the lingering grief within me. She devoted all her energy to this fight, all because she loved and valued life so much. That was what made my Felicia so special, so unique.

A Trip to Reconstruct the Past

David, Faith, Albert and I returned once again to NIH. On March 17, 2000, in springtime Washington, D.C., we entered the gates of NIH and looked for Building No. 10, where Felicia underwent high dose chemotherapy and autologous BMT. However, I do not know whether it was due to dreaded fear or the fading of memories with time, I actually lost my way along a route that ought to be very familiar to me.

I said to my three children, "That's strange. It used to be possible to locate No. 10 by simply following the numbers on the buildings." Memories from five years earlier, when Felicia and I fought cancer together in the hospital, suddenly started flooding back to me, and I thought to myself, I must have been emotionally stirred.

Indeed, there were some changes to the roads because of the construction of new buildings in NIH. Finally, the children and I found ourselves in front of Building No. 10. David looked up at the blue sky. He was quiet all this while; I knew this brought him back to the times he accompanied his mother in her battle. Albert strode in with brisk steps; he could not wait to reach the prayer room on the top floor, because that was where Mom prayed. Faith said to herself in reflection, "The first time when Mom came here to have her checkup, I accompanied her. Back then, we still didn't know whether the doctors would allow Mom to participate in the clinical trial as a patient."

That day, we had an appointment with Dr. Windham H. Wilson, the head physician. At nine o'clock in the morning, the whole family was already standing in front of the National Cancer Institute building. Every step forward brought lingering poignant pauses of thoughts, feelings and memories, and that described my sentiment of my return to NIH.

Dr. Wilson was already waiting for us at his office. He gave us a hearty greeting. After Felicia passed away, Dr. Peng-Wang returned to NIH to attend a conference and she took the opportunity to inform the doctors and nurses who had taken care of Felicia that she had succumbed to her sickness. They were sad, they also remarked to Dr. Peng-Wang in a heavy-hearted tone that Felicia was the most extraordinary patient that they had ever encountered, and that they would never forget her. They would also never forget the fact that Felicia was among the breast cancer patients with liver metastasis who had survived the longest after undergoing high dose chemotherapy and autologous BMT. The sorrow and empathy shown by the physicians and the nurses certainly touched Dr. Peng-Wang.

NIH was an important stop in our trip of rediscovery. Our friend, Professor De-Mao Chuang had set aside all his work at NIH that day to share with us his reminiscences of Felicia at NIH. Here, Felicia faced the most arduous three months of her life, and here, the glory and splendor of her life shone through. And it was here that I was able to feel even more acutely the most beautiful aspects of her, especially her unparalleled resolve and tenacity. Felicia was like a spiritual guide; she took me along to the highest state of emanation of true human spirit that is both profound and eternal.

Testimony of a Lifetime of Fighting Cancer

Inside his office, Dr. Wilson pulled out Felicia's file. He spoke to us in a tone like he would to his old friends, relating stories of Felicia's stay at the hospital. Beside me, the children were all listening raptly. The pungent smell of disinfectant and medicine permeated the environs of the room, transporting us back to the past. We turned back the clock to Felicia's struggle for life five years ago.

Before she checked into the hospital in late June, Felicia went to visit her university classmate, Bing-Yi Ying. Upon learning that Felicia had come to undergo a dangerous operation, Bing-Yi Ying was extremely concerned. She was religious, hence she would find every spare moment to visit the hospital and pray for Felicia. In the journals that Felicia kept to record her treatment, she took copious notes about every aspect of her daily routine during the treatment. She naturally also penned a great deal about the love, care and concern of her friends and acquaintances.

Looking back, Bing-Yi Ying recollected that even in sickness, Felicia was always impeccably dressed and neatly groomed. Felicia, who was a good conversationalist, would ask Bing-Yi Ying strings of questions about religion. Felicia herself did not have a religious faith, and in the face of the most critical phase of her treatment, she continued to demonstrate her great thirst for knowledge by probing a field that she had not previously delved into. This earned Bing-Yi Ying's deep respect for Felicia.

Felicia started to keep a daily record of her medical treatment from the day she first arrived at the hospital. She wrote down all the details concerning her medication, her body's responses to the treatment, the feedback from the medical caregivers, and her daily diet. The entry was done at every hour interval. On days when she was feeling well, she would insist on writing it herself; and, when she was feeling her worst, the children or I would write on her behalf. Felicia's medical treatment record is the testimony of a life that fought against illness, and the documentation of a painful treatment process. Until the time of her death in July 1999, she left behind eight volumes of journal painstakingly written and archived by her.

Creative Spirit

Like Felicia, I do not have any religious faith, and I do not have any religious affiliation. But when I was young, I read the Bible avidly, and I remembered I had a pen-pal who was a Christian minister, and with whom I exchanged views about religions. I never believe that man is born on this earth to redeem the wrongs of a past life, and I also do not believe the challenges and obstacles encountered in this life is the consequence of the past life, because Felicia and I both hold the conviction that our responsibility is to create and leave something useful behind for mankind. That was the reason why we chose science and research as our career.

Though Felicia has left the earth, she left behind many unforgettable memories, her spirit, and her wisdom. A biblical quotation by Job, which I read when I was young, left a strong impression on me: "For there is hope of a tree, if it be cut down, that it will sprout again, and that the tender branch thereof will not cease. Though the root thereof wax old in the earth, and the stock thereof die in the ground; [yet] through the scent of water it will bud, and bring forth boughs like a plant." (Job 14:7–9).

Another passage in Job goes: "And surely the mountain falling cometh to nought, and the rock is removed out of its place." (Job 14:18). This time Felicia's treatment was like a rockslide or a forest of trees set aflame. Like a butterfly undergoing metamorphosis, emerging from its cocoon and shedding its skin layer by layer in a crucifying fire, the one hundred days of treatment were painful beyond words. And how she, who sought survival and life on the verge of death, diligently recorded each test of life during that painful treatment — word by word, sentence by sentence. Ah! Spring silkworms spin silk until the very last minutes of their lives. Felicia knew that she wanted to make a contribution that would last beyond her lifetime, and though the pain she endured during the process would disappear in death, what she went through was truly unfathomable!

15

High Dose Chemotherapy

Dr. Wilson slowly unfolded his recollections of Felicia's painful one-hundred day experience at NIH, beginning from the day Felicia was admitted into the hospital.

Felicia's Violent Response to the Clinical Trial

Wan-Chan was scheduled to take care of Felicia during the preliminary stage of this experimental treatment. She accompanied Felicia to the hospital in late June. Before beginning the treatment, Felicia had to undergo a physical examination and take Interleukin-1, a drug used to heighten the effect of high dose chemotherapy. The purpose of the medical check was to confirm that Felicia could take Interleukin-1 at the appropriate time.

Felicia and I both studied and understood very well the treatment procedure beforehand. From the NIH experiment record, we learned that this initial phase of the procedure would not be too tough or painful for the majority of patients. That was also the reason why I arranged Wan-Chan to look after Felicia then. However, Felicia's reaction to Interleukin-1 was unexpectedly severe.

Interleukin-1 is a type of cytokine. Before undergoing high dose chemotherapy, it is necessary to receive two weeks of injections. The drugs that Felicia would receive in high dose chemotherapy treatment were

Interleukin-1 and three types of anti-cancer drugs — Ifosphamide, Carbonplatin, and Etoposide (ICE). Because this drug combination had not been tested previously, the preparatory preclinical stage was extremely important.

After just one dose of Interleukin-1, Felicia started experiencing shivers all over her body; she was also running a high fever. From a clinical point of view, her response was deemed quite severe as the majority of patients do not experience such severe reactions to the drug. But Felicia started to feel discomfort since her first week at the hospital. That caused the medical staff to question immediately whether she would be able to go through high dose chemotherapy and autologous BMT.

I was extremely concerned and worried about Felicia's reaction to Interleukin-1. I called her from Taiwan almost every day. If she was not feeling well and was unable to answer the telephone, Wan-Chan would update me on her condition.

Dr. An-Li Cheng, Felicia's main attending physician in Taiwan, and I both knew the cause of Felicia's severe reaction. From the outset, Felicia was determined to use adriamycin, the strongest medicine available at the time, in order to rid herself completely of cancer. Afterwards, when the breast cancer spread to the liver, the gravity of the situation forced doctors to use potent anti-cancer drug combinations such as CAFL to save her life. All drugs leave residues in the body, and because Felicia had already been treated with the strongest medicines available, there was naturally a great amount of accumulated drug residue. Thus, when Felicia was injected with Interleukin-1, the chemical substances from previous treatments could have reacted with this new medicine and incited a violent response.

Dr. Wilson, the main attending physician at NIH, and I discussed Felicia's physical condition. He suggested that perhaps she should not continue with high dose chemotherapy and autologous BMT. After all, Felicia's condition was quite stable after the traditional chemotherapy. Dr. Wilson hoped that Felicia and I would have a detailed discussion before making a decision whether or not to continue with the treatment.

Of course, I knew Felicia would not be willing to give up even before raising the issues to her. As I expected, she said she had already made up her mind to travel to NIH to receive the new treatment. She had known beforehand that it would be an extremely dangerous procedure. As a patient, she would not back out just because she had encountered difficulty. Thus, she felt that other people, including her physicians, should give her as much support as they could to help her complete the treatment.

I relayed Felicia's opinion to Dr. Wilson who gave her words much thought for a long time and finally agreed to continue with the procedure. But he felt the second dosage had to be decreased since Felicia had had such a strong reaction to Interleukin-1. After the second dosage, her condition would be assessed to determine the best appropriate timing to start the high dose chemotherapy and autologous BMT.

The second dosage of Interleukin-1 was still extremely painful for Felicia. She suffered from shivers and a fever that would not abate — even her arms and legs felt scorching hot as if they were on fire. But Felicia knew that she had to grit her teeth and bear it; otherwise, her trip to NIH to receive treatment would have been completely in vain. Although the second dosage of Interleukin-1 was just as painful as the first, the duration of the reaction was slightly shorter than the first round. Looking back, I would think Felicia endured not because of the decreased dose, but in large part it was her determination to conquer the first hurdle.

Because of the severe reaction of Interleukin-1 on Felicia at preclinical stage, the dates originally scheduled for high dose chemotherapy and autologous BMT were pushed back. At that point, Wan-Chan had already stayed at the hospital for a full two weeks, and she had to return to work. Next, it was my responsibility to take care of Felicia. I knew that it would be a fierce battle of life and death, and I had to be by her side to give her strength and confidence.

Extracting Bone Marrow

The physicians waited until Felicia's fever had subsided and she had recovered sufficiently before continuing with the rest of the treatment. First, Felicia had to have her bone marrow cells extracted. They would be tested to confirm that there were no cancer cells and then frozen. During this period, Felicia wrote her treatment journal diligently. An endless stream of encouragements from her friends and former classmates in the

United States who came to visit her, boosted her morale. Some friends who knew that Felicia had a craving for Chinese food brought over noodles and other Taiwanese snacks, which she ate delightedly. Felicia often said she was deeply touched by the love and concern everyone had shown her, and that had galvanized her determination to put up a tough fight for a beautiful victory, or else she would let everyone down.

Finally, everything was ready. Felicia's physical condition was also ready for the treatment. The first step in the treatment was to extract bone marrow. It was July 5, 1995. This was the beginning of a period of excruciating pain. That day, I saw Felicia struggling to endure the pain. But through it all, she did not utter a single sound, nor shed a single drop of tear. But my heart was crying and wrenched in pain.

The physicians made eight holes on both sides of Felicia's hipbones and performed successive bone marrow extractions at two to three cubic centimeters for each extraction. That day alone they extracted a total of eight hundred grams of bone marrow. It can be deduced that more than two hundred and sixty-six extractions were made through the same eight holes. Though the extraction was done under an anesthetic, the two hundred over extractions naturally inflicted immense pain on Felicia. But she endured it all without shedding a tear, she swallowed in silent the sharp pain of needle piercing the bone.

Bone marrow must be frozen quickly. But even frozen bone marrow has its expiration date, so the next step in Felicia's treatment could not wait. A dosage of ICE was administered the very next day. Approximately five grams of each medicine, or twenty times the normal amount, was administered.

Felicia recorded every detail of the Interleukin-1 treatment as well as the intermission time during which she waited for high dose chemotherapy. Because she perpetually ran a high fever, Dr. Wilson had to postpone the bone marrow extraction. When Dr. Wilson finally announced that Felicia could begin the next stage of treatment as soon as her fever subsided, she was extremely excited. Her writing in the journal was full of expectation and hope. She was truly ready for the first test. But even though she was brimming with courage and optimism, she knew the battle had only just begun.

Wrestling the Poisonous Drug

The wounds on Felicia's hipbone where the extractions were made still hurt badly, but Felicia had already begun to take chemotherapeutic drugs. The first day after the intravenous dosage of ICE, Felicia once again experienced chills. As she did not experience fever, her condition was not considered that serious.

Hospitals in America do not allow family members to remain overnight in patients' wards, I could only stay with Felicia every day from seven in the morning to eleven at night. By eleven o'clock, I had to leave; even being a physician could not exempt me from the hospital rule. The day when Felicia started the chemotherapy treatment, her condition was expected to experience major transitional changes. Much as I wanted to remain by her side through the night, and the hospital could not make it an exception for me to stay overnight, I had to steel my heart to leave the ward.

That night, I did not sleep well. The next morning I immediately went to the hospital. I saw Felicia, and I fell into a deep shock. In one anecdote from the Chinese classical history of the Warring States Period, General Wu Zi-Xu's hair turned white overnight. In Felicia's case, her hair completely fell out. Not only that, her skin also turned from pale yellow to dark brown overnight. Her lips were parched and charred, and her entire body was discolored and blackened like an African. The state Felicia was in was analogous to a scene out of the *wuxia* martial arts novels I had read in my younger days. When a person was fed poison, they became black all over and their lips charred. Felicia looked exactly like what I imagined in those novels. In actual fact, high dose chemotherapy was a poisonous drug that killed cells indiscriminately all over the body. This treatment had ravaged Felicia's body beyond recognition.

Felicia said she was in a lot of pain; she tossed and turned the entire night, constantly feeling like she wanted to throw up. Every slight turn she made, a clump of hair would fall out. When she woke up and felt her head, she realized that all her hair was gone. The nurse came and swept her hair away to tidy up the bed. It was at that instant her head started to spin.

Nausea and vomiting were not the only side effects she experienced. Her mouth felt dry and her tongue parched. Her throat felt as if there were ten thousand needles piercing it all at once. It hurt so much that even talking was difficult. She told me it felt like there were armies of ants attacking the nerves in her fingernails and toenails. The needle-like sensation burned like fire. I could imagine how much pain she must have been putting up with.

The medicine used in high dose chemotherapy could not be allowed to remain in her body too long; it had to be washed out within a day, or else it would kill her along with the cancer and bone marrow cells. So on the second day of the treatment, the physician immediately inserted a large IV drip to wash out all of the medicine. This enabled her to receive the high dose chemotherapy and also sustain the strength needed to stay alive.

Felicia overcame one battle, but another one followed almost immediately. In one night, the drug had ripped her entire body apart; now, the IV drip that washed out the anti-cancer drugs compounded Felicia's pain. Lying on the hospital bed, her body weak and emaciated like a strand of thread, Felicia endured an entire day of high-speed IV wash. Her heart was already over-burdened due to the high dose of anti-cancer medicine; the IV wash taxed her heart yet further. That day my anxiety intensified. Given the intensity of pain Felicia was already experiencing, how could she endure the high-speed IV wash?

Suffering Excruciating Stomach Pain

As expected, by afternoon the poison had already wreaked havoc to the entire inner wall membrane of her entire digestive tract from mouth to anus. Felicia started to have diarrhea. The pain from the violent purging of the bowels was like having one's intestines disgorged. I supported Felicia by hand one little step at a time to the toilet; she collapsed onto the toilet bowl like cotton candy. The fluids discharge was like a faucet gone awry. When she finally stopped excreting water, I supported her to shuffle slowly back to bed. But as soon as she laid her head onto the pillow, she would struggle to get back up again. Her blackened cheeks bore a greenish tint, and bouts of cold sweat clung to her body. Her icy, shivering lips trembled as she said she needed to go to the bathroom again.

That afternoon while Felicia was receiving the IV drip, she experienced five to six episodes of diarrhea. The nurses and physicians came to check on her and said that her condition was really too serious. But the physicians were unwilling to prescribe medicine to stop the diarrhea, because the IV was administered for the purpose of washing out the ICE. An extremely high amount of anti-cancer medicine remaining in her body would attack her other organs and bring even greater harm to her. So Felicia had to endure the bouts of wrenching abdominal pain. Ah! It is easy for an outsider to empathize with the situation, but to the patients themselves, the pain is truly intolerable.

By evening, Felicia's diarrhea seemed to have receded, but there was barely any strength left in her. She was drained. After I helped her to take a shower, I fed her something to eat and noticed that sores had formed on her lips and mouth, which was one of the side effects of high dose ICE. I already knew that was going to happen, but I had not expected Felicia to develop these symptoms after just two doses. That was also the point when her diarrhea was the most severe. Felicia knew what she needed now was nourishment to regain strength, so she forced herself to eat. It was certainly difficult, as the sores on her tongue and lips made each mouthful a huge ordeal. I sought out the attending physician, and he gave Felicia some morphine. With each spray of morphine, and in, a small morsel of food, another spray, and in, another tiny morsel, this went on until she finally finished her meal.

That night at eleven o'clock, it was time for me to leave once again. Felicia's diarrhea had depleted all her energy. She lay on her bed exhausted and lifted her hand with difficulty and waved listlessly at me, signalling me to hurry and leave. Taking care of patients is indeed extremely tiring, but wasn't what Felicia went through ten million times more painful? I could do nothing but to obey the hospital rules. I was really unwilling to leave, but all I could do was to request and remind the nurse to be extra careful at night to check on Felicia's condition and instruct Felicia to buzz for the nurse should she need help. I repeated this reminder several times before dragging myself reluctantly out of the hospital.

At night, what would be her condition like? I could not sleep, as if I was on pins and needles, but there was nothing I could do except to wait until daybreak. I made some rice porridge for Felicia, and Dr. Peng-Wang's husband, George, also woke up early at dawn to make me breakfast. I finished the meal hurriedly, carried the container of the rice porridge and rushed to the hospital.

Felicia was lying in bed. She looked worse than the night before. Her face was already discolored to a black hue due to high dose chemotherapy. Expressionless as though a deep frost froze her facial muscle, vestiges of suffering and weariness were written clearly all over her face. She could not speak audibly as she related to me the events of the night before in a soft, halting tone.

The night before, she continued to experience diarrhea. She was unwilling to trouble the nurse, so she forced herself to get up on her own. Heavens! Every step towards the bathroom seemed like eternity. She sat up, with all the strength she had, dragging the IV rack along with her, as she walked every step was a monumental effort. The pain in her stomach was like daggers slicing open her abdominal wall. But Felicia gritted her teeth, dragged her battered body to the bathroom step by step, and expelled everything in her bowels. The pain was excruciating.

Her body had taken in large amounts of IV fluid, which had to be eliminated together with the fluid already retained in her body. Because her intestinal wall was already worn thin to the point of rupture by the side effects of high dose chemotherapy, the experience of diarrhea was like having a sharp-edged knife scraping against the abdominal wall. The pain was beyond words. She was on the verge of collapse and encountered near-death experiences, many a times. And each time, she came back. Had it not been her endearing thoughts for her family, her children, me, and the people who encouraged her, she would not have made it. She told herself over and over again that she just had to make it. She must not pass out under any circumstances, because if she did, she might not regain consciousness. Under the extremities of torturous pain, Felicia gritted her teeth and endured until morning. She knew as soon as she caught a glimpse of the first ray of sunlight, I would soon be at the hospital. No matter what, she had to make it through.

The Unbearable Itch

I supported Felicia and helped her sit up. My heart went all out to her as I slowly fed her rice porridge. It was only the beginning of high dose chemotherapy. What sorts of difficulties would she encounter in the days ahead?

In the afternoon, Felicia was still experiencing nonstop diarrhea. Suddenly, a shadow of darkness loomed over her face. Her eyes and the expression on her face suggested that she was experiencing a deeper, more deadly pain. Her weak and frail hands reached out to her arms limply — it was obvious she was trying to hold herself back from scratching. Her eyes glistened with tears that threatened to fall at any moment. She said, "I'm itchy — itchy to the point where I can't take it anymore."

I looked at Felicia's hands, tightly clutched with layers of dead skin. High dose ICE had unleashed its might on Felicia's body by killing not only the cancer cells, but also the normal dividing cells, such as skin cells. Felicia's skin had started to peel because the dead skin cells were falling off, and this made Felicia so itchy that she could not help scratching despite her extreme weakness and fatigue.

Felicia could grit her teeth to overcome the grueling pain from the bone marrow extraction in her hipbone and the rupturing pain from the thinning of the intestinal lining; and she even managed to scrape through the ordeal of previous night which was a life and death struggle. But the itch all over her body was extremely difficult to endure. I knew she was already putting up with it, but the itchiness was simply unbearable that she ended up scratching her body very hard with both hands.

I told Felicia that she had to endure it, because if she broke the skin and caused it to bleed, it would increase her chances of becoming infected — especially in a few days, when her white blood cell count would drop rapidly. If that were to happen, there was no telling what would happen next. But how could the itching be stopped? The doctor dispensed ointment to stop the itch, but it was of no help, as the source of the itch was not on the surface of her skin, but inside her body. Seeing Felicia break out periodically in bouts of extreme itchiness brought an inexplicable itch in me too, as a person in good health then. The sight of Felicia with tears streaming down from her eyes and the resistance she put up to tear open her skin, left a deep crevasse in my heart.

I said encouragingly, "You have to endure it." I helped her up and carried her onto a wheelchair and wheeled her out of the hospital room to the lounge. I turned on the television, and let her watch, hoping to divert her attention so that she would not scratch her body. I made a mental note to myself to bring some Taiwanese videotapes for Felicia to watch the next day, so that she could forget about the pain which had assaulted her for the past few days, and at the same time overcome the side effects of high dose chemotherapy to proceed smoothly to the bone marrow transplantation procedure in the next phase.

I looked at Felicia. Her body had already been ravaged by the medicines. All her dividing cells would ultimately die, regardless of whether they were hair cells, membrane cells, skin cells, bone marrow cells or any other type of dividing cells. The death of each healthy cell was a new torture and hurdle. She was like a candle in the wind, struggling valiantly to sustain its weak life energy to fight and ward off the ferocious winds.

To speak the truth, at that instant, I came to understand her desolate desperation to defeat her disease. When life and death cross paths, that instantaneous moment culminates life to fast flashes of two dichotomous messages: one is the fleeting moment of weakness to forego the painful battle to end all pain, and the other is the resilience and resolve to survive.

Anyone would struggle with these two contradictory impulses, but not Felicia. Felicia was always like the great Don Quixote — as long as she felt the cause was worth fighting for, she would arm herself to put up a brave fight at all cost. Of course, this was also the reason why she had suffered so much through these treatments. Just think, the fifty-three chemotherapy sessions that Felicia underwent in her lifetime, there was not one single session that would not torment her consistently like the onslaughts of turbulent floods and vicious fire. Especially so in this particular instance of high dose chemotherapy!

The following day, Felicia was still scratching her skin until it bled. Clumps of dead skin cells fell off and onto the bedside like lint. They were thin, airy like balls of cotton breaking apart and falling away. Felicia had been tormented by diarrhea and itchiness for an entire day. By evening, her energy was completely spent and she lay lifelessly on the bed. So I placed a bedpan by the bed and told her that if she needed to go to the bathroom, she shouldn't walk to the bathroom by herself, but use the bedpan instead. At eleven o'clock, the nurses went to all patients' rooms to shoo visitors out; I too had to leave. Walking out of the main door of the National Cancer Institute, I was greeted by the light, warm breeze of the summer night. Exhaustion and anxiety loomed over me. When night descended, I was even more disquieted and worried about Felicia's medical condition and the suffering she endured. Since then every night in bed, I tossed and turned, unable to close my eyes to sleep, and I had to rely on sleeping pills.

At night, I would have nightmares, one after another. The dreams were random and unconnected. At one moment I was unable to find Felicia, at another a doctor would go on explaining something endlessly that I was unable to comprehend, and at yet another instant, Felicia was in extreme pain and crying out my name… It was like the unedited snippets of scenes from a movie presented in jump-shot sequence. The traumatizing dreamscape awakened me suddenly — covered in cold sweat — in the middle of the night. After getting up and looking at myself, I realized that I had developed rashes all over my body which itched until I could not help but scratch them. It was as though Felicia's itchiness had remotely transmitted to me and infected me.

Not Admitting Defeat — Gulping Back Blood and Teeth

Felicia, her face still looked tarred, woke up at dawn, saw me, cracked a bitter smile and said, "Morning has come." From her demeanor, obviously, she had not slept well either; it must have been another night of struggle. Felicia said although the diarrhea had got a little better, she was still in a lot of pain, and itchy all over. The bedpan was by her bedside, but even using it was difficult and took a long time that seemed forever, like the road to heaven. She had no energy left even to prop herself up. With great effort, she attempted to wriggle around and shuffle her feet until she was gradually able to get out of the bed. She was already covered in a cold sweat and out of breath at that point.

She looked at the bedpan in great distress and bitterness — what seemed to be a simple action that can be achieved in one single step by a healthy person was to her a difficult feat that would take eternally forever to complete. She felt a momentary weakness in her resolve to fight cancer, and tears flowed uncontrollably from her eyes. But then, the thought of the children and me immediately fueled her with a new source of strength. She motivated herself with her own motto: "Keep on going! Keep on going! You can definitely make it through; you can't let the pain get the better of you. This time, you have to return to health!" That was how her strong spirit would force her beaten body to endure the pain, the itch, and the ordeal of diarrhea which had her — body already thoroughly drenched in sweat — expended every last ounce of energy she possessed.

A healthy person can hardly imagine the unbearable pain that people with serious diseases must put up with during treatment. And a cancer patient generally can hardly imagine the tormenting hardship of high dose chemotherapy. In order to survive, Felicia confronted all hardship of assaults like a beaten and fallen fighter — she got up, gulped back her blood and swallowed the knocked teeth to endure all outcomes. After less than a week, Felicia was fragile like a thin strand of thread, hanging on precariously. The treatment had hit and tormented her beyond recognition, but she told herself vehemently not to give up. Felicia hoped her story of struggle could offer optimistic hope to other cancer patients in times when they feel disheartened.

Dreaming the Impossible Dream

I mentioned earlier Felicia's spirit was like that of Don Quixote. That brought me back to my recollection of the 1996 banquet held in celebration of the establishment of the National Health Research Institutes. Dr. Tai-An Cheng, a research fellow at the Institute of Biomedical Sciences, sang a song entitled, "The Impossible Dream." The lyrics of that song captures the valiant struggles and the poignancy of Felicia and the multitude of other cancer patients who are fighting their battles against their disease.

> To dream the impossible dream,
> To fight the unbeatable foe,
> To bear with unbearable sorrow,
> To run where the brave dare not go.
>
> To right the unrightable wrong,
> To love, pure and chaste, from afar,
> To try, when your arms are too weary,
> To reach the unreachable star!
>
> This is my quest to follow that star,
> No matter how hopeless, no matter how far,

To fight for the right,
Without question or pause,
To be willing to march into hell,
For a heavenly cause!

And I know, if I'll only be true,
To this glorious quest,
That my heart will lie peaceful and calm,
When I'm laid to my rest.

And the world will be better for this,
That one man, scorned and covered with scars,
Still strove, with his last ounce of courage,
To reach the unreachable star!

In order to prove the existence of heaven, Felicia was willing to stride forward to hell. No matter how difficult, she would fight to the very end till the very last breath and consciousness to reach the unreachable star. Ironically, for all cancer patients, reaching out to the farthest and brightest star in the sky was a convoluted battle of mind and flesh, and of life and death. The torments of chemotherapy and cancer treatment — Felicia put herself to test and had it all. She was like a guardian angel from heaven, entrusted with a mission to dissolve the pain of cancer patients with her true human spirit and all-encompassing love. The period when Felicia received high dose chemotherapy and autologous BMT, I witnessed how she bravely plunged into the fire, endured the scorching flames, and then re-emerged, reborned over and over again like a glorious phoenix. Again and again, she had close brushes with death, and narrowly avoided death during numerous critical moments.

But the pain that Felicia experienced — likened to sufferings in the furnaces of hell — was beyond words, how would other people possibly understand?

16

Autologous Bone Marrow Transplantation

We reached the chapel on the top floor of the hospital. The setting was similar to a church, but without a religious deity at the center of the altar — a design consideration taken to accommodate the different religious faiths of the hospital patients so that they could pray in peace. This soft, dimly lit prayer precinct exuded tranquility and peace. Felicia came here to pray, contemplate and seek solace, she prayed in anticipation to God to give her strength and support in her fight against cancer.

The Chapel and the Lecture Hall

As I entered the chapel with my children, we tried to imagine Felicia's feelings at the time. Did she feel powerless? Was she resolute? Was she bitter about the astringency of her experience? Or was she hoping the heavens would empower cancer patients with hope and the optimism to dream? Felicia did not have any religious faith, and she made few visits to the chapel, but the fact that she felt the inclination to pray at the chapel revealed how lonely she was, and how tough the going had been in her treatment journey. We were all behind her, giving her our full support, but in the end the burden of hardship and pain fell on her, which she had to endure in solitude with her flesh, body and mind. Her pain haunted her like a shadow that was impossible to sever.

The ambience was tranquil and serene. David walked up to the altar in the center of the chapel. Always the quiet and thoughtful one, David appeared even more staid, more solemn. I saw him gazing upward at the soft light above the main altar, which cast a lingering shadow behind him. David's contemplative silence was full of grief — a melancholic longing for his mother. Faith has the personality of Felicia; she always says what is in her mind. That day all of us were filled with thoughts for Felicia, but Faith — who has the attributes and takes after the personality of her mother — must have felt the resonations of her mother's feelings at that very moment in the chapel. Faith said that every time her mother came to the chapel, she found calm and peace in her heart.

I walked out of the chapel with the children. We looked out from the top floor of the hospital to identify the building which Felicia had walked to, to attend lectures. Felicia was still staying in the hospital for observation during her treatment period, she took her weary body on a fifteen-minute walk to attend a lecture at the NIH lecture hall. Back then, Felicia's physical condition was still quite critical. My good friend at NIH, Dr. De-Mao Chuang, said, "I recall the day when there was a scientific lecture. Felicia knew about it, and she actually walked fifteen minutes under the burning sun to attend the lecture. The auditorium was already fully occupied, there were no seats left and Felicia had to stand at the back of the room." Dr. Chuang saw her standing there in the crowd, looking frail and ill. Worried, he quickly brought over a chair so that she could sit down. But the determination and professionalism she showed in coming to the lecture made an indelible impression on Dr. Chuang, he had great respect for Felicia.

The lecture hall in the northeast corner of the hospital towered majestically before us. Felicia's attendance at the lecture discerned a different aspect of her state of mind at the time. The chapel and the lecture hall bore traces of Felicia's time at NIH, reflecting two very different emotions and mental states she experienced. Only the children and I could understand and experience how she felt then. The traumatic pain of her disease not only failed to triumph over her, but in a way, it let her realize that her hopes lay in her spiritual strength and resolve. She lived on with the strong conviction that as long as she held onto hope, her dreams would become reality.

As long as one does not believe that one has come to a cul-de-sac, then one will meet another crossroad, and a chance to move on. While Felicia was at NIH undergoing high dose chemotherapy and autologous BMT, we held onto the hope that there is a glimmer of hope at the darkest hour, and that one day we would emerge from the darkness and suddenly see the light.

Making a Trip to Death's Door

Felicia hoped that after enduring the medical treatment that was as painful and agonizing as being smelt in a furnace, she would be free of cancer forever. But it appeared that the disease was not ready to let Felicia go. Felicia's treatment was already painful enough to bring tears to her eyes, not to mention that it was life-threatening. Dr. Wilson still remembers that at that time, Felicia had a few close calls with death, especially during the high dose chemotherapy. Felicia's reaction to the medicine was stronger than that of all other patients.

Dr. Wilson stated that of all the clinical cases of high dose chemotherapy and autologous BMT that he had conducted, Felicia's reaction was the most severe, and he believed Felicia to be the toughest and most courageous of all the patients he had ever treated. The medical team had tremendous respect for her spirited fight against cancer, and her inquisitive and curious attitude, which constantly kept them on their toes. Also, they were impressed by Felicia's sharp acumen as a scientist which was evident in the concise focus of her line of questioning. That put the medical team in the right perspective on their responsibility and dedicated care to the patients. So Dr. Wilson felt the life's lesson Felicia imparted to the medical caregivers was not only her fighting spirit, but also many medical and scientific enlightenments about the profession.

Felicia was like a candle; she exhausted her lifespan to glow and illuminate others with her light. But ironically, she paid a steep high price for bringing brightness in other people's life. Felicia's white blood cell count dropped lower and lower, until the seventh day, it ultimately dropped to zero. With a zero white blood cell count, of course, one is susceptible to infection and disease; thus Felicia had to be isolated and quarantined. At that time, I had to disinfect, put on gloves and wear a mask over my mouth to get into the hospital room. Danger lurked close by, I was extremely careful. However, hospitals are essentially hotbeds for germs and bacteria, Felicia had an infection.

She started to experience fever and have all sorts of hallucinations. For example, after watching the movie "Empress Dowager" on videotape, she thought Empress Dowager had called her on the phone. And the entries in the medical journal which she faithfully kept records of became as inscrutable and illegible as the book of Heaven. Even the paintings hanging on the wall made her think of evil demons. It seemed as if her mind had gone haywire and erratic. Of the greatest concern was the high fever that would not subside. The doctors dispensed every kind of antibiotic they could think of, but none was effective.

The doctors were worried. If the antibiotics had no effect, it meant the germs would multiply and spread uncontrollably. Then Felicia's life would be at risk. I had meetings with the doctors every day so that we could try to solve the problem together. The doctors were stressed and felt enormous pressure; every time they saw me, their brows furrowed and they shook their heads. Felicia simultaneously underwent all sorts of tests. It had already been confirmed that her pneumonia was becoming more and more severe. Her high fever just simply would not go down, and she was losing her ability to think clearly. In the midst of this tense situation, Felicia was transferred to the intensive care unit.

Albert hurried over from school. He was originally scheduled to take care of his mother after the dangerous phase of the medical treatment, but Felicia still had not even cleared the first critical point of the treatment. I told an extremely anxious Albert, "This time Mom's condition is very serious; she might not make it." After transferring to the intensive care unit, Felicia's condition continued to deteriorate. My discussions with the doctors became more and more frequent. Tests of Felicia's blood revealed the presence of at least four different types of germs. Although we were already using the fourth line of antibiotics, it did not seem to have any effect on her pneumonia; in fact, the pneumonia seemed to aggravate. Albert and I were extremely worried — but aside from worrying, there was nothing we could do.

On Sundays and holidays, all doctors had the day off; only the chief resident doctor remained on duty. I paced around the intensive care unit anxious like an ant on a hot stove, I was unable to calm the agitation in my heart as I did not know and have an answer whether Felicia's pneumonia could be controlled. Then, a specialist of infectious diseases, Dr. Thomas J. Walsh, came over specifically to visit Felicia. He extracted some fluid from Felicia's bronchial tubes, took a culture, and brought it under the microscope to investigate the cause of the problem. That day was a holiday, and he had especially made time to come and examine Felicia.

Dr. Walsh immediately told me that he had discovered an extremely rare colony of yellow-colored germs in Felicia's lungs. Antibiotics were completely useless against this germ, so he suggested using sulfonamide, a type of medicine used to kill germs before antibiotics were developed. That was our last resort!

On that same day, the doctor immediately replaced the antibiotics Felicia was taking with sulfonamide. At that time Felicia was laying in the intensive care in a very serious condition. Her skin was extremely itchy, and the situation called for morphine to be administered to combat the pain and itchiness, but even morphine was unable to stop her discomfort. To make matters worse, the medicines caused Felicia to experience constipation and perpetual flatulence. Compounded by her pneumonia and high fever, Felicia was in a semi-conscious state. Despite that, she still unconsciously scratched at her itches and yelled out in pain. Her condition was unimaginably dangerous and unstable.

That was a period of torturous waiting that put a strain not just on the patient, but on the patient's family as well. Troubled and worried, I could not sleep. Just when my eyes were about to close to catch a few winks, I would suddenly wake up with a start for absolutely no reason. Whereas Felicia lay alone on her hospital bed in the darkness of the night, fighting her battle against cancer. My anxiety and her fighting spirit intertwined like an intricate web of net that locked us firmly together, inseparable. Going through the thick and thin together deepened our feelings for each other as husband and wife. I really wished I could help her shoulder the burden of her pain, but I could not. At night, sleepless, I tossed and turned as always.

On Monday morning, Albert and I got up early, anxious to see how Felicia was doing. Miraculously, her fever had receded; this meant sulfonamide was effective against the tenacious germ that terrorized her body. The medical caregivers heaved a sigh of relief. Albert and I hugged each other in joy. We were immensely grateful towards the infectious disease specialist who had saved Felicia's life.

A few days later, Felicia's condition improved and her life was no longer in danger, so she was transferred out of the intensive care unit. She saw Albert and me. Though she was unable to speak, her tears which welled up in her eyes spoke volumes. She knew that this life and death battle would be one of many that she had to fight to get through the treatment, and she had made it through after labyrinth of hardships.

Albert and I, together, took care of Felicia. Because she was extremely weak at the time, every day Albert wrote down what she wanted to say in the treatment journal. I took his place occasionally when the entry involved specialized medical knowledge. Felicia was extremely demanding when it came to her treatment journal. She wanted to review every entry that was written; it had to be written in great detail till she was satisfied. Albert and I "teased" her in a joking tone that despite how seriously ill she was, she still insisted on such high level of detail and perfection. But Felicia had her rationale of doing this; she felt she could be a typical case study as a cancer patient. If she could help other cancer patients with such a minimal amount of effort, then she would gladly do her part. Felicia's selfless action of putting cancer patients before self went to show her great compassion for them.

Inserting Bone Marrow

Altogether, Felicia spent ten days in the intensive care unit before she was transferred out. High dose chemotherapy had destroyed all her bone marrow cells, so there were no white blood cells in Felicia's body. Her recovery was extremely slow, but the extracted bone marrow cells had a certain life expectancy and they had to be re-inserted within a certain span of time, or they would die. So even though Felicia's physical condition was not ideal, the bone marrow had to be re-inserted on schedule.

Transplanting bone marrow is an extremely dangerous procedure which should be conducted under infection-free condition. The consequence would be disastrous if infections occur. Even if the procedure goes smoothly without contamination, whether new bone marrow cells would grow after the transplant operation is a question mark looming over the situation. The danger in Felicia's treatment was that, after the first test, there was no telling what was to come. Though Felicia and I had high positive hopes for the transplantation, in our hearts we felt a jittery unease — we were afraid of venturing out to face a deadlock on the road ahead, and get stranded with no route of turning back.

July 26 was the day of the bone marrow insertion procedure. Albert and I watched from the hospital room with mixed emotions. The procedure took two hours — a long, hand-wrenching wait. Fortunately, the insertion went extremely smoothly, but recovery still hinged on the patient's strength and determination. Felicia's great challenge to weather the various effects of the bone marrow transplantation lay before her.

The next morning, Felicia was right there in the hospital room waiting for Albert and me. Her face still looked blackened, with a pallid yellow tint. She looked exhausted. But as soon as she saw us, she smiled. We asked her how she felt, and whether she was in a lot of pain. She merely shook her head and said she hoped everything would go smoothly. To her, the pain was inconsequential, she had already learnt to endure the hardship.

My original plan was to stay and take care of Felicia during the two most critical weeks at the National Cancer Institute, but her treatment had dragged beyond the intended period due to the many serious complications, hence the two weeks I had scheduled had long passed. Felicia still remained in a critical condition, I would not leave her alone — no matter what.

My original schedule was to return to Taiwan in the middle of July, after two weeks in the United States. At that time, the NHRI extramural research department was conducting a grant review session, and I was scheduled to attend a meeting with sixty foreign and local scholars. I did not want to leave Felicia considering her condition, so I telephoned Dr. Shu Chien, the chair of the meeting, briefed him on Felicia's condition, and told him that my wish that he would explain to the scientific reviewers why I was unable to attend. Dr. Chien gladly obliged without further questions. He told the scientists and academics about Felicia's condition. Moved by Felicia's courage, determination, and fighting spirit, these academics wrote cards to encourage Felicia and convey their convictions that she would definitely triumph over cancer.

Receiving all those cards and letters with encouraging words embedded brought tears to Felicia's eyes. She was an emotional person with sensitivity and a compassionate heart — her eyes would be moist and glisten with tears in gratitude when she received an act of kindness. At that instant, the warmth of friendship and encouragement moved and overwhelmed her again that tears were her expression of gratitude. Felicia told me she would keep on fighting until the very end and would never give up for the sake of her family and friends.

The White Blood Cells Grow

Encouragement could boost Felicia's morale and spur her on, but it was still unable to reduce the risk and pain that she encountered during treatment. After the bone marrow had been transplanted, Felicia had to wait for it to grow. Felicia's white blood cell count still remained at zero, and danger lurked around her like a shadow.

The growth of white blood cells would trigger and stimulate reactions in the body. The high dose chemotherapy had caused considerable damage to Felicia's organs in the body; thus, as the white blood cells grew, she had to endure the discomfort of the adverse reaction without the administering of any pain suppressant. For example, she must refrain from taking morphine or other medicine when in pain, the objective was to encourage the growth of white blood cells in an undisturbed and unadulterated condition.

The tormenting high dose chemotheraphy had mentally prepared Felicia to endure the painful aftermath of the bone marrow transplantation, but it was another distressing torture that was analogous to being thrown into a hot furnace, ripping out her guts and dismembering her limbs. She had fallen into an abyss of suffering. Again.

Felicia felt itchy all over after high dose chemotheraphy because of the death of dividing skin cells. Now, Felicia felt another insufferable itch — but this time new cells were growing. No words could describe the intolerable itch. Unconsciously, her fingers scrawled over her skin and unintentionally, she scratched till her skin bled. Albert and I tried various tactics to distract Felicia's attention away from her itch. I borrowed some videos from George, wheeled Felicia to the lounge, and played the videos for her. Albert found some of Felicia's favorite music and played it for her. He sang his mother's favorite Chinese songs which she had taught him.

Felicia remarked that the itch this time was different from the previous bout; it felt like there were million colonies of ants crawling around under her skin, burrowing aimlessly and uncontrollably in her muscles, bones, nerves, and blood vessels. The burden of suffering was so heavy that she could barely shoulder it anymore.

Albert and I gave her our assuring encouragement that the itch was an indication of new skin cell growth, and that also implied the multiplying growth of white blood cells as well. That was a positive sign of recovery, and she had to hold out the discomfort of itchiness no matter what. Then, brave Felicia flashed a hopeful smile, picked up the medical journal and began to write slowly, "Today, I felt extremely itchy as usual, and unbearably itchy…" That were just a few words, but they expressed all her bitterness and suffering, which, alas, were beyond words.

What I admired most about Felicia was her resolute and positive spirit. Although Felicia had to put up with unspeakable pain, she was always positive and optimistic. She was willing and ready to put up a tough fight because of her passion for life, the deep feelings and attachment that she had for her family, me and the children. But, Felicia gave us much more, especially to the children. The strong willpower she embodied gave them many important lessons about life, setting the paradigm of lifelong learning. In times of adversity down the road, the children could take pride to look upon their Mom as a role model and a source of inspiration for her optimism and tenacity. An irony indeed. Cancer-stricken Felicia was instead our invaluable pillar of strength through her journey of pain, tears and hopes.

Despite her unbearable itchiness, Felicia's white blood cell count rose extremely slowly. A normal person's white blood cell count is approximately seven thousand per milliliter, and the platelet count, one hundred and fifty thousand per milliliter. The epidermal cells all over Felicia's body itched for almost four days, and almost every inch of her body was scarred. But her white blood cell count remained below one hundred. Albert and I grew very anxious, and distress signs were written all over our faces. Felicia was worried too; she knew that this would imply the bone marrow growth was far from ideal. If the bone marrow had problems growing, it would be difficult to decide what to do next.

We all realized what we could do now was to wait patiently, and with great faith and confidence. I told Felicia not to worry as it would affect and aggravate her recovery rate. Felicia was still diligently recording her treatment situation in the journal. During that period of waiting, she would also telephone her friends and doctors in Taiwan and America. My mentor Dr. David Goldthwait, her physician Dr. An-Li Cheng, and Academia Sinica members Dr. Chien Ho and Dr. Horace Loh all encouraged her and wished her well on the telephone.

Dr. Cheng clearly recalls the telephone conversation with Felicia who called him to briefly report on her medical condition, he heard her quiet sobs as she tried to fight back her tears. He knew Felicia very well; every time she was overwhelmed with emotion, tears would come to her eyes. What Dr. Cheng heard and could sense, from across the ocean, was the anguish and the heavy-hearted anticipation of a tough and iron-willed patient. Dr. Cheng reassured Felicia that the symptoms she experienced were as expected. He advised her not to become over-anxious, but be patient and wait. Being over-anxious would affect her mood and morale. He reassured her that in one or two days her white blood cell count would be expected to rise.

The doctor's comforting words were a booster in the arm. Felicia always had great faith in her doctors. She waited patiently. Rays of hope emanated and glowed beneath Felicia's dark-complexioned skin. And true enough, by the beginning of August, Felicia's white blood cell count rose to around four hundred, which signified that she was out of the danger zone. When Albert and I announced to Felicia the good news, she was in tears! She sat on her bed, face streaked with tears but those were tears of joy and jubilance…

The Platelet Count is Too Low

The white blood cell count had risen, but I was still concerned about Felicia's platelet count. Strangely enough her platelet count remained in the environs of a couple of hundred, far from the normal average. According to medical treatment standards, if her platelet count remained below one thousand, it was crucial to keep injecting platelets, otherwise the patient would be in danger. If a patient experiences clotting problems and loses large amount of blood due to a low platelet count, the repercussions would be frightening. The doctors and I had many rounds of discussions. They said they had already notified the blood bank to prepare blood for a transfusion for Felicia. I waited in anticipation for three days, but the doctors were not seen making any preparations to transfuse any blood into her. So I asked the doctors about Felicia's situation and found out that Felicia's platelet type was not available at the blood bank; they were, at the moment, doing a nationwide search of blood banks to find suitable platelets.

However, the doctors felt that if a transfusion of platelets became really mandatory, it could be conducted by mixing together different types of platelets from various donors. That I could not accept, because in the event of a hemorrhage, we would not be able to establish exactly which location in the blood vessels causes the bleeding. If, unfortunately, she had a brain hemorrhage, the most dangerous type of stroke, then it would be too late to do anything.

So I did a couple of things: I contacted David and Felicia's brothers and sisters in the United States, asking them to come and have their blood examined to see if their platelets were compatible with Felicia's platelet type to be used for transfusion. Felicia's eldest brother Herbert and younger brother Michael both rushed over. Her second brother Jing-Ren lived a little farther, so he had his blood examined at a local hospital.

Of course, as possible blood donors, David and Albert were the most desirable candidates, because there was a fifty percent probability that their platelet type would match Felicia's. But after the blood transfusion, Felicia's platelet count didn't rise. This implied there were antibodies in Felicia's blood which acted against and lysized the children's platelets, rendering the blood transfusion from the children ineffective. Among Felicia's three brothers, one of them whose platelet type matched Felicia's, was unfortunately a Hepatitis B virus carrier, so he could not donate his blood to Felicia. The other two brothers' platelet type was like David's and Albert's, and therefore would have no effect in improving the platelet count in Felicia. At this point, Felicia's condition had reached a dangerous deadlock.

Meanwhile, I telephoned to Taiwan's blood bank, and told a blood specialist there, Dr. Mary Lin, about Felicia's situation. Felicia's medical team in Taiwan, including Dr. An-Li Cheng and Dr. Pan-Chyr Yang, made emergency nationwide appeals to help search for Felicia's platelet type. After searching the whole country, they only found four donors whose platelet type matched Felicia's.

At that time, the United States Blood Bank had already contacted all the hospitals and confirmed that there were no blood specimens that matched Felicia's. I became frantic once again. According to the regulations of the United States government, there was a restriction imposed on donated blood brought into the United States from other countries, in view of blood safety. And even if importation were possible, the half-life of platelets was only four to five days. In that time frame, any action taken would be deemed hopeless. The situation was certainly dire.

The whole family once again sank into the depths of anxiety and despair. Felicia had already gone through so much suffering, instead of sparing her some moments of reprieve, she was constantly tested with treacherous situations. But Heaven ultimately forsakes no one. During this tense and uncertain moment, help came. A technician at the blood bank learned of Felicia's situation, and found out that his platelet type was seventy-five percent similar to Felicia's. He voluntarily donated five hundred cubic centimeters of his own blood. After the transfusion, Felicia's platelet count rose, indicating that his blood was compatible with Felicia's. On learning that Felicia's platelet count had risen, this Good Samaritan donated another five hundred cubic centimeters. After two transfusions, Felicia's platelet count rose to ten thousand. Although that was still far from normal levels, at least Felicia was out of danger.

Two Lives Inextricably Intertwined

This selfless technician instructed the blood bank not to reveal his name, to this day we still do not know his identity and we have not been able to thank him personally. But we are eternally grateful to him. After the blood transfusion incident, whenever Felicia was invited to travel to the United States to deliver her lectures, she would take the opportunity to encourage Asians in the United States to have their blood type tested and registered. She also advocated the establishment of a blood bank for Asian people.

At that point of time, David, Albert, and I were all at the hospital keeping Felicia company. We monitored her rising white blood cell count and saw her situation gradually stabilized. Her white blood cell count rose to eight hundred, and I slowly heaved a sigh of relief. Judging from her condition, her bone marrow was growing well.

It was not until Felicia's white blood cell count rose to above one thousand that I decided to leave the hospital. By then, I was already there for over a month, staying by Felicia's side in a tug-of-war fight against the disease, marching with her through the deepest ravines of her life, and fighting with her shoulder-to-shoulder against the unyielding Angel of Death. Needless to say, it was Felicia who suffered most, but I also felt the drain on my strength and spirit.

The doctors and nurses at the hospital advised me to have sufficient rest and take some time away from the hospital as David and Albert would be there and Felicia's situation was under control. They said that if I did not leave, I too might fall ill. I deliberated their advice for a long time and discussed with Felicia. She agreed that I should return to Taiwan because firstly, my work at NHRI should not be held back, and secondly, she hoped that I would be able to recoup some rest. So I passed the baton of responsibility of Felicia's care to the two children.

When I left NIH Hospital, Felicia's white blood cell count stood at one thousand, but her platelet count had not reached the normal level. I told Felicia not to worry, and reminded her to pay attention to her platelet count during blood transfusion. In the middle of August I left the NIH Hospital and returned to Taiwan. When I stepped into my office, all my colleagues were shocked at the sight of me. They said that I looked wearied and had aged a lot.

I looked at my reflection in the mirror, I was uncertain if I had actually aged, but seeing all my white hairs and comparing my appearance to what I used to look like when I returned to Taiwan back in 1988, it really seemed I had become a completely different person. In fact, the same could be said of Felicia. Years of incessant hard work and dedicated research as well as the burden of illness had left their traces — the tracks and lines of age — indelibly etched on her face. We had walked the journey together for over thirty years; the most quintessential and most arduous experiences of our lifetime had fused our lives as one. Time was proof of our true feelings for each other, and weathering innumerable struggles together with Felicia deepened my belief that our lives were destined to be inextricably intertwined forever.

17

Reborn in Fire, Arisen from the Ashes

Our whole family feels a strong bonding with the National Institutes of Health which holds our countless memories. We descended from the rooftop chapel down to the cancer ward and chanced upon the two nurses who had previously taken care of Felicia. They came to know that our entire family paid a visit to Dr. Wilson to reminisce and catch up on old times, hence, they too rushed their way here to meet us.

One of them was a long-haired nurse with large eyes named Karen. She told us she had a picture taken with Felicia. She still keeps it posted on the board in front of her desk. Among the patients she has taken care, Felicia left the greatest impression on her. Karen recounted her fond memories of Felicia during her hospital stay. She said Felicia loved to share knowledge about her scientific research, talk about her family, and narrate the journey of her fight against cancer. Felicia, in Karen's recollections, was a person full of passion and enthusiasm — if she encountered anything that she did not understand, she would persist to figure it out to get to the bottom of the issue.

There was no one but Felicia who, according to Karen, could still keep up a sunshine disposition and a fierce fighting spirit even after the high dose chemotherapy and autologous BMT. Hence, Karen had kept the photograph in front of her desk not only as a remembrance for

Felicia — a patient of unique personality — but also as an inspiration and a form of encouragement in life.

There was another nurse, Patty, who is rotund and always wears a warm smile. She recalled vividly Felicia's brief encounter with former President Bill Clinton on August 5. Patty mentioned inadvertently to Felicia that President Clinton would be coming to the hospital to visit a congressman friend. Felicia was in a critical condition at that time, yet she stood patiently keeping vigil by the door, eagerly awaiting Clinton's arrival. The wait stretched for at least half an hour. She reminded me repeatedly to snap a picture of her with President Clinton.

At that time, I was not in favor of her actions. I hoped she would have more rest. I certainly did not expect that when Clinton finally appeared, Felicia would hurry towards him to request for his autograph. Patty only saw Felicia rushing forward to speak to him but she had no idea how long Felicia had stood at the door waiting. It was only much later did I find out that Felicia had intented to have a conversation with President Clinton and she had prepared in advance what she was going to say. When Felicia saw President Clinton, she said, "Mr. President, I am from Taiwan. I hope one day you will be able to come and visit Taiwan."

I was not quick enough to take a photo of Felicia with President Clinton, but his bodyguards were able to capture that short moment on film. Soon after, David wrote to the White House to request the photo to be sent to Felicia in Taiwan. Felicia saw the photograph opportunity as a great honor and displayed the picture on a glass window in her laboratory along with all her other favorite pictures. Since then, Felicia received a Christmas card from President Clinton every year inquiring after her condition. Felicia's laboratory was full of mementos of our family photos which served as her greatest source of spiritual nourishment for the soul.

The children and I had a brief interlude in this American hospital room where memories of the doctors and nurses who took care of Felicia brought sunshine to the otherwise cold and frosty spring. Time never stops to linger and cling to the past, so we can only recollect and chase these memories that still bring pain and sadness to our hearts. Felicia's treatment at NIH was the most challenging and difficult, but the journey was full of meaning and profundity because we, the whole family, walked through the hardships of her life journey with her.

The Night Before Leaving the Hospital

Upon my return to Taipei, I talked to Felicia on the telephone every day. Her white blood cell count gradually returned to normal. Her platelet count was far from ideal, but at least it was better than before. Albert returned to school; David stayed at the hospital to take care of his mother for a while longer, but he too had to return to school. At that time, Felicia felt her strength and energy returning on an uphill ascent — which was an encouraging sign. And also, her friends in the Washington, D.C., visited her almost every day.

As long as she had regained some strength and energy, Felicia's sonorous voice could be heard from the hospital bed. Felicia recorded all the details of her friends' visits. Every single word and sentence carried the depth of her feelings and her appreciation for the noble friendship and kindness bestowed upon her. Sometimes when I read Felicia's manuscripts, I was transported back to the days when I saw her struggling stroke by stroke in writing down every little detail of the treatment. My heart involuntarily fills with poignant sadness. But as I read on when she wrote about someone bringing her some Chinese delicacies, or someone came to visit and had a wonderful conversation for the afternoon, a warm feeling immediately wells up inside me. To this day, the concern and kindness that our friends had shown towards Felicia during her critical moments remain with me in my heart.

Felicia stayed in the hospital for over two months after the bone marrow transplantation. She knew her physical stamina was returning, hence, as an outgoing person who could not tolerate being sedentary, she hoped to be discharged soon. But the doctors felt that although her situation had improved markedly, it was still inadvisable to let down their guard, so they permitted Felicia to leave the hospital only occasionally. On those rare occasions, Felicia stayed at NIH researcher Su-Chan Su's home. Su-Chan Su was, during her university days, Felicia's teaching assistant. As soon as Felicia exited the hospital doors, she was like a bird released from its cage. She was joyfully dining and shopping with friends and chatting happily with them until late into the night. Only after repeated cajoling from her friends would she finally decide to turn in early and rest.

That was Felicia. She fought hard on the verge of death in exchange for every breath of life, she did not want to waste a single moment and she wanted to live life to the fullest. The doctors saw Felicia was on a smooth, steady road to recovery so they finally decided to grant her short-term discharge from the hospital temporarily on the condition that she still had to come back for frequent examinations and regular checkups. Felicia was ecstatic when she heard the news. I, on the other hand, was worried when she told me that she was allowed to leave the hospital. I knew that her platelet count had not yet returned to normal. But all I could do was to remind her not to over-exert herself.

It was night-time. Felicia had one last platelet transfusion before the intended discharge. By this time, the nurse and Felicia knew each other well and they chatted while the nurse prepared the transfusion procedures. The blood transfusion was in progress, and the nurse left the room.

As soon as the nurse was gone, Felicia felt a sudden impulse akin to an electrical shock in her body; in that instant, her body became cold and she began to shiver. A thought flashed through her mind: something was grossly wrong with the platelets. She knew there was no time to spare and immediately pressed the emergency call button. The doctor rushed over. Upon seeing Felicia's trembling body and her lips turning blue, the doctor immediately pulled out the tube that fed platelets into her body in order to save her. In this short span of time, Felicia practically lost consciousness.

This was an unforeseen medical error and negligence in the treatment. If Felicia had not responded promptly and quickly, she would have undoubtedly lost her life. Felicia once again survived a life-threatening situation. It goes without saying — she had to remain in the hospital bed the next day and rest rather than discharge from the hospital.

Felicia often said, "If I had another ten years, I would have no regrets." But Felicia treasured every moment because she knew death would come to her any moment, and the fleeting, ephemeral nature of life would mean she could lose her life in a split second due to any unforeseen circumstances. In her diary, she wrote, "Every day at dawn, when I wake up to see the cheerful, glorious sunshine, I know, God has given me another day on this earth, and my heart is filled with immense gratitude."

How an acutely ill patient fares in the journey of treatment and recovery is defined by that one moment of thought. One could choose to wallow in the depths of despair, thinking of oneself as the most unfortunate person on earth — or one could choose to persevere relentlessly, telling oneself that life is short which makes it all the more important to treasure every minute and every second, make the most of what one is given, and fulfill the value and worth of one's life. Felicia was certainly grateful for the time that God had given her. As long as she had one more day to live, to be with her family, and to encourage fellow cancer patients, then all the ordeal and pain from the treatment were definitely worth it. And that spurred her aspiration to be discharged from the hospital, as she had already laid down her life's goal for the days ahead.

Weakened Heart — Readmitting to the Hospital

The platelets incident prolonged Felicia's stay, but she finally received permission to leave the hospital. She split her homestay time between two friends who lived in the area: her high school classmate Bing-Yi Ying and my good friend Dr. De-Mao Chuang. But every two or three days she had to go back to the hospital for routine follow-ups and monitoring. This time when Felicia left the hospital, she thought, God had certainly given her the greatest blessing. Her good old self — outgoing, active and effervescent personality — was back.

Meanwhile, in Taiwan I was busy with the planning of the establishment of NHRI; I also had to fulfill my duty and responsibility for the Institute of Biomedical Sciences. Though busy, I made it a point to communicate with Felicia once a day. Like a child let out of school, she was actively involved in all sorts of activities. At this juncture, I was, instead, more worried for Felicia whose enthusiastic involvement in activities might jeopardize her health. So I always cautioned her to get ample rest, and not to go overboard and ignore what her body was telling her.

After Felicia and I returned to Taiwan in 1988, we had originally planned to invite my parents to live with us. However, my father had been bedridden for several years due to a stroke. My elder brother and sister-in-law took really good attentive care of my parents. When we first returned to the country, our housing matter was not finalized, so we decided to postpone our plan to move my parents in to live with us. During holidays, Felicia and I often took my mother out, who by then was approaching ninety. Sometimes we would take long walks in the suburbs, and at other times, we would enjoy our dine-outs together. During the period I was in the United States with Felicia for her treatment, I had not seen my parents for a long, long time. Hence, upon my return to Taiwan, I made time on weekends to take my mother out.

One weekend, I took my mother to Yangmingshan and updated her on Felicia's medical condition. That morning at around eleven, from the top of Yangmingshan, my mother and I gazed into the far distance — vast expanse of greenery unfolded before us with clouds fleeting languidly in the blue sky. I took my mother's arm, and we admired the luxuriant greens on the slopes. At that point of time, I thought of Felicia and wondered how she was doing. Longing to hear her voice, I gave her a call on my cellular phone.

Felicia picked up the phone. She sounded bright and boisterous as usual, but at the same time, she sounded a little out of breath. I asked if she had been continuing her treatments and medical follow-ups at the hospital; she said she had followed the doctors' instructions and gone to the hospital for examinations as scheduled. I asked whether the doctors had made any observation about her heart. Felicia was a little taken aback, and replied after a moment's pause that they had not.

I told Felicia to make a quick trip to the hospital, because her gasps for breath even when talking signified something serious and critical. I was worried that her heart had been damaged by the high dose chemotherapy. This was a serious side effect which should not be taken lightly. After hanging up, my worries were not alleviated. I took my mother's arm. I did not dare to reveal my thoughts to her, because she would no doubt get worried. My mother missed Felicia, mentioning her name all the time, and she was counting down to the day when Felicia would recover and return.

Separated by oceans, mountains and continents, standing atop the Yangminshan on a bright sunny morning with my mother, our thoughts were with Felicia. I thought longingly of my wife and hoped she could overcome this difficult period, return home, remain healthy and live happily. I am sure on that same day, Felicia, though far away, would have the telepathic feeling — our anticipation for her return to home one day. I remembered a stanza from the poem of Shao-You Chin which my high school teacher, Chong Wang, had taught us, "Resigned but at peace, allowing oneself to be swept along with the water to the end." Here I am, already sixty. Long past the youthful age, I am no longer ignorant of life's bitter and sorrowful moments; thus, I am able to understand the meaning of this phrase. Ah! I await Felicia's return.

Felicia went back to the hospital to be examined. She called me — she was admitted to the hospital again. Because of the toxicity of the medicine used in high dose chemotherapy, her heart was severely damaged and there were signs of failure. So, the doctors compelled her to be re-admitted into the hospital. This time when Felicia returned to the hospital, she was all by herself; there was no one to take care of her. However, fortunately, she was in Washington, D.C., where she had friends like Bing-Yi Ying, Su-Chan Su, Man-Yu Lin, my good friends Drs. De-Mao Chuang and Long-Shiong Hsu, my colleague Dr. Jacqueline Peng-Wang and her husband George Peng, and NTU physician Chi-Hsin Yang, who was in NIH at that time for training. They visited her to show their support and concern constantly. Felicia was appreciative of the help and devotion of these friends and she remembered their kindness in her heart. She said she drew her strength from their friendship. She would never want to be a cause of worry to her friends and thus she was determined to get well soon to be able to share the warmth of their friendship again.

The Meaning of Love

Soon after, Faith also made a trip to Washington. Faith was then working at Taiwan's Ministry of Foreign Affairs and contributing to its efforts to join the Asia Pacific Economic Council (APEC), hence she was the last of the three children to accompany their mother through the treatment. Also, her work prevented her from staying with her mother for a long time; she stayed for about a week or so before she had to rush back to Taipei to take care of APEC-related matters. But during the week-long sojourn she spent with her mother, Faith felt distinctly the perseverance and optimism embraced by her mother to make the most out of her life, and that impression remains with her till today.

Because of the treatment, much of Felicia's hair fell out, and her skin turned to a dark hue. The National Cancer Institute has a special service for female patients who undergo chemotherapy where patients are taught how to groom themselves to improve their external appearance, particularly in dealing with baldness and skin discoloration as a result of the chemotheraphy. Felicia knew about this special service and she definitely would not give it a miss. Hence, Faith accompanied her mother through these classes where she saw her learn how to put on a head wrap, apply makeup, and wear a wig.

In the past when Felicia underwent chemotherapy, she used to wear a wig to work. Given the opportunity to learn more sophisticated grooming tips, Felicia was all geared up to participate. Seeing her mother enthusiastically picking up tips on how to dress up and manage her personal appearance despite her illness, Faith was deeply comforted with blooms of joy in her heart. Faith was positive that Mom's optimism would conquer the painful disease. She knew Mom wanted to return to Taipei looking her best — full of life and energy.

At that time, due to Felicia's weak heart condition, she could not sleep well, often waking up after one or two hours of sleep. She would make notes about her treatment in the middle of the night, and sometimes, update her diary. The life-and-death struggle had renewed her perspective about life, and she developed a clear train of thought about life. She reflected upon her life and reaffirmed her understanding about the value and significance of life. She wrote in her treatment diary, "From this moment forth, I must cherish my life all the more, really live and savor life, and live a life I enjoy."

My niece, Ming-Hui Chen, is a devout Christian. She is also an evangelist. While in the hospital, Felicia telephoned Ming-Hui and asked her why she believed in God. Ming-Hui shared her view with Felicia for almost two hours. Felicia listened carefully and later wrote in her diary, "Ming-Hui explained to me the meaning of 'love' in religion's context."

Felicia was not one who embraced hedonism; instead she was a person who understood the meaning of "love" and that realization led her to the answers and knowledge of how to enjoy life. Felicia often said, "Enjoying life is about putting all of one's emotion, heart, and energy into making the most of life's love and passion." This was what Felicia had really achieved in her lifetime thereafter.

Felicia stayed at the NIH for over three months. The doctors were very careful and on high alert, because high dose chemotherapy had damaged the main organ in the human circulatory system — the heart. Her stay was, this time around, not as difficult as the previous one during which she underwent treatment, but the medical care professionals were stricter with her, as they all hoped she would be able to recover and return home healthy.

Returning to Taiwan and Continuing Follow-up Examinations

Finally, the hundred days of treatment was completed and drew to a close. Felicia returned home in the beginning of October. I went to the airport to pick her up. Seeing her weaving in and out of the crowd in brisk steps to reach me, I was all smiles from ear to ear — it was the same Felicia in her effusive effervescence. I believe no one in the busy throngs, except I, would know that this energetic woman was actually a cancer patient who once teetered on a thin line between life and death.

The feeling was like seeing a familiar swallow fly home. I felt an inexplicable sense of happiness. I saw Felicia tremble slightly the moment she stepped into the front door of our house. It occurred to me that Felicia was, at one time, teetertottering on the precipice of life but she walked back; and the treatment was devastating and yet, at the same time, strangely life-giving. As I reflected upon our future together, I thought, our mutual trust and interdependence were so strong that nothing could separate us.

After returning to Taiwan, Felicia contacted Dr. An-Li Cheng right away to arrange for a medical checkup to be done. Dr. Cheng conducted a thorough examination; Felicia could not wait to hear the results. She asked Dr. Cheng, had her condition not improved a great deal compared to the time before she left for the high dose chemotherapy and autologous BMT?

Dr. Cheng smiled and told Felicia that of course her present condition was much better than her previous condition. Now she only had a few black spots that measured half a centimeter in diameter; these black spots might be already dead or simply calcified cancer cells. He and the team would have to rely on long-term monitoring and observation to assess future development and treatment.

Dr. Cheng's reply alleviated Felicia's doubts. She dearly hoped that the cancer cells could be kept at 10^5 level, in which case her body immunity could naturally keep the cancer cells from growing, and she could eliminate her nightmare of recurring tumor growth.

In fact, Dr. Cheng had his doubts about the effectiveness of the treatment, but he never told Felicia or me. He only mentioned this after Felicia passed away.

Dr. Cheng used to work in Felicia's laboratory. Because he was her student as well as her physician, they had built a strong teacher-student relationship. Hence, Felicia's trust in Dr. Cheng far exceeded the faith a patient would have in his or her doctor, and every word he said had a strong impact upon Felicia. For the same reason, Dr. Cheng chose to speak positively of Felicia's treatment results at that time. He held a different view of her post-treatment condition, but he discreetly modified his prognosis for a positive outlook. This was the strategy that he decided upon even before Felicia returned for her follow-up examination.

Too High A Price to Pay

While I was doing research to write Felicia's biography, I had a long talk with Dr. Cheng so as to understand Felicia's condition at the time of the follow-up examination. He revealed that after examining the ultrasound and PET scan, he had already derived his judgment regarding the effectiveness of the treatment. To ascertain his conclusion, he compared the scan with those taken before the treatment. He found that there was no obvious great difference. In other words, Felicia's trip to NIH and the life-and-death ordeal she went through during the treatment did not alter or substantially improve her condition as compared to her treatment at the NTU Hospital. In his heart, Dr. Cheng thought, the suffering that Felicia had gone through might come to nought and for nothing. If Felicia had lost her life or even sustained damage to other organs, that would really have been too high a price to pay.

But Dr. Cheng held back the truth. He knew that Felicia had taken a great risk to seek remedy, and she regarded the treatment as the only way to completely rid of the cancer cells in her body. If he told her the truth, it would be a huge blow to Felicia — perhaps a really serious one that would cause her to lose her fighting spirit. Strength of mind and hope were what kept Felicia going. If truth had to be revealed to Felicia at that instant, even a person tougher than her might not be able to take the blow.

Dr. Cheng locked up these worries and thoughts in his heart for four whole years. Felicia had already reached the limit in the amount of medicine that she could accept in her body. Furthermore, her internal organs must have also suffered tremendous damage due to chemotherapy, any future treatments would only do further damage to them. However, he kept these reservations to himself. In face of his teacher, Felicia, who was always hopeful and optimistic, Dr. Cheng inevitably felt a sense of helplessness.

No matter what Dr. Cheng had in his mind, he gathered that Felicia had to go through a period of rest and must not receive any further treatment after she went through the treatment that put a strain on her body. Hence, Dr. Cheng arranged for Felicia to return to NTU Hospital every month for an examination so that he could monitor her medical condition. Dr. Cheng recalled Felicia was at her happiest and most carefree then — until her cancer recurred.

When Felicia decided that she wanted to go through the high dose chemotherapy and autologous BMT, I collected many material that discussed the clinical results of these treatments. I already knew then even if the treatment were successful, the cancer might return after two years. Four years later when Dr. Cheng confided in me that he had kept quiet about the truth and his feelings about the treatment, I had, to some extent, suspected just as much. Today, looking back, we both feel that Felicia really paid too high a price to undergo the treatment.

Dr. Cheng said if mankind were more knowledgeable about cancer and possessed a clearer idea about how to treat it, he would definitely oppose his teacher to go through such a harrowing treatment, in which people virtually "die and come back to life." After Felicia passed away, I read in an NIH news report: "High dose chemotherapy and bone marrow transplantation are not as effective as anticipated; NIH is considering whether or not to continue this clinical experiment."

A Courageous Warrior

Sometimes I wonder, "If Felicia knew that today's medical knowledge had advanced to a stage that refute the effectiveness of the medical treatment she underwent, would she have regretted her decision?" I am not Felicia; I am unable to reply for her, but I know Felicia's personality. As long as she had decided on something, she would not complain and would never have a tinge of regret and reservation.

Long ago when she went to the United States to get her Master's degree, and I continued to study medicine in Taiwan, we were separated thousands of miles apart by the vast ocean. She was young, attractive and accomplished; there were many desirable suitors who showed an interest in her. But Felicia kept her promise and returned home so that we could realize our dream of building a life together. The forty-two years together — which we experienced the vissicitudes of life and went through thick and thin — cannot be explained simply in a couple of sentences.

Felicia chose to receive high dose chemotherapy and autologous BMT at NIH with the full awareness that the treatment might not be effective. Her primary objective was to cure herself completely of cancer, but she was motivated to do it because of her truth-seeking spirit as a scientist. She hoped that her own participation could add on and substantiate the body of clinical data available, and furthermore, enable the medical community to further understand the possibility of high dose chemotherapy and bone marrow transplantation as a cancer treatment.

Felicia, the courageous warrior! I am the dearest person to her, the one who truly understands her, and the one who is best qualified to speak in praise of her. I am convinced that if, up in Heaven, Felicia were to know that the time we weathered together at the NIH and all the increasingly difficult treatments she was to face thereafter have become scientific knowledge that benefit other cancer patients, then she would certainly smile and nod knowingly.

SECTION V

FIGHTING TO THE END

18

Cancer Strikes Once Again

The children and I left the National Cancer Institute and the kindly medical professionals who had fought side by side with Felicia through the high dose chemotherapy and autologous BMT. The past was like a dream and yet not a dream. The past was a valuable memory keepsake for our family — a real, true journey filled with poignancy and gratitude. Life's memories are such — we relive them to realize their value, significance and meaning, and perhaps perceive the rights and the wrongs. This was an unusual journey through which Felicia had led our whole family.

Enjoying Life after Being Reborn

For one and a half year after high dose chemotherapy and autologous BMT, Felicia went to the NTU Hospital for regular follow-up examinations. Dr. An-Li Cheng described this duration as the golden period in Felicia's post-treatment medical history. During this period, the medical team monitored Felicia's condition very closely, but did not administer further treatment. Felicia's body and health also recovered fairly well. Felicia returned to Taiwan with a weakened heart due to the damage caused by high dose chemotherapy. The physicians knew she was forced to readmit to the NIH Hospital because of the condition of her heart. So after her return to Taiwan, Dr. An-Li Cheng kept a particularly close watch on her heart. To his surprise, after only two months, Felicia was able to go hiking again!

In addition to hiking, Felicia made time for and participated in every activity or event. Whether it was flower arrangement, folk dancing, volleyball, movies or concerts, Felicia was equally active and enthusiastic. What impressed people even more were her outstanding achievements in scientific research. Since our return to Taiwan in 1988, Felicia accomplished breakthroughs in every area of her research, including the anti-cancer mechanism of Vitamin K3, the anti-cancer mechanism of the adeno-associated virus and its use in cancer therapy with gene gun technology, and the functions and mechanisms by which anti-cancer drugs operate to suppress cancer metastasis. Her colleagues in the laboratory remarked that to this day it is impossible to forget Felicia's tremendous focus and exacting demands she placed on herself and others in the laboratory.

Vitamin K3 became the first anti-cancer drug to enter clinical trial in Taiwan. At present, NHRI is planning a phase II clinical trial. I am particularly proud of these accomplishments because Felicia managed to achieve them at the time when she was being afflicted by cancer.

With regard to research, Felicia was extremely serious, persistent and precise, especially in her attention to detail. In her opinion, building a solid foundation is key to success — only with a well-laid basic building blocks defining the structure, would there be a detailed action plan for the subsequent phases derived. At first, her co-workers in the laboratory felt stressful from the demand for such meticulousness and her insistence on not letting even a small little English spelling mistake go uncorrected. Dr. Wen-Hsiang Chang, a postdoctoral fellow whom Felicia regarded very highly, once discussed her research standards with her.

Wen-Hsiang Chang said, "Professor, each and every individual's ability is different. And, each person has different career expectations. How can you expect everyone of them to measure up to the same standard?" Felicia replied, "I know! Although everyone has different abilities and different aspirations, scientific research has strict standards, not one of which can be compromised. Even if I know that some people are unable to meet this standard, I still have to uphold the benchmark which might even bring out their latent potential. In reality, I could already foresee that some of them may be unable to meet the requirements, but as long as they do their best, I won't be angry even though they fail to measure up. As far as I'm concerned, this is the attitude and ethos with which an experienced researcher should instill and nurture in his or her students." After explaining her logic and viewpoint, Felicia cautioned Wen-Hsiang Chang not to share this conversation with their colleagues in the laboratory, for fear that they would take a relaxed and laid-back approach and not try as hard.

That was Felicia's view on how things should be done. There is a common saying that goes, "Good teachers never tire of instructing their students." Felicia undoubtedly possessed this honorable attribute — she had the interests of every students in heart, offering them directions and good advice. Felicia's body gradually recovered during that one-and-a-half year period. She often worked in the laboratory until late at night, and I always ended up reminding her that in the first stages of recovery from a major illness, rest is extremely important. But my words had no effect on Felicia; she was too enthusiastic about life, and her mind was always preoccupied with the conceptualization of new research plans. To suppress her desire to do research was a difficult task indeed.

Our family life also became more active and lively as a result of the positive turn in her physical condition. During her healthy golden period, we explored the small mountain roads of Taipei suburbs, participated in competitions and sports events organized by NHRI, and immersed ourselves in the rich sensory experience of the Jian-Guo Flower Market. There were also our common loves — music, movies, and family get-togethers. From every involvement and participation in the activities, Felicia derived life's contentment and bliss. I, too, became lighthearted and carefree in my outlook.

The Good Times were Short-Lived

Felicia's body gradually recovered, and we decided to invite my parents to move in with us. My ninety-year-old mother had always wanted to live with us. Felicia had always understood and, of course, agreed with my intention to take care of my parents in their old age. So when Felicia started to feel she was making good recovery, she brought my mother home and made every effort to fulfill her filial duties as a daughter-in-law. This period of time was perhaps my mother's happiest days. But our days of enjoying meals together as a family and living under the same roof did not last long.

Cancer is a difficult disease, hard to deal with. In a routine examination in May 1996, Dr. An-Li Cheng discovered that the four or five black spots in Felicia's liver showed signs of growth. He immediately telephoned and informed me, saying that Felicia's cancer could be preparing to strike again. That meant the high dose chemotherapy and autologous BMT Felicia had undergone a year and a half earlier had only suppressed the cancer; the cancer cells had by no means disappeared.

Although the medical team knew that this news would be a great blow to Felicia, she still had to be told. They broke the news to her, adding that at present they were still observing, and that she should still go back to the NIH Hospital in July for her scheduled follow-up examination for the final word and opinion on her medical condition. Indeed, Felicia was extremely disappointed and dejected as she listened to the doctors' prognosis. The doctors' words reflected their heartfelt good intentions and tactfulness. By the 1990s, Taiwan's cancer diagnosis and treatment capabilities were already on par with the international standards, and furthermore, the medical team was composed of the top doctors in the country. Their opinions should not be doubted and taken lightly. And according to their analysis, Felicia's cancer had returned to torment her, and haunt her like a ghost.

My mother knew that Felicia's medical condition had once again made a turn for the worse, she too began to worry. My mother is a warm-hearted and traditional woman. Worried that her old age would be a burden to her son and daughter-in-law, she felt she should not impose on us and add to Felicia's burdens at that critical moment. At that time, we had a live-in maid. Usually when Felicia had to be admitted into the hospital for tests, the maid always went with her, but one day, she told the maid to remain at home and take care of my mother. She packed her own belongings and went to the hospital alone. My mother could not bear to see that Felicia's thoughts were still focused on taking care of her, the mother-in-law, despite being extremely ill. So that night, my mother gathered up her belongings and was prepared to move out. It brought pain to my mother's heart to see Felicia still worrying about her in spite of her own illness.

This little anecdote about my mother moving in with us clearly demonstrates Felicia's generosity and benevolence, and her sincerity to fulfill her filial duties to the mother of her husband. My mother has always treasured this memory and Felicia's compassionate love in her heart.

Vacationing in the Netherlands

Although Felicia still held onto a slim thread of hope in her heart, the harsh cold reality dealt a heavy blow on her and dampened her spirits for a period of time. I knew how Felicia felt; she had spent all of her energy fighting cancer and had endured many painful treatments, especially high dose chemotherapy and autologous BMT. Bracing herself with the hope for a complete recovery, Felicia braved numerous close brushes with death, and when she finally managed to escape and thwart the jaws of death, she could not avert the fate of a repeated attack of cancer on her life.

Such is life, full of setbacks. I could understand Felicia's disheartened feelings, and I wanted to take her out to cheer her up and release the burden in her heart. At that time I was invited to attend and deliver a speech at a scientific conference in the Netherlands. So I took this opportunity to take Felicia to Amsterdam, the capital of the Netherlands, for a vacation.

The beauty of Amsterdam lay in the colorful and vibrant blooms of tulips set against the clear blue sky. The picturesque sight, akin to a cascade of richly colored ribbons from the sky, created a "heaven-on-earth" experience. On the rolling green fields, windmills stood resolutely like a valiant warrior on his defence, but the vigilant pose also belied a gentle demeanor — the turning of the windmill blades was like a soothing breeze rustling a canopy of leaves. With Felicia by my side, we walked into the surreal beauty of this picturesque scenery, which we took delight in appreciating, but with a tint of sadness undulating in our hearts.

I knew what Felicia was thinking. She was thinking that she had worked so hard to carry on living because of her endearing love for every beautiful living being on earth. Most importantly, our family's strong unbreakable bond and her passion and determination to do scientific research — these were reasons why she was unwilling to give up, why she was reluctant to leave this world prematurely. But life does not turn out the way one wishes; such is the sad reality of life.

I took Felicia's hand and said, "The meaning of life lies not in its duration, but in its value and depth. Our lives are intertwined, we have realized and shaped the dreams we held in our hearts. How many couples in this world do you think share this kind of happiness and profundity of love?

And together, we have raised three children. Our children are the crystallization of our pure love and having them is the most splendored thing that had happened in our lives. The lifelong pledge of love we promised and made to each other gave enriching and beautiful touches to our lives.

I told Felicia that she should not be discouraged, and she had to continue the treatment. With the rapid advancement of modern medicine, the day would arrive when a complete cure was available and she would be able to outlive the day if she had faith and persisted to fight.

Felicia nodded her head vehemently. My words were partly an encouragement to Felicia and partly our anticipation and belief. I really hoped that cancer treatment methods would make a dramatic leap forward to provide patients with the best treatment quality and even the chance for a complete recovery. But my heart was filled with fear and doubt whether Felicia's body would be able to hold out in future treatments after many rounds of chemotherapy sessions. Her physical condition would become weaker and weaker through the course of each treatment. How much more pain could she take before she was able to escape from cancer's vicious claws?

Felicia and I shared our deepest feelings during the Netherlands trip. I was sure Felicia would muster up the strength she needed to face the challenges of the future treatments. We certainly did not choose to tread on this path, but since God had given us this test, we could not avoid them, we had to face them head-on.

Becoming a Volunteer in the Fight Against Cancer

Before Felicia returned to NIH to be re-examined, the medical team was already analyzing and deliberating on what medicine they should give her to continue cancer treatment. At that time, the newest and latest anti-cancer medicine was Taxol which was an extremely potent drug. As Felicia had already undergone many chemotherapy treatments, the doctors were weighing and evaluating the issue whether Felicia would be able to withstand Taxol's side effects.

While the doctors were racking their brains, Felicia likewise grasped her precious time to make the most out of it. When the cancer recurred for a second time, Felicia had a new outlook on how she should live her life.

In reality, while she was hospitalized, Felicia was already a model cancer patient. Every time a patient refused treatment and was not cooperative with the medical caregivers due to the immense pain of the treatment, Felicia inevitably became a source of assistance whom the medical caregivers would turn to. She would approach the patients to offer her advice, encourage them and share with them the experience and journey of her struggle with cancer. So the medical professionals regarded Felicia as their best volunteer.

Felicia held her first public lecture entitled, "Struggle against Cancer: The Experiences of a Cancer Researcher and Patient" at the Bureau of Telecommunications in May 1996. During the lecture, she recounted the years of hardship enduring the ordeal of cancer treatment. As a scientist who researched on anti-cancer drugs, she knew and understood fully that the road ahead in making breakthrough discovery in research laboratory and conducting medical research in clinical trials would be long and full of obstacles. However, if scientists and medical care professionals were such dedicated and committed to persevere in their cancer research and treatment, then how could she, as a cancer patient, give up so easily?

The response to Felicia's lecture was overwhelming. From then on, Felicia became a volunteer and activist in the fight against cancer. She made appearances on television, and she spoke at her alumni association, in social communities and hospitals, communicating anti-cancer messages to the public. She was even more actively involved in offering encouragement to fellow cancer patients to stand up bravely to fight cancer.

Undergoing Taxol Treatment

In July 1996, Felicia returned to NIH for a follow-up examination. The results of the examination confirmed that Felicia's cancer had recurred. The doctors in the United States and the medical team in Taiwan concurred with the decision to use Taxol, the newest, strongest and most effective drug at the time. However, in this treatment, the patient had to be administered Taxol continuously for ninety-six hours. An opening of five millimeters was created in Felicia's neck, and an IV catheter was inserted through the jugular vein which passed through the superior vena cava, and entered into her heart. In this way, the medicine would be injected into her heart and circulated throughout her body. During treatment, Felicia had to wear a pump from which medicine would flow into her body for four consecutive days.

Wearing a pump on the back was the method used to administer Taxol in Felicia when she was at NIH. If Taxol proved to be effective, she would have to continue the treatment, but she could not possibly wear the pump all the time and not removing it, thus the problem of injection of the medicine must be resolved. So before Felicia returned to Taiwan, the doctors implanted a subcutaneous intravenous injection device under the clavicle, the long collarbone located above the first rib, in order to facilitate subsequent Taxol treatments.

Felicia received the first course of Taxol treatment at NIH and responded fairly well to it. So upon her return to Taiwan, the medical team continued with the treatments.

As Taxol treatment required an intravenous injection every month, Felicia had to wear her carry-on IV pump for ninety-six hours each month. Her co-workers in the laboratory teased her jokingly that she looked and became more fashionable carrying a cool-looking purse every day to work.

Felicia did not feel bitter at all about her condition. Quite to the contrary, she would share her experiences with the research team and use herself as a living example for teaching. As for her colleagues' light-hearted observation that the pump looked like a fashionable purse, it was her colleagues' way of using laughter to encourage her, because they could see how difficult the treatment was.

Taxol had a significant positive effect on the cancer cells in Felicia's liver. Her tumors gradually diminished in size, but she also experienced and suffered from extremely severe side effects, such as serious peripheral neuritis in her extremities.

Felicia started to experience numbing in her hands and feet, and even the slightest movement of her finger joints brought her excruciating pain. The pain in her hands was still bearable, but because the legs and feet support one's body weight, when Felicia attempted to stand up, the pain hurt so much that she was not able to straighten her back.

Ultimately, Felicia had to go to work in a wheelchair. Every day, I would push Felicia to the Institute of Biomedical Sciences for work.

Her treatment was an extremely painful ordeal but Felicia knew that Taxol was the only way to suppress her cancer. So she was prepared to continue with it no matter what, because she had many unfulfilled wishes and dreams.

The Eldest Son Ties the Knot

Talk about Felicia's wishes, her children's marriages were her largest worry as a mother. Our eldest son David was already thirty-two years old; he had an elegant and high-achieving French girlfriend named Christelle Bousquet. Christelle graduated in law from the University of Paris in France, and was a practicing lawyer. The two of them met in the University of Cambridge in England, while David was doing his postdoctoral research and Christelle, a Master's degree in law. Felicia and I had both met Christelle and felt that she would be an ideal life partner for David. After Felicia's cancer relapsed, I mentioned to David that if Christelle was "the one," then perhaps he should consider getting married.

That fall, David and Christelle came to Taiwan together to live with us. Faith and Albert also took time out from their busy schedules and hurried over for Christmas vacation because they knew that their mother's cancer had recurred and hoped to spend as much time as possible with her. As soon as Felicia saw the children, all her pain and suffering seemed to disappear. She and the children talked until late into the night. It took continuous persuasion on my part before they would go to bed. The power of love and family bonding had already disintegrated and melted away Felicia's pain.

I found a few opportunities to have long talks with David. At that time, David had just accepted a teaching position as assistant professor of chemistry and chemical engineering at the Colorado School of Mines in Golden, Colorado. I told David that he was making a head start in his career and it would really be the time to consider tying the knot if he and Christelle were truly and deeply in love. I shared with him that when a person has his own family, then he is more stable, and this would enable him to devote all of his energy to his career… Of course, the main reason was that his mother had become ill again; this time, it remained doubtful whether or not she would be able to withstand and survive the painful treatments in the future. But if he and Christelle got married, not only would

Felicia have one of her wishes fulfilled, and perhaps it would also motivate her to continue fighting cancer bravely. Felicia vowed to herself that she must live long to see and cradle her grandchildren in her arms.

David took my advice. He and Christelle talked the matter over very carefully and decided to get married to make a lifetime commitment. I felt reassured and comforted that David had found such an intelligent and refined wife. Felicia, of course, was ecstatic; she told the doctors to postpone her scheduled treatments because she had to make preparations for David's wedding soon within a short span of time, and she would resume regular treatment after David's wedding.

Felicia had always loved and enjoyed lively gatherings. But this gathering in particular held special meaning for her because it was her eldest son's marriage. She became the wedding planner for David and Christelle, taking care of practically all aspects of the wedding such as the choice of wedding rings, the wedding gown, photography, reception venue, and the program for the ceremony. But perhaps the most touching moment was her sincerity and determination in inviting her older brother Chi-Ching to attend the wedding. Since leaving the country thirty-seven years ago, Chi-Ching had not set foot on Taiwan. She called her older brother, saying that according to the Taiwanese custom, the eldest uncle of the groom on the mother's side is considered the most important guest at the wedding, and no matter what, he had to return to Taiwan, attend David's wedding, and sit at the head table. Chi-Ching accepted. Looking back, Chi-Ching recalled his trip back to Taiwan. Certainly, he came back to attend David's wedding and visit his family home and his motherland which he had not seen for thirty-seven years. Actually, his thoughts were with Felicia, knowing that her body was gradually becoming weaker. Visiting Felicia for a family reunion was thus his ultimate priority.

David's wedding was set for January 1, 1997 at the Hyatt Hotel in Taipei. Christelle's parents and her brother flew in from France. That evening, about six hundred guests attended the grand and solemn wedding ceremony, which was celebrated in an East-meets-West fusion style. David and Christelle were resplendent in their traditional Chinese wedding gowns — the groom in a mandarin jacket and long gown, and the bride in an elaborate phoenix-shaped crown and cape. In the presence of the delightful guests, the couple exchanged the wedding vows, sealing their promise of a lifetime commitment to each other.

I remember clearly the blessing Felicia gave to this newlywed couple during the wedding. In her words, she spoke from her experience, drawing analogy from our marriage. She said that we had upheld our marriage vows for over thirty years. Despite coming from different family backgrounds and our personality differences, for thirty years we were united as one, and we had blissfully raised a family together, all because of our mutual commitment and determination. It was also our belief that no matter how difficult life's journey would become, as long as the couple is of one united heart, any obstacle could be surmounted. Love forms the foundation of marriage, but in time of adversity, mutual support and trust are values that can help us weather through the odds. Such is true love — impregnable, unconditional and all-encompassing. She hoped that David and Christelle would remember her words: No matter how tumultuous the road ahead of them might become, as long as they believe the home they build together could, figuratively speaking, withstand torrential storms, and as long as they hold hands to brave their difficulties together, their love will grow, and their relationship will strengthen, and they will live happily ever after without regrets.

Felicia's words stirred me immensely. I believed David and Christelle understood how Felicia and I honored our commitment to each other. Felicia and I certainly had our differences in terms of personality and family background, and indeed, we did have some problems in communication. But the unshakable faith and strong love deeply rooted inside our hearts were like fortresses impregnable to external conflicts — we stood by our belief and the vows we made. The sweet and bitter experiences, the struggles, and the meeting of mind and soul — these, I believe David and Christelle will come to understand and experience themselves one day in their lives. Life is never smooth-sailing, but with strong family bonding and support, all difficulties could be weathered and overcome.

Taxol's Side Effects

The lively wedding celebrations finally came to an end and it was time for farewell when everyone went their separate ways. The newlyweds returned to the United States, and Albert and Faith returned to school. Felicia's eldest brother Chi-Ching Chen and his wife Shi-Chen Wu, younger brother Hsih-Kuan, and younger sisters Wan-Chan and Shin-Yin, who flew in to attend the wedding, had also returned to the United States. Felicia felt a sense of loss. Looking into her eyes, I understood how she felt — when the song performance ends, the seats are empty and the audience disperses. With her close kins gone back to their homes, loneliness and a sense of emptiness crept inside Felicia, who cherished family togetherness. Her forlorness was heightened as the challenges of a more difficult treatment loomed upon her.

Felicia's treatment was postponed to accommodate her wish to plan and prepare David's wedding, but Dr. An-Li Cheng thought that she should resume her treatment as soon as possible and thus he pressed her to do so. Just one week after the wedding, she resumed the Taxol treatment.

Taxol treatment is extremely effective, but it also causes severe reactions in patients. It was Felicia's premise through years of cancer treatment, to be treated with the most potent anti-cancer drug available to stop cancer cells from destroying her health. However, the extensive use of anti-cancer drugs had caused increasingly violent reactions in her body, as a result of the accumulation of the toxins from the treatment — the level had already reached the optimum. If she were to be administered with more potent drugs, the treatment would induce far greater pain and sufferings.

Taxol damages the peripheral nerves in hands and feet. When the treatment began, Felicia's hands became so numb that she could not even button her clothes, so stiff that it hurt even to type or write. Despite the pain, Felicia went to work in wheelchair every day as usual. Her co-workers in the laboratory were motivated by Felicia's conscientious attitude and that spurred them to work hard. The cancer research team's group morale was thus heightened and they were confident that their teacher Felicia would get better, and that they would accomplish many more exciting scientific discoveries under her mentorship. Felicia's illness became a source of inspiration to the team, and the team members bucked up and intensified their pace of work. Felicia's student Wei-Chen Liao said, "We knew there is still a gap and disparity between laboratory results and clinical trials, but we have in us the passion and energy that drive us on to persevere and work hard as we hope what we do might one day benefit our teacher."

Felicia already knew how difficult the treatment would be. However, she and the medical team did not expect the side effects of Taxol could be so severe. In reality, only twenty percent of patients in the clinical trial experienced numbness in the joints, and furthermore the pain was known to be within the tolerable limits of these patients. Felicia's pain was not simply confined to numbness in muscles and joints, hers was such an excruciating pain that her hands trembled, and her palms were covered in abscesses and blood. The skins on her palms and the soles of her feet cracked and peeled, layer by layer, down to the epidermis, exposing blood vessels. The pain was beyond the level of threshold of any average person could endure. Eventually, the pain reduced Felicia, a person of high mental strength, to be wheelchair-bound. That went to show how much pain she was putting up with.

Besides the pain in her hands and feet, Felicia suffered from inflammation of the membrane in her mouth, stomach, and intestines. She gritted her teeth to bear through the pain in order to stay alive. Dr. Cheng recalled, that year, every month when Felicia received Taxol treatment, she was suffering from torturous pain — an ordeal which was akin to the process of shedding the mold and skin in metamorphosis. Dr. Cheng was deeply affected by Felicia's ordeal. Each time he administered the treatment, he always thought to himself, "Nobody but Felicia could endure such tormenting ordeal. Any patient would choose to discontinue the treatment if he or she experiences such severe side effects. But Felicia just doesn't give up; she even continually reassures doctors by saying, 'Do what you need to do to treat me, and don't worry about my body's reaction.'"

The reason Felicia was able to endure it was quite simple: She recognized the value and significance of life, and she wanted to do all she could to be of some contribution to society. She loved her family and her friends, so she was determined to survive no matter what it took.

From July 1996 to August 1997, she underwent nine sessions of Taxol treatment. Each and every treatment she underwent brought her severe physical pain and wreaked havoc to her health, but Felicia took it bravely. Try as one might, the severity of pain could not be put into words. I hoped after Felicia underwent all these hardships, she would be reborn, and emerge from her cocoon as a butterfly, and return to the embrace of a beautiful and enriching life. But deep down I knew after all these treatments her body was becoming more frail and weaker.

19

Trying Medicine after Medicine

After a year of Taxol treatment, enduring extreme pain and suffering, cancer growth in Felicia seemed to have been suppressed. But the doctors and I well knew that cancer cells gradually and eventually develop resistance to even the best medicines. In other words, the doctors themselves were unsure how long they could continue using Taxol to suppress tumor growth.

A year later, the cancer cells in Felicia's liver once again started to spread and multiply. Although extensive chemotherapy and the strongest anti-cancer medicines available had almost completely eradicated the weaker cancer cells in Felicia's body, what survived the weeding-out process of numerous chemotherapy sessions were the more aggressive types, and their tough resilience was evident. Felicia's immune system, on the other hand, was weaker than ever as a result of long-term chemotherapy.

Dr. An-Li Cheng and the medical team once again started considering the possibility of using new medicine. In fact, at that time, the medicines that Felicia could choose from were rather limited, and judging from Felicia's present condition, it was not possible to wait for the next drug discovery to treat her. So while the medical team was considering which medicine to switch to, they continued to use Taxol but changed the dosage and the method by which it was administered. In the past, Felicia received a monthly injection of Taxol but it became once a week. The new treatment method was tougher on Felicia, but after a month, the tumors showed signs of shrinking. There was ultimately still a ray of hope, and Felicia's face glowed with joy.

That period of time was also one of the most exhausting and physically damaging for Felicia. The increased frequency of Taxol treatments put a tremendous strain and burden on her mind and body. I still took Felicia out to have her favorite Japanese food; she knew that she absolutely had to eat well and take in proper nutrients to gain the strength to fight her illness. But her mouth and esophagus were inflamed and covered with ulcers, eating was extremely difficult. In order to eat, she first had to apply a drop of anesthetic to her mouth, then eat a mouthful of food, she had to repeatedly numb the pain with anesthetic until she finished the meal. I don't know how the food would taste like in her mouth, but no matter what, she was determined to finish the food and not waste it.

To finish just one meal was already extremely difficult, what was most distressful was the side effect of severe vomiting induced by chemotherapy. Very often, soon after we stepped out of the restaurant after dining, Felicia would throw up the food that she had just eaten. When I saw her leaning over the gutter drain expurgating everything she had just consumed, my heart was filled with despair and anguish.

The Loneliness of Cancer Patients

Felicia endured all ordeals and sufferings in order to survive — her determination to live was strong and unshakable. As her close and dear one standing by her to give her the support she needed, I did not blame Heaven nor did I bear a grudge against men. But Heaven was indeed cruel, inflicting her with difficulties and challenges to finish even a simple meal. For those people who are fastidious about what they eat, I am just wondering, would they feel guilty the next time they face a plate of food if they have seen how painful Felicia's ordeal was to even put a morsel of food into her mouth? This is simply because there are unfortunate people in the world who have trouble consuming even a single meal.

To be able to eat is a blessing. After Felicia fell ill, the pleasure of enjoying food was already deemed a luxury for her. From July 1996, when Felicia started receiving Taxol treatment, her health deteriorated like the setting sun. Not only was she unable to eat a proper meal, her physical pain and uncertainty about the unknown future were also worries heavy in her mind.

Felicia knew I was tied down with my heavy workload. She was also unwilling to let the children worry, but everyone has his or her moments of weakness and loneliness. In front of her laboratory research team she always cut a strong, dominant figure. Deep in her heart lurked the abysmal sadness and hurt which she suppressed and never let out. So her confidant was Dr. An-Li Cheng who was most knowledgeable about her medical condition.

Dr. Cheng said Felicia broke down in tears in front of him when she felt powerless over the physical and mental hurt she suffered, and how in desperation she wanted to stop and eradicate the threat of cancer. But she herself knew what the outcome was to suffer from cancer. In fact, she even had an idea of how long she could hang on and keep going, given her present condition.

That was the loneliness of a cancer researcher who had a good understanding of cancer, and also fought a desolate battle against cancer. Dr. Cheng listened to Felicia quietly, he knew no amount of comforting words could bring solace to his senior. And then, in his heartfelt words, he said, "Considering these factors — your medical condition, the severity of your cancer, and the treatment therapies you underwent, you have already set an unprecedented record with your fight against cancer. You should be proud." Then, Felicia would break into a tearful smile, she picked up her courage again to confront the ongoing battle and she regained perspective of her self-worth. Soon after, Felicia bounced back, offered support and encouragement to her other comrades in cancer. The valley of her low spirits did not defeat her, instead it served as a source of inspiration for her.

Searching for New Medicines and Treatments

Changing the method of administering Taxol enabled Felicia to withstand the drug's violent side effects for a little over two months. Felicia received a total of twelve Taxol treatment sessions — which was a record number of treatments known to have undergone by a cancer patient. However, as the side effects grew increasingly severe, she had to stop taking the medicine for a new alternative anti-cancer treatment. That was in November 1997, Felicia came to the bottleneck for an alternative treatment again, after the torments of Taxol treatment.

The seemingly infinite space, endless sky, and horizon in the distance — what do all these mean? Meng-Die Zhou wrote a poem, "On a Ferry Boat," which goes:

> Man is on the boat
> The boat is on the water
> The water is at the horizon
> The horizon is
> The infinitely happy and sad moment when life ends.

Having experienced this sense of infinity in Felicia's years of fighting cancer, I do not know if we should accept the voyage that Mother Nature has determined for us simply because the boat is on the water, or whether we should control the boat, steer it forcibly against the current, and continue to battle aggressively. Felicia and I are like oarsmen in the boat; although the waves are tumultuous causing the boat to rock wildly, we encourage each other to boost our morale, and tell ourselves that we have to navigate and tide over the dangerous situations.

As Dr. An-Li Cheng put it, from September 1997 onwards when I stood by Felicia in her fight against cancer, that was virtually the last stand and defense. At that time, the options for an alternative anti-cancer drug was running out and Taxol was practically her last resort. The medical team tried all means to find a new drug suitable for Felicia. But they were not confident of finding a new alternative and they were unsure for how long would the drug suppress her cancer.

In January 1998, the doctors decided that since Felicia's cancer had always been confined in the liver and did not demonstrate any signs of further migration, they could execute a liver transarterial immunochemo-embolization (TIE). In TIE, a catheter is passed from the femoral vein in the groin, through the hepatic artery and into the liver. It uses a special substance with glue-like properties to block blood vessels inside the liver from passing nutrients to cancer cells; the cancer cells then stop growing due to a deficiency of available nutrients.

However, the liver TIE performed at NTU Hospital was not successful. Felicia's tumors continued to grow, and the situation was quite critical. The medical team had to re-analyze and investigate the problem and explore using new medicines to suppress cancer.

In February 1998, Felicia started to take a type of new cancer medicine, a 5-FU called Capecitabine that could be administered orally. She took a large dose of Capecitabine with Leucovorin, Gemcitabine, and Cisplatin in order to suppress cancer growth. In the beginning, the prescription appeared to have some effect.

At that time, Capecitabine was one of the latest anti-cancer drugs which was not imported into Taiwan yet. In fact, it had not even been tested and approved by the Department of Health, and Felicia's condition was so critical that the timeframe to import the latest drug may be deemed too slow, too late. The cancer cells in her liver had to be suppressed quickly, or her life would be at risk.

Capecitabine was manufactured by Roche, the Switzerland-based international pharmaceutical company. The then director of the Taiwan branch of Roche, Dr. Jong-Kai Chen, used to work at NHRI. He offered his assistance to make a telephone call to Switzerland to inquire about the distribution network of the medicine. He was informed that Hong Kong happened to have a batch of the supply, so he made a hurried trip there and made the necessary arrangements to bring back the medicine himself. Whereas back in Taiwan, Dr. Oliver Yoa-Pu Hu, director-general of the Bureau of Pharmaceutical Affairs, was also extremely helpful. Based on a regulation in the pharmaceutical administration law, a new drug can be given the authorization for import if it is supported by documentations or reports that prove its benefits to patients. And this made it possible for Dr. Jong-Kai Chen to bring Capecitabine into Taiwan.

The Effectiveness Gradually Dwindles

To patients suffering from the terminal phase of cancer, this drug indeed spelled a ray of hope to them. Statistics showed an effectiveness rate of a mere fifteen to twenty-five percent which was considered low, but to the terminally ill patients, the percentage symbolized a chance to fight. Felicia was extremely fortunate to have the opportunity to try Capecitabine, but its effectiveness lasted for a mere two months during which her energy level sunk lower and lower after each treatment.

Dr. An-Li Cheng remembers the treatment period after Taxol, during which Felicia was perpetually changing medicines and treatment methods and he described the process as a moving picture with rapid-changing scenes and visuals that unfold before one's very eyes. As a cancer specialist, he knew new medicines prove their effectiveness in the beginning, but for a brief momentary period — this put Felicia to emotional test and challenge again. When cancer cells first come in contact with new medicines, they are not accustomed to the drug and die off quickly. But when new drugs are administered for a prolonged period, the cancer cells come to understand the drugs' actions and gradually develop a resistance to them. By then, any larger amount of dosage would not be able to suppress cancer growth. The new drug eventually becomes ineffective, the tumors continue to grow, and the next imperative move is to switch to another drug and start again with a new course of treatments. The highs and lows become increasingly close together and like a line graph, the gradient goes steeper; in other words, with each new drug, the effectiveness period gets shorter and shorter. Tumors that are previously suppressed will grow again once the drug effectiveness is gone. It is only a matter of time when the search for effective new medicines is exhausted.

The doctors on the medical team, to say nothing of Felicia, were absolutely clear about what the final result would be. She was, after all, a scientist who researched on anti-cancer drugs. So Dr. Cheng described this period as a tough battle, a tug-of-war in mud. Both the doctor and patient felt a great deal of pressure — especially the patient, in addition to enduring all the ordeals of the treatments, she still had to deal with the anxiety and stress of responsibility in her heart. The magnitude of the physical strain and emotional stress that Felicia underwent is truly beyond the endurance threshold of a healthy, able-bodied individual.

The Determination to Learn to Dance

Due to the countless chemotherapy sessions, discoloration spots which looked like burn marks covered her cheeks. Her eyes were gleaming with vigor as always, but traces of fatigue of her protracted fight against cancer — locked between her eyebrows — could be faintly perceived. Her weariness was especially magnified from the strong reactions and side effects of the chemotherapy regimen, which people around her might not have noticed but I know, all her limbs and bones were in pain. In fact, only the doctors and I understood the suffering she endured, she hid and masked the physical pain with her carefree and cheerful laughter. But Felicia was not one to be beaten easily; the more difficult the treatment became, the more determined she was.

At our thirtieth wedding anniversary dinner, which is also called the "pearl" anniversary, Shu-Chi Hsu-Weng, the wife of Zi-Chiu Hsu, former director-general of the Department of Health, performed a rendition of Hawaiian hula dances. That evening, Felicia enjoyed herself immensely. Also, she and Shu-Chi Hsu-Weng discovered that they were distantly related and before long, the two of them became good friends despite their great difference in age. Felicia had always been interested in music and dance, so in 1997 she set up the Taipei First Girls' School Alumni Dance Club. Every Saturday afternoon, the dance club members would have their dance lessons and socializing sessions at the house of their instructor Shu-Chi Hsu-Weng.

Each time after her chemotherapy session, Felicia would make her way to her dance instructor Hsu-Weng's house for lessons. Her instructor could not bear to see Felicia over-exert herself physically and advised her to rest more. But Felicia said she was already used to the pain and discomfort of chemotherapy. Dancing and immersing herself in the beautiful music had enabled her to relax and forget the agony of chemotherapy, so this could only be good for her. Rain or shine, virtually every Saturday afternoon, Felicia went to Shu-Chi Hsu-Weng's house for her lessons and practices in folk dancing from around the world. She drew on the energy from her University of Minnesota days when she made her morning run as a daily regime, and for dancing, she adopted the same philosophy too to persevere.

Felicia kept close watch on her treatment results and doctors' prognosis. She knew she could not afford to make a single mistake; she had to be very cautious in order to hold back the attack of cancer. For two months, Capecitabine had been quite effective, but this also meant that Felicia had to put up with the severe side effects of the drug.

Felicia had been treated with Taxol for more than a year. Her peripheral nerves had already suffered extensive damage. With the addition of Capecitabine, another strong powerful drug, an explosive torrent of all the side effects wreaked havoc to her body, inflicting pain and suffering that were beyond words. The cracking of the skin on her hands and feet became extremely severe; thus she wrapped bandages around all her joints. The soles of her feet — too horrifying to look at — were covered with cuts and cracks which bled and were clotted up in streaks of dried blood. In order to walk and move around, she had to dress the wound of her feet with bandage, and then put on shoes with soft padding. Under such agonizing pain and condition, she persisted to learn dancing, to visit the Zoo, the botanical gardens and the countryside on a wheelchair, and even attempt mountain hiking.

The Internal Struggle of the Doctors

To endure is to survive, and to hang on for any last glimmer of hope. But even Capecitabine, the newest anti-cancer medicines at that time, ceased to be effective after only two months. Felicia's tumors had grown larger and that was an indication that the cancer cells had already become resistant to Capecitabine.

Felicia's treatment after September 1997 was like one long drawn-out battle — both the doctors and the patient were under immense stress. In April 1998, when the medical team announced that Capecitabine was no longer effective on Felicia, their disappointment and helplessness were no less painful than the ordeal that Felicia went through. As Dr. An-Li Cheng put it, the doctor-patient relationship is that of mutual understanding and concern. Though his mission as a doctor is to cure patients, he must also take into consideration their quality of life, which is to dispense treatment not only to alleviate their suffering but also to ensure the dignity and sanctity of human life, and to uphold the patient's self-worth. So it hurt him like a knife pierced to his heart to see Felicia struggling so valiantly to endure the treatments and to wait in anticipation for a new cure.

Felicia would ask him persistently, "Are there any new medicines? What medicines can I still try? I don't fear pain; as long as the medicine is effective, I can withstand any amount of pain." Felicia never lost hope; she was always hopeful for new drug discovery. The doctor felt torn apart, because the kind of pain that Felicia endured was already far beyond what an average person could tolerate.

The Side Effects Intensify

In April 1998, Dr. Jacqueline Peng-Wang found a new anti-cancer drug from the United States called Lipodox. Dr. Cheng administered it together with Capecitabine in the hope that this combination would suppress the cancer cells, and Felicia received a total of five treatment sessions.

Felicia's body became weaker and weaker. Every time, when the side effects of a new drug kicked in, her intense suffering was analogous to ascending a mountain of blades barefooted and being thrown into a vessel of hot oil. She hung on and endured the agony simply for the results of the medical examination. If the report yielded that the new drug was effective, she would brim with confidence and hope. She constantly encouraged herself by psychological tactic that as long as she worked hard, God would give her a chance at life. So no matter how much she suffered or how her body had been ripped apart and devastated by the chemotherapy, Felicia faced each new day the same way she would during her healthy days.

Felicia said each day she woke up and opened her eyes to see the beautiful world around her and feel herself breathe, she would feel happy and thank God for giving her another day. It was an ecstatic happiness of welcoming and embracing a new life. So she went to work as usual, made notes in her treatment diary and planned trips that the family would take together when the children returned from the United States. With each day came a new life which she embraced with joy, Felicia's smile remained bright, cheery and carefree.

The liveliness and sparkle in Felicia's eyes never lost their intensity; the pain and suffering that spanned more than a decade had only strengthened the determination in those deep, twinkling bright eyes. But I knew her body was becoming extremely weak, and furthermore, her treatment was becoming increasingly more difficult.

The new medicine was effective for a short span of time, but the pain afflicted was also extremely severe and the side effects took on a multiplicative toll on her body. As Felicia previously received strong treatments which already did great damage to her body, the new drug treatment triggered all previous reactions and side effects, very much like the action of stair-climbing which is an accumulative and building-up effect until at such point, the amassed effects mercilessly wreak damage on the patient.

Felicia was not spared the strong drug reactions resulting from the new medicine, and their side effects were even more extreme. She was in so much pain that she had to rely on morphine, but even morphine was unable to quell it. She suffered from insomnia and was on sleeping pills prescription to make her sleep. But she never skipped her research work, meetings, and discussions, and she never missed a single word when editing the papers and reports of her students or research assistants. She embodied the true spirit of "seize the moment" and from within, she manifested the essence of living life to its fullest.

Rejoicing Too Soon

After the third treatment session, Felicia went to the hospital for a follow-up examination, and actually discovered that the thirty or forty tumors in her liver had miraculously and completely disappeared. Felicia was extremely excited on learning the news. She thought the new drug was really effective against the tumors in her body. She broke the news enthusiastically to everyone she knew, and her children. That was the period when she was feeling upbeat and in good spirits. Her smile of relief and contentment was infectious.

But Dr. Cheng and the other doctors on the medical team did not dare to let down their guard. They performed a more detailed examination and found out the reasons why the previous ultrasound did not reveal the tumors: ascites (abnormal amount of fluid in the abdominal cavity) had blocked the scan, creating the false impression that all the tumors had disappeared. In reality, Felicia's tumors were still in her liver, and what made the doctors most worried was that the new medicine lost its effectiveness to suppress tumor growth. The tumors did not shrink, instead they appeared to be gradually growing larger.

No matter how strong Felicia would seem to be, her confidence was dented, this incident of false hope caused her spirits to sink to an unusual low. I saw and sensed her disillusionment and dejection. Even though she did not say a single word, I could imagine the deep pain she experienced.

On sleepless nights, Felicia would go to the laboratory to continue her work. She would write papers and correct student reports until late into the night. Time and again, the countless tormenting treatments, the endless renewed hopes, the recurring disappointments, and the constant self-encouragement to face up to repeated challenges — these had hit Felicia's emotional state dramatically. Sometimes, she would say to me that there was not much time left so she needed to do as much as she could to accomplish her goals; at other times she would sigh wistfully and hope to be given another ten years, during which she would be able to achieve more in scientific research, continue her anti-cancer volunteer work, and see her children raise families and build careers.

The Willpower to Attend the Wedding in France

Every day since her passing, I would light an incense stick. Curls of smoke — which is, figuratively, the soul of Felicia — waft in the air. I have long talks with her, telling her everything that has happened since she left this world. The falling ashes from the incense reminded me the final two years in Felicia's life fighting cancer. Felicia was just like the incense stick that glows and gives off heat. But her light and heat were gradually depleting in the wind, slowly dying off in flickering glow, and dissipating in the wisps of smoke. In my heart lies the infinite compassion and regret for Felicia and her resolute spirit. Looking back, the treatments only prolonged her life, but I gave her the absolute support for every decision she made, because in all moments of life and death, I was her unwavering shoulder for support.

The new drug combinations drove Felicia up to the wall, to the limit in terms of the pain she could endure. The side effects were so severe that she had to be admitted to the hospital for treatment. Felicia hated hospitals. At that time, David and Christelle planned to return to France during their summer vacations to hold a church wedding, during which Christelle's family hoped to introduce David and our whole family to all their relatives and friends. Felicia regarded this as an extremely important family affair. Under no circumstances would she be absent from her son's wedding in France. But the side effects of the medicines caused serious skin inflammation and laceration to her hands and feet, it was difficult for her to walk even a single step. So after extensive discussion, we decided that she had to stay at the hospital and receive treatment, and I would attend David's wedding in France.

Felicia was extremely unwilling to accept the decision, but she was unable to convince me and reluctantly agreed. On this trip to France, other than David's wedding, Felicia and I had originally planned to attend the "France-Taiwan Symposium on Cancer and Viruses." Felicia was scheduled to give a lecture at the meeting and we cancelled the lecture as well.

I set off to France alone, and of course, I was worried about Felicia's emotional state. Unexpectedly, less than two days after I had left, Felicia told Dr. An-Li Cheng that she was determined to take leave from the hospital to go to France and attend David's wedding. Dr. Cheng did not agree. At that time, Felicia's platelet count was extremely low. The doctor was worried that she would suffer internal bleeding as a result of her low platelet count, thus putting her life in danger. But Felicia was insistent, on the one hand, she telephoned the maid and instructed her to prepare her clothes, and on the other hand, she begged Dr. Cheng to prepare the required daily dosages of medicine to be administered orally and by injection. She said she could handle it herself.

Dr. Cheng cautioned her time and again that she was putting herself to risky situation. If anything were to go wrong and with no doctor available nearby to attend to her, who knew what might happen. But Felicia was very adamant on leaving the hospital. Dr. Cheng just stood there shaking his head helplessly, thinking that he understood the personality of this patient, who was both his teacher and friend, too well; if she had her mind set on something, nothing could stop her. He had no choice but to go along with her wishes. Another reason Dr. Cheng gave in was that Felicia assured him that she would monitor her condition and carry out the injection therapy every day. She would also visit a French cancer center near Paris where she had previously done research and was quite familiar with the people. She would then consult the experts there for their opinion about her disease.

The doctor finally gave his approval to let her go, and Felicia lugged her suitcase excitedly, straight from the hospital to the airport. At the Chiang Kai-Shek International Airport, she even requested the service attendant to allow her to board the airplane in a wheelchair. I received the news in France; Felicia would be arriving soon. When Felicia arrived at the Paris Charles de Gaulle International Airport, the children and I were already there waiting for her.

We had not expected that Felicia, who emerged from the dense crowd of passengers, would cut a lively and animated figure brimming with energy. When the children caught sight of their mother's smile, they embraced her tightly and joyously. Their mother had overcome innumerable difficulties to come to France to attend David and Christelle's church wedding. That meant a great deal to both of them. And miraculously, Felicia did not display even a single sign of exhaustion upon arriving in France, because in Taipei she was indeed severely ill. Her children were her entire world, she loved them so much that she forgot her pain and suffering which were cached and hidden away like a genie — there one moment and gone the next.

Completely Different as if Body and Spirit are Divided

The week Felicia spent in France, she talked, laughed, and participated in all types of activities. On the day of the wedding, she wore a red *chi-pao*, or the traditional Chinese dress. She watched endearingly as the bride's family gave Christelle to David, and the two of them exchanged marriage vows in front of the minister. Felicia's eyes were filled with tears. She had come to France because she did not want to miss this sacred moment of her son and her daughter-in-law in the church. Felicia was the saintliest and happiest of all mothers.

An alfresco reception followed soon after the wedding. On the lush green lawn, Felicia — looking beautiful and dainty in her red *chi-pao* — stood out bright and prominent. I saw her cheery red silhouette moving breezily among the guests with whom she had hearty talks. She walked in brisk footsteps as if she was not in the least bit of pain. At the party held that evening, Felicia changed into a purple evening gown. David took his mother's hands and together they danced. Her smile was like a blossoming flower in the spring dew. Although that night was David and Christelle's wedding party, where the spotlight was on the newlywed, I still felt that, Felicia was the most beautiful woman that evening. I had fallen into the embrace of her charming, radiant smile; we held each other close and danced. We saw our grown-up son and his wife smiling as they wove in and out among the dancing couples before us. We watched David's pretty wife, Christelle, dotingly — the couple would soon start their bright future together. The two of us, on the other hand, were about to turn sixty. Felicia was still battling her illness. I didn't know how much longer I would have her, but at that moment, it felt like forever. The party lasted late into the night, but Felicia looked not the least bit tired — she had completely forgotten the pain of her illness.

After the wedding, I went with Felicia to the French cancer center to seek the opinion of the experts regarding her future treatment options. Because Felicia had already undergone too many treatments, her body had built up resistance to all medicines that were administered. The problem was indeed very tricky. After the French oncologists gained a fuller picture about Felicia's condition, they said it would not be advisable to try various medicine in huge amount, as a complete cure would be extremely difficult. They suggested that a single medicine to be taken orally would do.

That week, Felicia injected herself with anti-cancer medicine daily. Christelle's father, Professor Bernard Bousquet, made special arrangement for Felicia to have blood tests in the laboratory to confirm that her white blood cell and platelet count were not too low. At night she would bandage her cracked feet. Her finger joints hurt so much that they shook when she put on clothes or attempted to hold a pen, but that week the side effects disappeared and were gone with the wind. She could put on her clothes easily without the least bit of difficulty.

I knew Felicia relied on her determination and perseverance to keep going. Before returning to Taiwan, she would undoubtedly be able to maintain the same high energy level. And true enough, one week after the wedding celebrations were over as Felicia and I were to return to Taipei, and as soon as we stepped into the departure hall of the Paris Charles de Gaulle International Airport, Felicia could take no more — she limped, her hands went stiff, and she lacked the strength to even pull her suitcase. I borrowed a wheelchair and pushed Felicia onto the plane. As soon as we boarded the plane, Felicia's cheeks immediately sagged, as if she had completed and gone through a long, treacherous and arduous journey. She was truly tired, and fell into a deep sleep…

20

The Last Stage

Dr. An-Li Cheng recalls Felicia's treatments administered from October 1998 to July 1999, when Felicia finally departed from this earth, were less regimented.

Felicia's treatment had hit a wall. The medical team knew that Felicia had long since reached and surpassed the limit of the medicines that was allowed, so any new medicine that she was put on trial would add on to more severe reactions. Generally, for most cancer patients who have reached this stage, the physicians would not prescribe further medication, because the pain would greatly reduce the quality of their lives. But Felicia insisted on continuing the fight; she was determined to try any new drug no matter how much pain she had to undergo.

The medical team and the French oncologists were of the same opinion that Felicia should just concentrate on one single medicine to treat her illness so that the damage done to her body would not be as great; the best that they could hope for was to maintain the present size of the tumor and suppress their growth. The medical team opted the treatment with Lipodox and stopped Capecitabine, because Capecitabine's side effects were really too severe; it even caused the skin on Felicia's feet to crack open. However, after only two sessions of Lipodox, the doctors realized that it had no effect, and immediately discontinued it.

Clinging to Life Through Sheer Will

Dr. An-Li Cheng knew that, at that point, the effectiveness of medicine was of little significance. At that last stage of cancer, Felicia kept the flame of life burning through sheer determination.

February 1998 was the seventieth anniversary of Academia Sinica. Felicia was invited to speak about her career as a scientist and her personal journey of her fight against cancer. It was spring, bitterly cold and the rain fell endlessly, and the attendance to the celebratory event was sparse. But that afternoon the lecture hall at Academia Sinica's Institute of Biomedical Sciences was packed with two to three hundred audience. Among them were the president of Academia Sinica, Yuan-Tseh Lee, and his wife. Felicia's voice resounded sonorously in the lecture hall. She spoke for a full two hours unreservedly about her fight against cancer and explained in depth the various types of cancer treatment — surgery, radiation therapy, chemotherapy, immuno-therapy, and gene therapy — which she had extensive knowledge. On the podium, she was a teacher of great patience, tirelessly imparting knowledge, and passionately sharing her experiences and new findings of cancer with her audience.

Most importantly, she offered her advice to the cancer patients never to give up as only they could help to save themselves. An optimistic and positive outlook, confidence and perseverance would help deal with the pain of cancer better. She also advised patients to have faith in their doctor and adhere to the treatment regimen, and not blindly adopt alternative folk medicine. She shared her experience that one could still find value of life despite illness, that is, by returning to the normalcy of daily life at work, in family and community.

The audience in the lecture hall stayed rapt and hung on to Felicia's every word as she narrated her emotional thirteen-year struggle against cancer. She spoke with energy and enthusiasm. My heart was filled with gratitude and admiration. I had Felicia's strength of character to thank for, if not, the laughter and happiness in our family life would have long since disappeared, because the children and I would have been dragged into the agony and despair of her battle with cancer. For Felicia, her deep love for her family was the pain suppressant. Because she loved us, she took on the pain of cancer alone, and did not want the children or me to worry.

On the podium, Felicia was unusually boisterous which incited the anxiety and concern of Drs. An-Li Cheng and Pan-Chyr Yang who were in the audience. In fact, Felicia was on a special permission to be discharged from the hospital to make this speech. The two doctors knew her physical condition had deteriorated and were worried that Felicia would overexert herself, so during the speech they kept a close observation on her. On seeing that Felicia had spoken for two hours and was still intent on carrying on full steam ahead, Dr. Cheng told the professor who emcee-ed the event that she could not keep on speaking, and that her condition would worsen if she continued to do so. But there were many people in the audience who wanted to ask questions; Felicia warm-heartedly answered each and every one of them. As a result, at that speech, Felicia stood for three hours without a break. At last, she asked me to come to the podium and thanked me for taking care of her. The audience wanted me to speak. I gathered my thoughts and said that Felicia was an extraordinary person with the strongest determination, and in fact, the one who should be grateful was me; if it were not for Felicia's strength, I would not have the resolve to march on, not to mention to do anything for our society and country.

The doctors were the most concerned and on high alert of their patient's condition. After the lecture, Dr. Cheng and Dr. Yang whisked Felicia back to the hospital. They were already mentally prepared for the expected turn of condition, they were worried that Felicia's body would suffer from negative physical reaction. And sure enough, the doctors' anxiety was well-founded. That night, Felicia's blood pressure dropped to forty, she went into a coma and shock, and was immediately transferred to the intensive care unit. At that time, it was practically impossible to measure her blood pressure. Her condition became extremely dangerous.

After a night of frantic rescue efforts, Felicia was revived. The next day when Dr. Cheng came to check on Felicia, he lectured her severely, because the chain of events that happened the night before were really too dangerous. All it would take was just one mistake, and the consequences would be unimaginable.

But no one could stop Felicia from realizing the mission she harbored in her heart. She felt that she was the best person to help cancer patients regain faith. No matter how exhausted she was or how low her energy level had plummeted, she would do her best to share her experiences with anyone who needed her help. Whether the people who sought her help called her via telephone or were from their hospital bed, Felicia would advise them that determination and optimism were the best weapons to fight the battle, and never to despair.

In fact, each time Felicia saw the results of her own medical report, she, as a scientist, fully knew what the report meant and she would say to Dr. Cheng, "I know that I don't have much time left." She said she was like a candle in the wind facing the peril of being extinguished by a sudden gust of wind, any moment. Despite knowing her condition was dire, she tirelessly continued the search for ways and means to prolong her life.

All Chemotherapeutic Agents Prove Ineffective

Lipodox was deemed ineffective against her tumors in December 1998. The doctors were at a complete loss, and finally decided to explore the possibility of administering Capecitabine as a single drug rather than in combination with other drugs. Felicia's response to the drug was drastically extreme, her two hands hurt so much that she could not even hold the chopsticks. But after two painful treatments, it became apparent that the tumors still continued to grow, so the doctors gave up on Capecitabine as well.

It was January 1999. The doctors and I held frequent conferences, desperately finding a way to keep Felicia alive. At that time, there were already forty to fifty tumors ravaging half of Felicia's liver. My teacher, Professor Rui-Lou Song, was an authority on the liver. At that time, he was honorary president of Sun Yat-Sen Cancer Center. I went to Sun Yat-Sen Cancer Center specifically to seek an opinion from him about Felicia's condition. My teacher said if the tumors spread to more than two-thirds of the liver, it would be life-threatening. According to his experience, if the tumors continued to grow, he estimated Felicia had at most three months to live.

Felicia and I did not believe in sitting and waiting for one's demise, that simply was not our philosophy. We still had to find that thread of hope for Felicia's survival. Flowers blossom in full bloom but they will wither one day; I told Felicia and myself that she and I were comrades in life and in death. If Felicia really had only three months left, then it would be now more than ever, the two of us had to rely on each other for support to fight this battle which we would never surrender.

In January 1999, the medical team tried Navelbine once again, along with a high dose of Methotrexate. At first, the treatment seemed to have some effect, but the doctors were clearly aware that the good news would not last long. Felicia was already extremely weak. A high dosage of anti-cancer medicine acted against her body with extensive damage like a raging, violent storm. Felicia, however, insisted on continuing the treatment. She never gave up hope.

The Navelbine and Methotrexate combination treatment session only lasted until February 20. The medical team realized that not only were the treatments ineffective in suppressing the tumors, they instead appeared to be multiplying. Dr. An-Li Cheng said to me with a heavy heart, there were no more medicines that could yield any effect on Felicia. Giving her more medicine would only add to her pain, and the foreseeable thing to do is to seek alternative treatment method. Even though this was a long expected development, in my heart I was struggling with pangs of despair to hear the doctor utter those words. The news that I least wanted to hear had come from her doctor's lips. I shuddered, it was like having a bucket of icy cold water dumped on my head.

The Possibility of a Liver Transplant

During those three years after Felicia's cancer recurred, the intensive, strong treatment had successfully contained the cancer cells inside the liver. Upon the advice of my teacher, Professor Juei-Low Sung, and Dr. Andrew Huang, president of Sun Yat-Sen Cancer Center and my former classmate in medical school, we started to consider the possibility of a liver transplant.

Given Felicia's present medical condition, the medical team thought the risk of such an operation was extremely high. However, they also felt that at this point, it was possibly the only chance that Felicia had. Thus they devoted their energy into investigating the success rate of liver transplants in cancer patients.

Felicia completely understood her own situation. Not giving up was the belief she upheld in her battle against her illness. Medicines had proven to be ineffective, there was still the possibility of a liver transplant. She set her mind to adjusting her mental state and physical condition so that the transplant operation would have the greatest chance of success.

Felicia followed the passion in her heart to strive her best in realizing her aspirations — as a scientific researcher, as wife and mother and even as a seriously-ill patient. That was what described Felicia's personality — she was true to herself and action, and she took to a romanticized, idealistic outlook to realize her aspirations. Setting her sights on a liver transplant, she was determined to take care of her body in top form so that the transplant could take place.

March is the season of flower blooms at Yangmingshan. Fiery red flowers blossomed in abundance, creating a lively scene with the verdant greens bringing out the crimson of the blossoms. We held hands and ambled along the mountain path. The narrow, tree-lined paths were just like in the old days, and the green hills as beautiful as before. We reminisced the days when we were young and the day trip we took along the North Coast on a bus from Taipei en route to Yangmingshan, and continuing to Jinshan, and then from Jinshan to Keelung on foot, before returning to Taipei by bus. We were young and full of energy then, and our steps brisk and sprightly. Now we were already sixty years old. Felicia walked the journey of life with me and endured over thirteen torturous years of cancer. Time and tide consumed our youth; our appearances had changed, the only thing, however, that remained unchanged was our love, which grew stronger with each passing day.

I took several pictures of Felicia against the blooming flowers. Her smile shone brilliantly; every laugh line etched on her face was a testament to the beautiful years that we spent together. That day, Felicia's beauty reflected our lifetime of mutual support and dedicated commitment. Our marriage spanning over thirty years held the most genuine and deepest moments of our lives, and Yangmingshan had once again borne witness to our love and commitment.

Assessing the Feasibility of a Liver Transplant

The University of Pittsburgh performs the highest number of and most successful liver transplants in the world. In order to assess the feasibility of Felicia receiving a liver transplant, I contacted the University Hospital, explained to them the details of Felicia's condition and asked for their opinion. After understanding Felicia's condition, a doctor there responded by letter, expressing the opinion that a liver transplant was not necessarily the best alternative. First of all, Felicia was a patient in the last stage of cancer and the risk of the surgical procedure was much greater than in other patients, and even if the transplant was successful, Felicia's cancer might still resurface and threaten her life. Second, in the selection of liver transplant candidates, doctors are obliged to consider patients' medical conditions because suitable donors for liver transplantation are limited, and the doctors have to choose patients whose physical condition are most suited for receiving transplants. Even if there were a liver compatible with Felicia, according to medical ethics, the doctors were obliged to give the liver to the patient with the greatest chance of survival. However, the doctor also wrote from the perspective of a medical practitioner that he would not give up on any patient. He added, if we could, on our end, find a liver suitable for transplantation, he was willing to perform the surgery on Felicia.

In fact, Taiwan's liver transplantation technique was internationally recognized. My teacher, Dr. Juei-Low Sung, recommended Dr. Chao-Long Chen of Kaohsiung Chang Gung Memorial Hospital who had already performed liver transplantation on over sixty patients with a success rate of over ninety percent. The medical team also suggested that if Felicia had already decided to have a liver transplantation, perhaps she should first meet Dr. Chao-Long Chen and let him do a thorough evaluation of the feasibility of such a transplantation.

In March, Felicia and I flew to Kaohsiung to consult Dr. Chen. We hoped he would tell us what he thought Felicia's chances were of having a successful liver transplantation.

Dr. Chen listened carefully and came to understand the efforts that Felicia had expended to fight cancer over the last thirteen years. He then said that although he had performed over sixty liver transplant operations, the operation itself was still considered as one of extreme high risk, especially given that Felicia's physical condition was far from ideal. However, he admired Felicia's resolve, so he was willing to take the risk of challenge in performing the operation.

But Dr. Chen also said that at present there were not many people who opted to donate organs when they passed away. According to past records, every two months, there would be a healthy liver suitable for transplantation, but whether or not the liver would be compatible with Felicia was another question. In other words, the possibility of a liver transplantation ultimately was still a waiting game.

Thus our top priority was to stop the cancer cells in Felicia's liver from spreading. If the cancer migrated outside her liver, then changing liver would prove useless and futile.

That night, we headed towards the Grand Hotel on Cheng-Ching Lake. The window opened to the lake before us, its stillness stirred by the faint ripples on the lake surface. The beautiful moon and a blanket of stars glimmered above us, casting silvery light rays on the water. I accompanied Felicia on her graduation trip after she graduated from college, and the Cheng-Ching lakeside was where we strolled and shared our thoughts and dreams. After she returned to Taiwan, our whole family had also taken a trip to Cheng-Ching Lake. However, our thoughts and feelings that evening were completely different from those previous trips.

We sat on the balcony. The shimmering lake was as captivating and breathtaking as before, just like the first time we came. I said to Felicia, "Let's go out for a walk." Felicia laughed and said, "We've already walked for forty years." Ah, yes! In the blink of an eye, it had already been forty-two years. From the time we first met till we got married, we committed ourselves to a lifetime journey together. Though we were no longer young, our love for each other had grown into vintage maturity and sweetness with the passage of time.

In the dark of the night, the lake exuded a beauty of mystique. We held hands under the pristine moonlight. I knew that in her heart, Felicia was still thinking about Dr. Chao-Long Chen's words: the imperative was to find a suitable liver in order to perform the transplantation. But how long could her body wait?

I said to Felicia, "Don't worry. If time runs out and we haven't found you a suitable liver, as long as mine is suitable, I'll give it to you." Felicia was extremely moved. She grasped my hand tightly, just like when we made our promise to be together for a lifetime, she was unable to speak for some time. That night, we lingered by the shimmering beauty of the lake, with the celestial heaven and earth close to our hearts. The picturesque lakeview in front of us, the light breeze that caressed us, the poignant heart-to-heart talks — roused inside us a wistful feeling. Felicia and I held the same hope — she would recover and we could continue to hold hands and walk an even longer journey together.

In order to stop the migration of the tumors in Felicia's liver, it was necessary to control the growth of the cancer cells in the liver. My classmate Dr. Andrew Huang said since none of the drugs had any effect on Felicia, and any medicine would cause her tremendous physical pain, he suggested Felicia to have another transarterial intrahepatic embolization (TIE) operation. The operation, which was called chemo-embolization (CE), would be different from the previous procedure. The CE procedure involved an anti-cancer drug as well as a gel substance causing blockage to enhance the anti-tumor effect. The plan was to have the operation at the Sun Yat-Sen Cancer Center, because Dr. Bo-Hsiang Chuang, the vice-president of the Sun Yat-Sen Cancer Center, was an internationally renowned TIE specialist. Sun Yat-Sen Cancer Center's repute in TIE operations is respectable, and it is also well-known for its very high success rate.

In March 1999, Felicia was admitted into the Sun Yat-Sen Cancer Center for the TIE operation. Because Felicia grew extremely weak, they only performed a TIE on the right liver lobe. Although the operation was performed at the Sun Yat-Sen Cancer Center, Dr. An-Li Cheng kept a close eye on Felicia's condition at all times. He knew that Felicia was in for a rough time. With the arteries in the liver plugged up, the pressure building up in the internal organs induced such insuppressible tightness and pain that the agony was vividly similar to the suffering Felicia experienced the pain when her cancer recurred. It hurt so much she could hardly sit up. Felicia endured the pain for that one last hope — the liver transplantation. At the Sun Yat-Sen Cancer Center, besides the special care from Professor Juei-Low Sung and Dr. Andrew Huang, my old classmate Dr. Che-Hsiong Chen and his wife, who recently returned to Taiwan and worked at the Sun Yat-Sen Cancer Center, were particularly attentive to Felicia and gave her a great deal of encouragement.

Felicia stayed at the Sun Yat-Sen Cancer Center for almost a month. After leaving the hospital, it was of course mandatory to continue close observation. The preliminary results were already out; not only had the tumors in her right liver lobe shrunk, they had also ceased growing. After the TIE operation, Felicia experienced pain and was running a fever, and due to the poor condition of her liver, she also suffered from acute jaundice. Felicia left the hospital physically exhausted, but she strongly believed her strength and perseverance could keep her going until the moment she would receive the liver transplantation.

During the month at the Sun Yat-Sen Cancer Center, Felicia worked from her hospital bed as usual. Every day, she edited the reports of her students and research assistants and telephoned to make sure everything was under control in the laboratory. I was also her postman, delivering messages for her, to and fro, between the laboratory and the hospital. Because of the pain in her liver caused by the TIE procedure, she was often unable to sleep. Even taking sleeping pills did not help, so night-time also became her work time. I advised Felicia not to work too hard, she would always say that she was not able to know how the wait for the liver transplantation would turn out. If the unexpected happened, then she would not have much time left, so it was all the more important for her to get everything done.

I understood how Felicia felt: though she had to hope for the best, she was also prepared for the worst; she just did not allow herself to express it in front of us. As a scientist, her faculties of reason made her clearer than everyone else regarding her own physical condition. That was certainly her most painful and agonizing moments.

Each time she was discharged from the hospital, she would always go to the office first so that she could check out on the state of the laboratory. Usually, after updating herself on the progress of the work, Felicia would convene a meeting involving all laboratory staff. This time around, when Felicia was discharged from the hospital, she went to the laboratory as usual. What made her colleagues in the laboratory sad was that her frailty and fatigue were discernibly obvious.

In the past, Felicia's voice was sonorous despite her condition. In meetings, she was always energetic. But at that time, when the research assistants were presenting their reports, Felicia dozed off, exhausted. That was the first time Felicia's co-workers witnessed her state of exhaustion and failing health. They finally realized that Felicia's condition was deteriorating, and they were in deep shock and grief. They let her sleep, undisturbed.

Wen-Hsiang Chang, Wei-Chen Liao, Nian-Tsu Chang, and De-Ping Sun had been working with Felicia in the laboratory for many years. It was not until this very moment that they saw the sickly look on Felicia's countenance. They continued their discussion in the meeting until their teacher woke up, and when she did, they advised her, "You're too tired; go home first and get sufficient rest…"

The Wait for the Liver Transplantation

I personally telephoned the chief superintendents of the Chang Gung Memorial Hospital, NTU Hospital, Veterans General Hospital and other hospitals requesting for assistance to find a suitable liver for Felicia. They had all agreed to do their best, but the opportunity for a suitable liver had not arrived. The tumors in Felicia's right liver lobe were under control as a result of the TIE operation performed at the Sun Yat-Sen Cancer Center, but the cancer cells in the left liver lobe were still spreading. In April, Dr. Chao-Long Chen telephoned to say there was a liver available, but he later discovered that this liver was not in good functioning condition, and so Felicia lost her first opportunity for a liver transplantation. The tumors in Felicia's left liver lobe continued to multiply ferociously. If there was no liver available for transplantation, it could really spell the end. Dr. An-Li Cheng was extremely worried. He told me that in his professional opinion, it would be a crisis that was extremely difficult for Felicia to make it through; she had three to six months at the most.

Felicia was clearer than others about her own situation. But she had already decided that she would hold on until a liver was available for transplantation; there was no way she was giving up now. But with the condition of her left liver lobe worsening, it became crucial to perform another TIE operation. In May 1999, Felicia was admitted to the Sun Yat-Sen Cancer Center again to have a TIE operation on her left liver lobe.

Because Felicia's reaction to the previous TIE operation was extremely violent, the doctors reduced the amount of anti-cancer drugs for the procedure. However, she still suffered from all the previous side effects, as well as pain resulting from the pressure on internal organs induced by the TIE operation. The severity of the reaction made it difficult for Felicia to eat and sleep. Seeing her suffering from such great pain, my heart hurt like stabbing wounds. I could not help but think of Dr. Cheng's words: "Given Felicia's present condition, the pain that she experiences from taking medicine already surpasses what her body can withstand."

But Felicia would never wave the white flag in surrender, she continued to grit her teeth and play tug-of-war with time, praying that God would enable her to hold on just a little longer for her last hope. The operation in May had put her through close calls with death experience; the pain afflicted was, figuratively, ripping and disintegrating her body into thousands of broken branches and fallen leaves, but the pain no longer bothered her. She simply wanted to know if the growth of the tumors had been suppressed, and whether the operation had bought her time to wait for the liver transplantation.

I understood what Dr. Cheng was telling me. Felicia was truly fueling herself on faith and determination, just like a candle in the wind, struggling and doing everything she could to burn brilliantly till the end.

The TIE operation on her left liver lobe in May was not as effective as the previous one on the right liver lobe. Felicia's body deteriorated like a looming sunset. The second TIE operation she had on the left liver lobe resulted in a severe accumulation of fluid in her pleural cavity. Sometimes it was so severe that, in one day, six hundred cubic centimeters of fluid was drawn and extracted. Tests on the fluid revealed the presence of cancer cells, indicating that growth of Felicia's tumors was not suppressed, on the contrary, cancer cells were spreading fiercely, widely, even outside her liver.

The Last Stand

To Felicia, that was the worst news possible. Even though she did not say it aloud, disappointment was written all over her face. Now it was really the medical team and Felicia's last stand. The doctors said she should start chemotherapy once again; at least it could extend her life.

In early July, Felicia was admitted to the NTU Hospital again and she was resolved to continue chemotherapy. The reason for chemotherapy was that cancer cells had been found in the fluid in her pleural cavity, and furthermore, the amount of fluid retention was constantly increasing, making breathing difficult. Every day, approximately five hundred to one thousand cubic centimeters of fluid had to be drawn out. The medical team planned to administer chemotherapy to help Felicia hold on a little longer.

It was already summer vacation. I telephoned David, Faith, and Albert and advised them to prepare to return to Taiwan as their mother's condition was critical. Because David was planning to apply for a research grant, he was working over-time into late nights. He told me he would return immediately as soon as he was done with the work. Faith had just graduated from law school and was preparing to take the bar exam, so she could only return to Taiwan after the exam.

Despite the severity of her illness, Felicia's bed was, as usual, stacked sky-high with the reports of her students and research assistants. Albert had already made plans to return to Taiwan; I said to Felicia that I wished David and Faith could hurry home too. She disagreed, saying that the children's careers were in fledgling phase, and she would not allow her own illness to affect the future of the children.

Felicia's passing in July was like an incomplete music composition, its dissonant and discordant musical notes lost in the oblivion like falling leaves floating soullessly in the wind. Before she checked into the hospital, she told her co-workers that her three children and daughter-in-law were all returning to Taiwan to spend the summer with her. After the chemotherapy, they would certainly go on a family trip. So she advised the staff to give her whatever they wished her to review as soon as possible, as this time she would be gone from the laboratory longer than usual.

This time when Felicia left the laboratory, she never returned.

July is the hot and humid month in Taipei; the air-conditioning in the hospital hummed quietly. Albert stayed at the hospital to accompany his mother; he saw her making telephone calls to the laboratory enthusiastically, carefully correcting each student's research plan page-by-page, and then telling him that after the treatment was over, she was going to have the next treatment session early, so that this time when his older brother and sister returned, the whole family could go traveling.

In the midst of the sweltering heat of July, my heart suddenly plunged into an abysmal cold. Dr. Cheng informed me that he feared Felicia would not make it this time as her condition was continually deteriorating. Although Felicia insisted on receiving chemotherapy, the dosage he administered was extremely small, as her body's organs would absolutely not be able to withstand the side effects of a large dosage. In reality, the chemotherapy regimen planned for Felicia was only to appease her.

July had always been the happiest month for Felicia, the period during which the children would return home for summer vacation. In order to make the most of her time with the children, Felicia would organize all sorts of activities. That year, because of her poor health condition, we planned to just travel within the country. Felicia had fond, vivid memories of her children's annual "pilgrimage" to home for a great reunion with her. On her sick bed, Felicia's eyes sparkled and her face glowed as she spoke of the entire family's travel plans. Her energy level was high as always. But only the doctors and I knew her true medical condition. Regardless of whether Felicia agreed with me or not, I was firm in my heart on the decision to tell our children and daughter-in-law to return to Taiwan immediately.

Because Felicia was ill for such a long time, I was already mentally prepared. But when the moment to face the reality that she was about to depart finally arrived, I was unable to hold myself together emotionally. Thinking that every time I saw Felicia's face might be the last, my heart bled. Was Felicia really going to disappear like a trail of smoke and dissipate into the misty oblivion? I was speechless; what could I ask of Heaven?

21

Death Summons

July, to us as a family, holds our painful grief that will never be cut off from our memories. July also mourns my painful personal sorrow that I will remember for the rest of my life, because it is the month Felicia departed from this earth.

Before admitted to the NTU Hospital, Felicia was constantly hoping for the opportunity to receive a liver transplant. In May when Dr. Chao-Long Chen of Kaohsiung's Chang Gung Memorial Hospital first called from his office to say that they had found a liver, Felicia did not expect to hear good news so soon. She packed her bags quickly, but before she made her airline ticket reservation to Kaohsiung, another call came from the hospital telling her that the blood type of the liver did not match. Poor Felicia had her hopes lifted the first instant, and then dashed the next.

At the Sun Yat-Sen Cancer Center when the left TIE procedure was performed on her, two calls came from Dr. Chen saying that they might have a liver and that they were conducting tests. They later discovered that the liver did not function well and the bilirubin level was too high and therefore, it was concluded that the liver was not suitable for transplantation. Thus, Felicia's hopes were dashed once again. Due to the left TIE operation, Felicia's jaundice became extremely severe; her pleural cavity had also accumulated large amount of fluid. The pain of the TIE procedure and the anti-cancer medicine's strong side effects brought her tremendous suffering, but she gritted her teeth to keep on going, in anticipation for the opportunity to have a liver transplantation.

The extensive fluid accumulation in the pleural cavity made breathing extremely difficult for Felicia. Furthermore, when she had the TIE operation at the Sun Yat-Sen Cancer Center, cancer cells had been found in the extracted pleural fluid. Her condition was constantly deteriorating at such a rate that she might not sustain for a liver transplantation. If the physicians did not administer chemotherapy quickly, a dangerous situation could develop any moment. On July 1, Felicia was admitted to the NTU Hospital for additional chemotherapy.

The Last Chemotherapy Session

The medicine administered for Felicia's chemotherapy treatment on July 8, Thursday, was a drug called Taxotere. The reason for choosing Taxotere was that its chemical structure is very similar to Taxol, a drug that had proven to be quite effective in Felicia's past chemotherapy experience. Taxol had been discontinued because her body was unable to withstand its side effects, but the doctors hoped that Taxotere would yield the same effectiveness as Taxol in fighting her illness.

But Dr. An-Li Cheng was certainly concerned whether Felicia's body would be able to withstand more medicines. And in my heart, could I not help but think the same? I was torn, but there were two reasons why I hoped the doctors would continue to give Felicia medication to prolong her life. First, Felicia's physical condition was critical and desperate, and it was necessary to suppress the spread of cancer cells. Second, I still harbored a shred of hope that a liver transplantation could take place.

The first time Felicia took Taxotere, she experienced a severe reaction. Besides vomiting, hair loss, and oral inflammation, the pain all over her body and the cumulative effect of past chemotherapy treatments had further weakened her body excessively. Dr. Cheng could not help telling Felicia that she really should not take any more medicine. She could no longer be able to withstand the harm inflicted.

Felicia continued to wait for the chemotherapy results. On July 10, after I finished work, I brought along several research reports from Felicia's laboratory and went to the hospital to visit Felicia. I relayed to her the messages from the researchers in the laboratory that they wanted her to take care, get more rest, and not to over-exert herself.

Stacks of papers were strewn on Felicia's bed and table. Her physical condition was extremely poor, but she was on the bed correcting student reports as usual. Seeing me, she said, "On your way back, you can take these reports back to the laboratory for me." I asked disapprovingly why she did not want to get more rest, she merely laughed and replied, "After resting, I feel worse, so it's better to work. At least it makes me more alert and reduces my pain." We talked for a while; I told her that Albert was on vacation and would be home the following Monday. Felicia became excited as soon as I mentioned the children, because she was making vacation plans to spend time with them.

As soon as I left the hospital, I felt the oppressive and sweltering heat of Taipei in July. In my heart, I thought though Felicia's body was weak, her energy level was encouragingly not too bad; perhaps she really could hold on until a suitable liver was found. Then again, perhaps I was just consoling myself. This time when Felicia checked into the hospital, I was constantly put on edge, nervous and uneasy, because I knew cancer cells were already detected in the fluid extracted from her pleural cavity. If the tumors had really spread, then a liver transplantation would be useless. This was the state of my troubled mind as I returned to the office and buried myself in my work to divert my worries.

On July 12, Albert returned to Taiwan and rushed to the hospital immediately to see how his mother was doing. Seeing Albert, Felicia was ecstatic; she engaged Albert in lively conversations about the family trip that we would take when his older brother and sister returned home. As usual, Dr. Cheng monitored Felicia's condition carefully after the first chemotherapy session. After analyzing her examination report, he said to me with his brows furrowed, "The first chemotherapy session was ineffective; the tumors in the professor's liver are continuing to grow."

The doctors briefed Felicia on the examination results. They knew clearly that Felicia wanted to understand every aspect of the treatment procedure, and it was impossible to conceal anything from her. Felicia was not in the least bit discouraged by the news that the first Taxotere treatment was ineffective; she was still determined to continue the chemotherapy. She said to Albert, "Not to worry! This time, the treatment was ineffective.

Next time, I want to increase the dosage. I still want to continue my treatment."

The Insistance to Continue Treatment

I could see the physician's concern in his eyes. Given Dr. Cheng's authority in his field, his anxiety was an unmistakable indicator that, figuratively speaking, the sun had set and the reality was gloomy. This time, though Felicia's energy level was still high, her voice was no longer as bright and sonorous as before. She still waited for the second chemotherapy session to begin; she was determined to eliminate all difficulties in anticipation of the reunion with David, Christelle, and Faith.

I went to the hospital every day to visit Felicia. Entering the hallway of the old building at the NTU Hospital, the smell of medicine pervaded in the air which acted like an invisible wall separating patients from the outside world. Felicia was waiting for me in her hospital room; Albert was there taking care of his mother. In my heart I felt a sudden pang of emotions; I hoped our children would return home soon.

I mentioned to Felicia once again, "Let's tell the kids to come home!" And as before, Felicia was adamant that the children should finish their work on hand. She had it planned that once the next chemotherapy session was over, the children would come home in time for the whole family to go traveling. Felicia pointed out that Faith had just graduated from law school that year and had to take the bar exam immediately which would mark the crucial stage in her budding career, and Felicia did not want her medical condition to affect her children's future. In addition, David was just drafting a research grant proposal; she would feel better if he sent out the proposal before flying home. I could not convince Felicia any further, so I had to give in reluctantly.

In hoping the children to come home, what I really wanted was time. But these were words that I could not say to Felicia, because that was tantamount to declaring a death sentence on her. Dr. Cheng kept telling me that Felicia's condition was extremely dangerous. Although she insisted on continuing chemotherapy, from a doctor's perspective, there was nothing to be gained from doing so.

I told Dr. Cheng that Felicia was expecting to go home after chemotherapy to wait for the children to return. If he did not give her the medicine, Felicia would feel that there was no remaining hope for her, and that would be a huge blow to her determination to live. Dr. Cheng had been Felicia's comrade in the battle against cancer for many years, he knew her personality too well. He thought for a long time and then finally said, "Okay." His tone was full of resignation. But Dr. Cheng still felt that they could only start the second chemotherapy session after her physical condition improved.

I knew Felicia's sentiments. No matter what, she wanted to suppress the spread of the tumors and wait for the liver transplantation. She still planned to fight through at least another five years and finish what she wanted to do. I told Felicia that the doctors were planning the second chemotherapy session for her. Upon hearing the news, her spirit was uplifted. In her heart, Felicia felt she had taken another step forward. As long as she continued with the chemotherapy treatments, it meant that she still had time to wait for the liver transplantation.

Passing through the long hallway to Felicia's hospital room, my thoughts were subdued; leaving the hallway and walking out of the NTU Hospital, my heart was full of sadness. Albert, who studied medicine, was also very clear about Mom's condition. But we comforted ourselves with the thought that Felicia had previously overcome many dangerous situations, we had pulled her away and saved her from the Angel of Death many times. Even if we felt beaten, in our hearts we still hoped that Felicia would be able to conquer yet another crisis, leave the hospital, and return home in good spirits, as she had always done.

July 14 was supposed to be the day that Felicia underwent the second chemotherapy session. Dr. Cheng had made all the necessary preparations, but when that day came, he hesitated and made no move to administer it, because he felt that Felicia's physical condition was still not fit enough for chemotherapy. Felicia was frantic. She questioned why he had not administered the medicine as scheduled and immediately telephoned me. I hurried to the hospital. Albert was in the hospital room; he helped his mother to sit up on the bed. Felicia said, "The second chemotherapy session must be conducted; the children are coming home soon."

Seeing the panic on Felicia's face, I was naturally torn. I knew how determined she was, so I discussed the matter with Dr. Cheng. Dr. Cheng emphasized repeatedly that he was worried that her body would not be able to take the medicine. I said, "You understand Felicia's personality; she's still fighting. If you don't administer her the medicine, she'll come to realize that even the doctors have all given up on her! That would be equivalent to pronouncing her to death sentence." Dr. Cheng was silent for a while before he said, "Then let's wait until tomorrow or the day after, when her condition gets a little better, before administering the medicine."

The Signs of Exhaustion

On July 15, Dr. Cheng felt that they could still wait one more day. That day Taipei was incredibly humid and hot. The air-conditioning in the hospital room hummed quietly, and dark clouds hung ominously low in the sky suggesting it was about to rain, but not a drop of rain was in sight. Felicia fretted over Albert remaining by her side in the hospital for so many days. She even suggested him to go out for a walk on Sunday. I knew she was starting to grow impatient about the wait for the second chemotherapy session.

On July 16, Dr. Cheng finally gave Felicia the second dosage of medicine. This time the dosage he administered was extremely minute, but he was still worried whether Felicia's body would be able to withstand the effects. That afternoon, Felicia slept soundly due to exhaustion. I went to the hospital to visit her as usual. As I passed through the corridor filled with people, it seemed as if they were moving to the drone of the air-conditioning. The past few times I visited the hospital my heart was heavy. The sluggish shuffle of the people in the hallway resembled immovable patients seriously ill for thousands of years, and one by one, they were adhered to the wall waiting for their disease to be removed from them. I tiptoed into the hospital room so as not to disturb Felicia. Albert was not there; most likely he went to the sundry store to buy something while his Mom was sleeping. The table beside the bed was full of Felicia's data sheets, papers, and documents. I helped to tidy the table, and absent-mindedly laid my eyes on a document that Felicia had faxed to the laboratory on July 4. This was what she had written:

Laboratory Colleagues:

While you are having the general meeting, I would like to take this opportunity to briefly describe the results of my examination report received on Thursday. They were as follows:

1) Blood: generally speaking, normal. Liver function was not good; no problem with kidney function.
2) Chest X-ray: evidence of fluid accumulation since May 21; it's dragged on far too long, not a good sign.
3) CT scan: fluid in the chest. Because the liver is enlarged, it is pressing up against the diaphragm. The lungs are filled with fluid, so breathing is difficult; the stomach is distended.
4) This morning (July 5) I'm scheduled to have another chest X-ray; after that the fluid in my chest will be extracted. The fluid will then be cultured and tested by both Dr. Yang and Dr. Cheng in their laboratories to determine if there are cancer cells present. If there are no cancer cells, a CE will probably have to be performed on the rear half of the right liver lobe (to be discussed later). If there are, it means that tumors might be growing in the pleural fluid (too much time has passed since the CE on May 21; it's not likely that it's reactive). The doctors are preparing to give me another chemotherapy session. This treatment will influence the possibility of my liver transplantation; at the very least it must be pushed back. Will know whether or not the pleural fluid contains cancer cells by Monday afternoon or Tuesday. I don't know when I can leave the hospital; it will depend upon the results of the examination today or tomorrow and whether or not the chemotherapy is continued. Everyone, please do not worry and continue to work hard. If you have any problems call or fax me. See you all soon!

From Felicia

In the letter, aside from describing her own condition, she emphasized that everyone should continue to work hard. My heart heavy, I put away the letter. Why did it feel so stifling and gloomy this afternoon? The door to the hospital room opened softly; I knew that Albert had returned. I said softly to Albert, "Mom has just taken the second dosage of medicine, so we need to be particularly careful." Albert nodded. At that point, Felicia woke up, saw us, and smiled wanly. She made no move to rise from the bed. I let her lie there. The telephone rang.

I answered the telephone. It was Wan-Chan on the line from Hawaii. She wanted to know how her older sister was doing. I described her condition briefly. Wan-Chan said she wanted to speak to her older sister. Normally, when her siblings called, Felicia would be ecstatic and be the first to reach for the phone. But today, Felicia responded in an unusual tone and manner, "I'm tired. I don't feel like talking. I'll call her when I'm feeling a little better." After hanging up, Felicia said that she was extremely uncomfortable, and that she slept very fitfully. I called the doctor on duty. He perscribed her sleeping medication. After Felicia had taken the medication, I waited for her to fall asleep before leaving the hospital room. When I left the hospital, I was confronted by the oppressive afternoon heat, and my steps were slow and heavy. The thought that I should make a call to David and Faith to rush home flashed in my mind again; I had never seen Felicia in such an unexceptional state of fatigue and exhaustion before. Dr. Cheng had been correct; even an infinitesimally small dosage was a huge burden on Felicia's body. A feeling of uneasiness lurked in my heart.

That evening, I telephoned David and Faith to inform them that their mother's condition was not good and that they should return immediately, if possible. The children were astonished and asked me disbelievingly, "Is the situation really that serious?" I had no way of giving them a definite answer. In the past, it seemed that Felicia had been in many more dangerous situations and made it through then, despite the many twists and turns. Of course, I hoped Felicia would be able to pull through yet again and leave the hospital. Ah! This would be our whole family's last strand of hope, we pinned all our hopes on Felicia's indefatigable determination.

That night, I tossed and turned in my bed, unable to sleep.

On Saturday, July 17, I called Albert from work. Albert told me that Mom had slept relatively well the night before, but he noticed she didn't speak at all, he figured that she must really be in a lot of pain. I told Albert that after work I would go directly to the hospital, but I felt extremely uneasy, and the unsettling feeling grew and intensified. Not long after, Albert called back to say that Mom's condition was not good. I hung up and rushed to the hospital.

Entering the room, I saw Felicia attempting to get up. She sat propped up sideways on the bed and said, "This time after receiving the medicine, I really don't feel well." Felicia's eyes were sunken. Because all her hair had fallen out, she was wearing a hat; deep wrinkles were etched in her forehead from the long years of struggle. It was a countenance of sickness, which I rarely saw in her. I asked Felicia once again about requesting the children to return home. She replied with a firm, "No." I said, "How about letting the children decide for themselves?" She did not say any more; there were tears in her tired dreary eyes. What was Felicia's feeling in her heart? She was rarely sad or in despair, but hearing me mention again that I wanted the children to come home, her heart must have surged with emotions, like a stormy tempest, unable to calm down. Of course, Felicia did not know that I had already telephoned the children the night before, telling them to return home immediately.

That afternoon, Felicia felt very tired. During those rare occasions when she spoke to Albert and me, her voice was soft and feeble. Though she herself was not feeling up to par, Felicia still repeatedly told Albert and me to go home and rest. She said her time would be spent sleeping in the hospital, and advised us not to worry. I knew that if we did not leave, Felicia would begin to worry and then toss and turn on the bed, and would be unable to rest well. I watched her till she had slept more deeply before leaving the hospital room for the night. Our home was empty and lonely. I was unable to appease my worries and my heavy heart. I was worried that Felicia would make a sudden turn for the worse. That night I could not sleep.

The next day, July 18, was a Sunday. I rose at dawn and hurried off to the hospital. The nurse said, "Yesterday the doctor prescribed medicine to help her sleep, but last night she still didn't sleep well." The doctors on duty also explained Felicia's condition to me in detail; they all thought that Felicia's energy level after this chemotherapy session was low and worrying. We could only wait until the chemotherapy took effect in order to ascertain the effectiveness of the treatment. Just as we were finishing our discussion, Felicia awoke. Seeing us, she smiled and said, "I'm a little tired, but it doesn't matter. After resting a while I'll be fine!"

Albert and I remained in the hospital room. Seeing her pallid yellow face, our hearts were heavy; we of course felt that the situation was not as rosy as Felicia believed to be. In July, the sun's rays are bright and overbearing, even at dawn, the scorching heat is a dizzy stifle. Albert and I could only wait in anticipation for Felicia to make it through this test.

Contracting Septicemia

In the afternoon, my mother was not feeling well, so I went home to bring her some medicine, and cautioned Albert to keep in touch with me at all times. Mother asked me how Felicia was doing. I made a brief reply; I did not want my ninety-two-year-old mother to worry. This time Felicia was admitted into the hospital for so long, our relatives were extremely anxious, especially my mother. She asked repeatedly to go to the hospital to visit Felicia, but I managed to stop her. I did not wish to see elderly folks worry, and I was even less willing to add on to Felicia's psychological pressure, so I always cautioned family members about letting their anxiety show through. That afternoon at around four o'clock, Albert telephoned me. He told me, in a panicky, frightened tone, that he feared there was something wrong about his Mom's condition, and I rushed back to the hospital.

Upon arriving at the hospital, I saw Felicia moving a little. She said, "It really is extremely painful; my body feels as if it's on fire." It was already six or seven o'clock at dusk. At that very instant, Felicia's whole body suddenly turned cold and she shivered uncontrollably. I felt Felicia's forehead. It was burning hot; she had a fever. A realization struck me — Felicia had caught septicemia. It was Sunday; the doctors were all gone. I hurried to find Dr. Yang and told him that there was a change in Felicia's condition. Dr. Yang rushed to the hospital quickly from his house and examined Felicia. He discovered that her right thigh had turned red and swollen. He knew that she had an infection, and immediately arranged to have her moved into the intensive care unit.

The more than fifty successive chemotherapy sessions that Felicia received over her lifetime had wreaked severe damage to her health. Now her body's immune system was virtually unable to fight off any bacterium, so it became crucial to administer the strongest antibiotics available to stop the spread of bacteria. Felicia changed into the garbs worn in the intensive care unit. The nurse took off Felicia's wedding ring and watch, and gave them to me for safekeeping; I put them in my pocket. Albert and I helped to set up Felicia's IV and checked the blood pressure, pulse and heart rate readings on the instruments. It was not until one o'clock in the morning that we left the hospital room.

It was already two o'clock in the morning on Monday, July 19 when we reached home. I telephoned David and Faith, informing them that their mother's condition was precariously dangerous and that they should fly home immediately. The two children panicked. They knew their Mom had already been sick for thirteen years and had even been through an abyss of misery with high dose chemotherapy at NIH. She had always been able to triumph and escape the clutches of death, but they were in disbelief that this particular chemotherapy session produced such an unexpected outcome.

The two children said to me that they would find and book the earliest flight immediately and inform me as soon as they had confirmed their flight schedules. It was a little past two in the morning when the children called to inform me their arrival time. David would arrive at Chiang Kai-Shek International Airport on the same evening at a little past eight, and Faith would arrive the next day after five o'clock in the morning. It was another sleepless night of turning and tossing on the bed. I was constantly worried that Felicia's situation would take a turn for the worse in the middle of the night, so I kept my eye on the phone by my bedside. Slightly past five in the morning, a call came from the intensive care unit. Felicia was having trouble breathing and she had to be hooked up to a respirator immediately. Felicia gave her consent. I asked the doctor to attend and handle it at once and I sped to the hospital.

Albert and I arrived at the hospital room at the intensive care unit slightly before six o'clock in the morning of July 19. The tube from the respirator was inserted into Felicia's trachea. Felicia was still conscious. Seeing Albert and me by her side, she nodded her head at us with a gratified look, and acknowledged that she knew she had been hooked up to a respirator, she also tried to reassure us that it didn't matter, and we shouldn't worry. My heart hurt like a stab wound. I told her that the children had already boarded the planes and were heading home; she had to hold on. At seven o'clock, Dr. Cheng arrived at the intensive care unit. Felicia was still conscious. Although she was not able to speak through her mouth, she made conscious effort to gesture with her hands. She pointed at the numbers on the respirator to indicate to Dr. Cheng that she be updated on her condition. Dr. Cheng told her, "Professor, please don't worry; I'll pay attention to it."

In fact, after Felicia saw Dr. Cheng, she relaxed and calmed down considerably; she knew that Dr. Cheng understood her physical condition, so she wanted him to make sure the other doctors and nurses in the intensive care unit would keep a close watch on her situation, which of course, he did. As Dr. Cheng left the hospital room, he told me in deep grief that although his teacher's mental state was still clear, he feared that her condition was deteriorating. If the septicemia could not be brought under control, he estimated that Felicia was already hanging onto her last day, or her last two days.

The cause of septicemia is bacteria. The bacteria multiply inside the blood and continuously produce poisonous substances. These poisonous substances latch onto the wall of blood vessels, rendering them unable to control the permeation of water. The water in the blood vessels then flows out into the body, causing edema. Normally, blood vessels are semi-permeable; the water in blood vessels and the body fluid outside the vessels maintain an equilibrium. But when the water inside blood vessels flows outward, the osmotic pressure of blood decreases, and a subsequent blood pressure drop will cause the patient to go into shock.

There are several keys to the treatment of septic shock. First, it is necessary to employ an IV to give patients sufficient fluid; second, it is necessary to give patients vasoconstricting agents. Constriction of blood vessels leads to an increase in blood pressure. These two steps enable patients to maintain a normal blood pressure. The third step is to give patients antibiotics to kill the bacteria spreading in their blood. But if septicemia patients are unable to control the acidification of blood caused by bacteria, then this will cause the entire treatment process to enter a vicious cycle.

The pH level of a normal person's blood is 7.0. When the poisonous substance latches onto the blood vessel, sodium ions leave the blood vessels and hydrogen ions enter the blood vessels, acidifying the blood. The acidification of blood renders the vasoconstricting agents ineffective; it then becomes necessary to give patients an injection of sodium bicarbonate ($NaHCO_3$) to neutralize the acidified blood. Subsequently, the vasoconstricting agents raises the blood pressure, allowing patients to maintain a normal blood pressure.

However, after sodium bicarbonate is used up, the blood pressure subsequently decreases, and the vasoconstricting agents are once again rendered ineffective. Thus, it becomes necessary to add sodium bicarbonate again, perpetuating the cycle. Felicia's situation was exactly like this. Because her blood pressure was too low, there was not enough oxygen reaching her brain, and she was already beginning to experience some dizziness and lose her consciousness.

That was the least optimistic condition one would want to see in a septic shock patient. Eyebrows knitted, forehead furrowed, anxiety was written all over on Albert's face and mine. Sometimes when Felicia appeared to be more alert, she would open her eyes and look at us, and then she wearily forced a knowing expression to acknowledge our presence, but her consciousness was no longer as lucid compared to the same morning. Albert and I kept on encouraging her, telling her that she had to continue fighting, now that her determination was the key to survival. Felicia nodded her head wearily as before. Throughout my life, I rarely experience hopelessness and disillusion. Now I sat inside the hospital room and sank into abysmal loneliness and fear.

The Demise of a Formidable Warrior

Every single words of what Dr. Cheng said hurt like ten thousand needles piercing through my heart. I knew Felicia's situation was extremely grave, but I refused to believe that this time she would not be able to make it. Yet, I am also a doctor and I was completely clear about Felicia's condition. That morning when I saw her, her arms and legs were swollen, the color in her face was completely drained, and her lips went purple. Her septicemia just would not improve; the water in her blood vessels continued to flow outward, and the increase in pleural fluid caused breathing difficulty. Furthermore, the acidification of her blood rendered the vasoconstricting agents ineffective, making it necessary to keep on injecting sodium bicarbonate. Her blood pressure would rise and she gained temporary consciousness for a short spurt. But after the effect of the injection subsided, her blood pressure dropped, and Felicia would once again sink into a hazy state. Her blood pressure climbed and plummeted but remained consistently below the normal range. The continuous injecting of water into her body would make her more and more swollen, forcing her heart and lungs to bear an even greater burden. Septicemia is a complication that cancer patients fear most. Having undergone over fifty chemotherapy sessions, the function of her organs became weaker after each session, and now her body was unable to defend itself against the attack of septicemia. The administration of medication could only serve to prolong her time.

"Felicia, don't give up," I prayed silently. My heart filled with hopelessness, I could find no words with which to ask anything of the Heaven above. I had accompanied and walked with Felicia through many difficulties and dangers. This time, I had lost the faith to win the battle with her. After Dr. Cheng left, Dr. Pan-Chyr Yang rushed over to monitor Felicia's condition again; he entered the intensive care unit and briefed the staff on administering medication. Seeing Felicia alternating between dazed and conscious states, he hung his head low and sighed. He said to me, "This time the question of life or death has really come to a head." He was deeply worried that Felicia was already at the stage of hanging onto her spent force and strength, like an arrow at the end of its flight, and he also feared that she might not even make it through that very day.

I was speechless. Trapped in disbelief, brutal reality, and the unexpected turn in the chain of events, I feared that Felicia would suddenly leave us and depart from this world and fall into the ravine of eternal loneliness. At a loss, I stood by Felicia's side, telling her incessantly that the children were coming home, and that she had to wait for their return. During those sporadic few moments when Felicia was alert, she would nod her head as if telling me that she understood, but most of the time, her blood pressure remained alarmingly low, and she sank into a state of semi-consciousness. The doctor added sodium bicarbonate to the IV to increase her blood pressure, but even then it was only possible to bring it up to 50 or 60 mm Hg. At that moment, tubes of every kind were inserted all over Felicia's body, and instruments of every type were placed next to her bed.

The display panels charted rapidly changing trajectories of lines and the monitor screens flashed a chaotic string of fluctuating numbers. Albert and I kept vigil next to Felicia, hoping that she knew we would never leave her, hoping that she would fight back bravely for us and pull through.

At around twelve o'clock, Wei-San Wang, an old friend of Felicia and mine, came by the hospital. In the morning, he called me to inquire after Felicia's condition. In my anxiety and emotional turmoil, I told him that Felicia's situation was not good. He rushed over immediately.

Wei-San was the classmate of Felicia's younger brother Hsi-Kuan and a lifelong friend of Felicia's family. He regarded Felicia as his own older sister, and he had been friends with us for over thirty years. When Wei-San came over, it happened to be visiting hours at the intensive care unit. He was so anxious to see Felicia that I let him go in first. At that point of time, Felicia was already unable to speak and constantly floated in and out of consciousness, but she knew that Wei-San had come to see her. Having her trachea connected to the respirator, Felicia was in deep pain; tears welled up at the corner of her eyes. Wei-San was torn upon seeing Felicia. I was distraught. Words were beyond us to profess our immense sorrow, which we expressed through the meeting of our eyes.

I fell into deep anxiety. Every single moment was torturous; how I hoped that in the next instant Felicia would be awake. But I knew that was just my wishful thinking, a fool's dream. I did not know what I should do to help Felicia pull through. As I thought of the children who would be flying in from faraway places, I wanted to cry but had no tears left.

Mobilizing the Hemodialysis Machine

At a little past two in the afternoon, Dr. Shu-Hsiun Chu, the former vice-superintendent of NTU Hospital and a former classmate of mine, arrived at the intensive care unit to examine Felicia. He saw Felicia's condition and told me that I should be mentally prepared; this would probably be it. At that time, Felicia was almost completely in a state of semi-consciousness, and in addition, because water was constantly being added to her body, she was bloated beyond recognition. I said to my old classmate, "The children are already on their way home. No matter what, it is necessary to enable Felicia to hold on until the children get here. But because Felicia's entire body is swollen, the pressure on her heart is already too great. I'm worried that her heart won't be able to take it and something will happen." As Dr. Shu-Hsiun Chu was a leading authority in cardiology, I asked his opinion on how to reduce the burden on Felicia's heart.

Dr. Shu-Hsiun Chu called an emergency meeting, asking for input from specialists of every field. The meeting ended at around three o'clock when Dr. Shu-Hsiun Chu had an urgent discussion with me. He suggested using a hemodialysis machine to remove excess water from Felicia's body.

A hemodialysis machine filters out poisonous substances from the blood of patients with kidney problems. So the doctors suggested using a hemodialysis machine to extract blood from Felicia's body, cleanse it, and then pump it back into her body. By using the machine to reduce the water content of her blood, not only the burden on Felicia's heart would be decreased, her blood pressure could be stabilized too. The swelling would also be alleviated to some degree.

I thought this would perhaps be the only way to prolong Felicia's life and gave permission for a hemodialysis machine to be used. At a little past three, another machine was added to the array beside her bedside. After an hour, her blood pressure gradually stabilized; although it was only about 60 or 70 mm Hg, at least it did not alternate between the highs and lows. Albert and I both heaved a sigh of relief albeit slightly. It was about ten minutes to five in the afternoon when NHRI secretary-general Winston Yu rushed over to visit Felicia. I told him that Felicia's condition was fraught with grim difficulties.

Departing This Life, Departing From the World Forever

It was evening. The scene outside the intensive care unit was a flurry of movements — the pacing and anxious look of the visitors, and the brisk and quick footsteps of medical staff attending to emergencies. The hospital was a real, vivid portrayal of the comings and goings of life and death. Those who have never experienced the passing of their loved one would not be able to understand the powerlessness and despair of the family members, whose beloved one suffers on the brink of life and death.

Winston Yu was in the hospital room with Albert and me. Noticing that Felicia's condition began to stabilize, he asked us if we had our dinner.

I replied that the two of us had not eaten anything since the night before. Albert and I were drained and exhausted. Winston advised us to take care and have our regular meals regardless of the situation, so that we have the energy to handle the difficult moments. Seeing that Felicia's situation seemed to have stabilized a little and thinking that Albert should also eat something, I said to Albert, "Let's go eat something and then come back."

I briefed the medical caregivers with some instructions, and reminded them to keep a close watch at all times. I picked up my cellular phone, and walked out of the intensive care unit with Albert and Winston. Our footsteps were heavy. We walked along the corridor and were approaching the door of the hospital when my cellular phone suddenly rang. The call came from the intensive care unit informing me that Felicia's heartbeat had stopped; they were trying to resuscitate her. Albert and I immediately sprinted back and dashed into the intensive care unit.

By then, artificial resuscitation had already been completed; Felicia's mouth and nose were covered in blood. Her heartbeat had returned. The doctors had employed defibrillation and artificial resuscitation to revive Felicia, but the electric shock seemed to have damaged her internal organs and ribs. That, Felicia was in immense pain, was expressed clearly on her blood-stained face, which was convulated in spasm. Albert and I embraced her body. We were in tears and were inconsolable. I told the doctors not to do it again, and to take away the hemodialysis machine as well. If her heartbeat stopped again, a drug injection to stimulate her heart would lessen her ordeal; she was already approaching the end. I was unwilling to let Felicia suffer so much towards the end of her life; I just wanted to let her go peacefully.

It was already past seven. Albert and I stayed by Felicia's side, each of us holding her hand. I told her that we were going to accompany her as she walked the last stretch of her life's journey. I said to Felicia that to have her as my lifetime companion was the most fortunate thing to have happened in my life. I was both grateful and thankful for what she had done for our family in her lifetime, and I did not have any regrets for the forty-two years we spent together. I would be waiting and one day we would certainly be reunited in Heaven.

Albert and I remained by Felicia's side. We saw her blood pressure dropping, lower and lower. The doctor came and gave her an injection to stimulate her heart, but there was no way to bring her back. Felicia was unable to hold out any longer for David and Faith. Albert and I held her tight. Her blood pressure fell lower and lower, and her breathing weaker and weaker, until there was no response registered on the respirator. Felicia had stopped breathing. Albert and I could not help but embraced Felicia. We cried inconsolably, in deep grief. We could not bear to leave by her side.

Felicia departed from this world on July 19, 1999, in the evening at half-past eight. I asked the nurses to cleanse her body carefully and remove all the tubes. When I left the intensive care unit, my brothers and sisters had all heard the news and rushed to the hospital. I asked the husband of my younger sister to buy an instant camera for me, and requested my younger brother and sister to go to the house and bring back some of Felicia's clothes. At nine o'clock, I entered the intensive care unit once again and saw that Felicia had been washed clean. She was in peace. Upon seeing her closed eyes, sadness and grief again welled up inside me. I embraced Felicia, kissed her face, tears running down mine. My younger sister's husband got hold of an instant camera for me, and I took a picture of Felicia. David and Christelle arrived at the hospital then. But their Mom was unable to wait for them.

David never expected that upon arriving at the hospital, his Mom would have already passed away. He and Christelle cried their hearts out. I said to Albert, "Let's go out, and let David and Christelle talk to Mom alone." Outside the intensive care unit, Dr. Yang and Dr. Cheng had also arrived. I asked Dr. Yang to make necessary arrangements for the mortuary and mourning hall. Dr. Yang reassured me that he would take care of everything. At that moment my younger brother and sister had returned from the house with Felicia's clothes. Tears flowed profusely as I took Felicia's clothes and shoes into the hospital room. David, Christelle, Albert and I dressed Felicia and put the shoes on her. We mourned and looked at Felicia's face again. She looked tranquil and at peace. Her serene face told us that she, in Heaven, knew that we were protecting and watching over her.

Slightly past eleven, all the arrangements for the mortuary had been made. The four of us accompanied Felicia to the mortuary. Before she was placed in the refrigerator, we each took an incense and prayed. That was the first time we prayed in reverence of Felicia. A trail of blood trickled down from her nose. My heart wrenched in deep grief as I wiped the blood gently off her. The four of us cried as we pushed Felicia into the refrigerator.

That was the first night after we lost Felicia. Heaven had no more words for my grieving heart. The children and I returned to the house listlessly. It was already past midnight. I sat on the bed for a long time, dazed and lifeless. Felicia's sweet fragrance seemed to linger in the air, but she was already gone. From that moment onward, I had to accept the cruel reality that Felicia was no longer with us.

One inevitably feels the loss of an eternal separation and the longing that comes along. I asked Heaven for an answer, but received none. I tossed and turned the entire night, my eyes brimmed with tears. As soon as day broke after four, our whole family went to the airport to fetch Faith home. Faith came out, saw us, and started to cry immediately. She knew that Mom had departed. Faith embraced all of us, tears streaming down her face. She kept on saying, "Take me to see Mom." We headed straight to the NTU hospital mortuary.

Opening the refrigerator door, we saw Felicia in a peaceful repose. Our whole family embraced and cried together. Faith cried and murmured repeatedly, "Mom, I've come too late." She caressed Felicia's face and said, "I want to help Mom shape the eyebrows and I want to share small talks with you." The other children and I left the mortuary and let Faith to have some private moments with Felicia. Now, the whole family was learning to live with the truth that Felicia was no longer with us. Ah! How difficult to live with the cruel reality!

The Funeral

Inside the NTU hospital mortuary, a simple altar had already been set up for Felicia. In my heart, I made conversations with Felicia: "Do you know that the children have all returned?" But Heaven remained silent without a word. The children and I returned to Nankang and made arrangements for the funeral service. I discussed the formality of the funeral with the children. I said to the children, "Mom didn't have a specific religious affiliation, but after she became ill, whenever she passed by a temple or shrine, she would always pray earnestly, and implore Heaven to give her the strength to fight cancer. And according to traditional Taiwanese customs, most people choose a Buddhist funeral. Mom was born a Taiwanese, and she died on the soil of her motherland, so I suggest that the ceremony be handled according to traditional Taiwanese customs."

The children respected the viewpoint and trusted that Mom's funeral would be a solemn service honoring her life. That day I made preparations for a traditional Taiwanese funeral. The children and I shared the wish that Felicia would have a safe and smooth journey to Heaven.

On Tuesday, July 20, the day after Felicia passed away, we received a call from Dr. Chao-Long Chen. He said that there was a liver suitable for transplantation into Felicia. But I could only tell him, devastatedly, that Felicia had passed away the previous evening. Felicia persisted with great perseverance to wait, but this time even she could not avoid the summons of death. I did not know whether or not this was fate. Perhaps, Heaven knew that Felicia had gone through tremendous suffering in the past thirteen years, and thus showed compassion onto her to allow her to return to Heaven. In Heaven, she would no longer suffer from pain and illnesses, she would not be forced to endure the excruciating ordeals of treatment, and she could finally free herself from the clutches of illnesses.

Felicia's funeral was set for August 3 for two reasons: first, to adhere to the Taiwanese customs that no funerals to be held during the month of July; and second, because the children were not able to stay too long. The children and I made the unanimous decision to go for cremation for Felicia. This was also in accordance with Felicia's wishes; she had mentioned it to me once during a hiking trip at Dajianshan. She said Taiwan is small; if everyone chooses land burial, not only would that contribute to a scarcity of land, and land burial is also deemed not as clean as cremation. Now, the least we could do was to let Felicia go peacefully without any obstacles.

The funeral was conducted under the direction of a monk. The children knelt down according to the customs. Although our daughter-in-law Christelle is a Christian, she also prayed with incense, knelt down, and bowed her head along with the other children. Felicia must have been smiling up there in Heaven, thinking what a good wife David had found. I went to Felicia's altar every day, offered her incense, and spoke to her. To think that she was now gone after decades of companionship brought tears to my eyes — it was a grieving sadness that could not be described in words.

The public funeral service was held on August 3 at half-past eight in the morning. I specifically scheduled a time-slot for a final reunion with Felicia. From seven to half-past eight, the children and I gathered close by her side. We voiced our thoughts and sadness at Felicia's side. Uncontrollably, we cried and were in embrace with each other. Felicia lay peacefully in her coffin. I surrounded her with her favorite flowers and photos; among them were photos that we took together at Yangmingshan in front of two intertwining, thousand-year-old trees. Years of harsh weather had withered the leaves and branches, but their trunks remained locked together. In front of the old trees was a wooden placard which read, "Two Hearts united in Eternity." In the picture, Felicia and I stood side by side. I burned the photo, with a conviction that she would know the feelings in my heart.

I caressed Felicia's cold face and gently kissed her lips. After closing the lid of the coffin, my eyes brimmed with tears. The transparent coffin cover now separated Felicia and me. The children weeped silently and tears streamed uncontrollably from their eyes. I was in tears. Felicia was really gone. Heaven knew that Felicia had not given up even in the last moment. She had lived her life to the fullest and now she was ready to embark on a new journey. I would never see her again; she and I could only meet in our dreams.

It was a solemn closing at the funeral service. We chose an auspicious time for Felicia's cremation. Our whole family, relatives and family friends accompanied Felicia to the crematorium. It was noon; the sun shone brightly and the air was oppressively humid. Our whole family prayed to Felicia once again. The auspicious time had finally arrived. Felicia's coffin was sent into the ferocious flames of the cremation oven. Locked in embrace again, we cried. All we have of Felicia, in the future, will be only her bone ashes. It took just one fire and the body which had been subjected to thirteen years of suffering due to illness was reduced to ashes. And by the same fire torch, Felicia was separated eternally from us. Luxuriant leaves and flowers will wither one day, just a flame splinter, a large, roaring fire engulfs and reduces them to flying ashes and swirling smoke.

That day we collected Felicia's bone ashes and placed the urn at the Xin-Dian's Long-Quan Cemetery, which would be the temporary resting place for her. We planned to move her to the Wu family tomb in Lin-Kou a year later.

In Remembrance of Felicia

After Felicia passed away, I was physically and mentally exhausted and I was feeling extremely depressed. There was a feeling of emptiness in my heart. After the funeral, David, Christelle, and Albert left and went back to the United States. Faith was concerned that I was too distraught and would not be able to part with my sorrow, so she stayed in Taiwan for a month to keep me company. I had the photos of Felicia and incense urns prepared for the children, hoping that upon their return to the United States, they would offer her an incense every day in remembrance of her. I also offer and light an incense to Felicia every morning and evening, telling her about everything in my life after our parting. After forty-two years together, and thirty-seven of these as husband and wife, to lose her in a flash of a moment sent my emotions spiraling into a bottomless abyss.

Constantly thinking of Felicia, a feeling of depression enveloped me. Sometimes, I took Faith down to Long-Quan Cemetery to talk to Felicia. To face those days without Felicia was truly difficult.

I knew that if Felicia in heaven were able to see what was happening here on earth, she would not want to see me in such a depressed state. So I told myself that I had to bring myself out of this stalemate; I should not let Felicia worry about me. I understood her wishes: over the many years in her battle against cancer, she kept a detailed record of the entire treatment in the hope that one day it might help other cancer patients. In addition, if her unique life story could serve as an inspiration to disheartened cancer patients, Felicia would nod her head in contentment and smile. I told myself, one step at a time, I had to finish what she had wanted to do in her life.

I took over Felicia's research on cancer metastasis in the hope that I could carry out the project with the same earnest pursuit of truth that Felicia embodied. I published a commemorative anthology, *Song of Life — Dr. Felicia Chen's Commemorative Volume*, enabling Felicia's friends and family to express their feelings for her in writing. Felicia was a member of Zonta, an international women's organization. Two members, Shu-Fang Su and Zhong-Qi Liu, who held her in great esteem, generously donated money for a documentary film on Felicia's life to be made. In order to shoot the footage for this film, director Hsiao-Di Wang, producer Li-Ming

Huang, and our entire family took a trip to retrace the steps that Felicia and I had taken in our life journey.

I hope the story of Felicia's struggle would continue to live on; thus I embarked on a personal mission to write this biography. Her entire life, such extraordinary, unique and filled with genuine passion, and her positive values and her love for her friends, her family, her children and her husband — all of these are worthy of being published.

It has been over a year. I do not feel that Felicia has left me; rather, I feel that she is even closer, because her spirit and vigor reside in my heart. We became one, long ago. Over the last year or so, I have made some difficult adjustments, but as long as I think that Felicia is watching over me, I do not feel alone.

The light from the lotus lantern never goes out, and feelings do not die. Though Buddhism offers no thoughts on the matter, I firmly believe that the love between Felicia and me will not die as a result of the divide between death and life. Our love is also the reason that I am able to walk out from the abysmal depth of sorrow and write about my feelings for Felicia, word by word.

In an instant time passes. One cannot wrest back the vestiges of the past; only with eternal love can we avoid emotional scars and relive the sweet memories. Felicia, how have you been? The children and I offer you incense every day. The smoke from the incense curls up and rises to Heaven, and I yearn to tell you everything that has happened, one after another. The years pass by without a trace. No matter where you are, in Heaven we will meet again soon.

This evening, I would like to tell you my heartfelt thought — may we and our beloved ones, living far apart, live long and healthy, even if we are thousands of miles apart from each other, we can still share the beauty of the same graceful moon at the same time together.

September 20, 2000
Mid-autumn

Epilogue

After Felicia passed away, there was a period of time when my memory was completely blank. Our whole family prepared for her funeral ceremonies with heavy hearts. Felicia passed away on the night of July 19, 1999, at half-past eight. We conducted a service for her on August 3, at nine o'clock in the morning. According to Taiwanese customs, I prayed daily in the mourning hall where Felicia lay, and we had mourning ceremonies which took place every seven days. Despite the scorching summer heat in late July, my heart was frozen in an icy winter shroud. Although I went to work at the office every day as usual, I was just an empty shell devoid of soul and spirit. To this day, my memory of the time when Felicia suddenly left us draws a complete blank, like a disk with memory space being deleted and erased.

What makes me most regretful is that I lost Felicia's wedding ring. At seven o'clock on the evening of July 18 when Felicia was transferred to the intensive care unit, the nurse changed her clothes for her, removed her ring and watch, and gave them to me to keep. That day my mind was in an unsettling chaos. I knew that this was our wedding ring, so I wrapped the ring in a piece of tissue paper and put it in my pocket. That night when I returned home it was already two o'clock, and I was utterly exhausted. I had a premonition that the danger Felicia was in this time would be extremely difficult to overcome. Many thoughts went into my mind, so I could only remember putting Felicia's ring in a drawer, as I desperately rushed to telephone and contact the children.

After Felicia's funeral was over, Faith stayed by my side to keep me company. At that time my emotional state had slightly calmed down in quiescence. I constantly encouraged myself that although Felicia was gone, I have to go on living, because I am the only one who could finish the work that she had set out to do. So I steeled myself to spring into action. I started to plan the tasks I would do for Felicia, and looked through her treatment diary, notes, and other documents. It was then that I remembered the wedding ring. But the strange thing is, though I looked everywhere, I couldn't find it.

I practically left no stone unturned in my search, rummaging through all the drawers, yet our wedding ring seemed to have vanished without a trace. I think of the times I had together with Felicia, and all the experiences we went through. To us, the ring symbolized our lifelong promise. How could I lose it? Felicia has left; could it be that the ring she loved most had vanished like smoke and dissipated like the mist? With the loss of my Felicia, I sank into absymal melancholy. With the irretrievable loss of the ring, I was plunged into a depression. Two years has passed, I still have not found the ring. I do not know whether this was a coincidence that the ring had departed with Felicia too?

I stood in the solitary light on a dark night, cutting a single lonely silhouette. The children had returned to the United States. I had to face the days ahead alone without Felicia. Every morning and evening, I would light a stick of incense, and let the swirling smoke convey my gentle whispers to Felicia. Besides my thoughts, I told her to entrust me to finish what she had wanted to accomplish. With that mission in mind, I would then be able to find the strength to re-emerge from the deep grief. In my remaining years, I am not just living for myself, but also for Felicia. I wanted to be conscientiously proactive and optimistic like Felicia.

Before she passed away, Felicia made notes about her struggle and fight against cancer. She had archived eight large volumes of medical records. She recorded in great details each time she was admitted to the hospital for treatment — the treatment process she went through every day, and the situations and side effects that resulted from the therapies. These records became the primary source from which I wrote her biography, especially during the period when I was in deep sadness and my memory was a complete blank. Her every word and every sentence were deeply etched in my heart, comforted me in my time of sorrow, and enabled me to recall everything that happened — by piecing together again the fragments of memories in Felicia's and my life — in the dark stillness of the night.

Memories are like scars — when one thinks of them, one becomes saddened all over again. Felicia's and my life are still in continuation. Even though she has already departed, she still lives on in my heart. As I arrived at this realm of realization, I came to feel that Felicia has not really gone. She has simply gone to another place to wait for me, to prepare a warm house for our future reunion. Thus, though in my heart I was overcome with grief, I will recover in time and actively plan to accomplish the missions for Felicia.

My original idea was to write about Felicia's extraordinary life, but while writing I discovered that her life was so unique, there were many cherished episodes and events in Felicia's life that I was unable to narrate and write in complete detail in the biography, such as her research career, her research team, the family and friends she loved, the medical team that cared for her, and her relatives who miss her — these constitute the many splendored facets about Felicia. It is inevitable that some details or events were omitted or incomplete, so at the same time as I was writing Felicia's biography, I also planned to publish a commemorative book for her. In the commemorative book, I have compiled the thoughts and feelings of Felicia's friends, advisors, colleagues, and medical caregivers, making up for what has been left out from the biography.

With this concept in mind, I started to invite the writings of friends and colleagues and organize Felicia's pictures, her handwritten manuscripts, and so on. Life after Felicia's passing was bleak, desolate and unbearable, but I gradually became alive once again as I realized the role I could play was to accomplish Felicia's unfinished work. Because I had lost her, I felt hopeless and forlorn, but it was also through the loss that my heart acquired a new spark of vitality and the flame of life began to burn again. In my life, I certainly cannot do without Felicia.

It came as a coincidence at the time that two ZONTA friends, Shu-Fang Su and Zhong-Qi Liu, decided to use their own funds to support the filming of a documentary on Felicia's life and her difficult struggle against cancer. The motivation for this beautiful act actually originated from

Felicia herself. She was a member of the international ZONTA organization, and had previously spoken on her fight against cancer at a ZONTA meeting in Taipei. It was from this speech that Shu-Fang Su had so much respect for Felicia's efforts. ZONTA is an international organization with focus on promoting women's health and rights. Because of Felicia's dual identity as a cancer researcher and cancer patient, ZONTA hoped she would be able to find time to visit their organization in California and deliver her lecture. Felicia naturally accepted the invitation to commit her time for any charitable or social causes.

It was unfortunate that Felicia — at that time undergoing treatment in the hospital — had to cancel the speech appointments with ZONTA on two occasions. The second time happened when Felicia was at the Sun Yat-Sen Cancer Center undergoing an arterial embolization procedure on the left lobe of her liver. At that time, Felicia's medical condition was extremely critical, and it was impossible for her to leave the hospital. However, Felicia, who was always serious about work and never left any loose ends, continued to take to heart about missing the lecture appointments even after she left the hospital. She felt apologetic towards the organizer for the cancellation of two lectures due to her medical condition.

The organizer in Taiwan who made the arrangements was Shu-Fang Su; in the United States, the contact person was Zhong-Qi Liu. Before Felicia joined ZONTA, Shu-Fang already knew that she was the older sister of her former classmate Wan-Chan. The year when Wan-Chan and Shu-Fang attended Taipei First Girls' High School together, Felicia's picture still hung on the school's honorary roll. It made the greatest impression on Shu-Fang, and furthermore, she naturally felt close to Felicia because she was the older sister of a classmate. Felicia and Shu-Fang also went to Shu-Ji Hsu-Weng's house together to learn Hawaiian dance. After Felicia passed away, Shu-Fang said to Zhong-Qi that they should do something in memory of Felicia.

This led to the trip that our entire family, as well as producer Li-Ming Huang and director Hsiao-Di Wang, eventually took to the United States. The project was completely funded by Shu-Fang and Zhong-Qi. The trip to revisit our life in the United States enabled our whole family to reminisce Felicia's life as well as retrace the path that our family had taken to arrive at where we are today. The trip was a walk-through of our life journey — the bitter experience of separation and the warmth of family togetherness. And also the many memory-sharing interview sessions with our dear friends wove together our thoughts and feelings for Felicia that speak volumes of reminiscence, joy and happiness, poignancy, retrospection and requiem. The children and I are thankful that Felicia gave us this unfathomably beautiful life, but Felicia's absence on this trip was certainly emotionally difficult for us!

Our interview schedule and itinerary were extremely tight. From March 12 to March 21, 2000, we visited and covered the Albert Einstein College of Medicine in New York City, our old home in Scarsdale, the SUNY Stony Brook campus, our old home in Long Island, Yale University, Case Western Reserve University, our old apartment in Cleveland, the National Institutes of Health in Bethesda, Maryland, Cornell University, our old home in Ithaca, and just before we wrapped up our trip, we were fortunate to meet Dr. Frank Gump, the doctor who performed mastectomy on Felicia, in New Jersey. Within a short span of ten days, we had completed our journey of memories which brought us roving to different states like in a dreamscape. Our schedule was tight, but everything went remarkably smoothly. Even producer Li-Ming Huang and director Hsiao-Di Wang said that unbeknownst to ourselves, we must have had Felicia's blessing.

Every phase of Felicia's and my life was intricately linked to our academic and research career. The joy and challenges of raising our children, and our return to our motherland, all these came into fruition because of our guiding principle — our lifetime ideal for scientific research — which we firmly uphold. To be able to return and travel on the trodden roads, and to have my children accompany me in exploration of their growing years, was certainly a rare and precious experience. It was also because of Felicia, her strength and her spirit that our entire family was able to take this beautiful trip. On this trip, I relived every single detail of the twenty-three years together with Felicia when we were away from our mother country. In the midst of sorrow and loss, there was warmth, because Felicia had given me an enriching and meaningful life. Through this trip, I learned to cherish deeply the encounters and events in our life, and I also gradually learned to let go of the painful loss of Felicia. At long last, I realized that Felicia had not really left me; she had already taken roots in my heart long ago.

Memories are effective prescription for sorrow and grief. After returning to Taiwan, I threw myself into writing. The editorial work and compilation of material for the commemorative book on Felicia were in good progress. In addition, the National Health Research Institutes and the Institute of Biomedical Sciences at Academia Sinica jointly organized the "Professor Felicia Chen Scientific Symposium and Memorial Service" on July 19, 2000, to commemorate the first anniversary of her passing. I am extremely thankful to have had the opportunity to do my part for Felicia, giving her all of my heart and soul. Our love, deep like the ocean, gave me the strength and motivation to redeem myself and live life again. And also, the inspiring strength and true spirit of Felicia had created a great impact on me.

Now as I ponder, I realize it is certainly the most difficult phase of my life. Nursing the wound in my heart, I discovered that Felicia has not departed from the world. She became my beacon in life long ago. I also believe that she would want me to live on bravely and passionately.

On July 19, 2000, the first anniversary of Felicia's passing, *Song of Life*, Felicia's commemorative anthology, was published through funding by the Health Sciences Foundation, and *A Passion for Life*, a documentary on her life, was also completed. Many distinguished overseas scientists participated in the scientific symposium and memorial service, and among them who spoke were Professor Don McCormick, Felicia's mentor at the Cornell University; Dr. Dipankar Chatterji, one of Felicia's postdoctoral students at SUNY Stony Brook; Dr. Gordon Hammes, a member of the U.S. National Academy of Sciences and my mentor at the Cornell University; and Dr. Jean-Bernard Le Pecq, Felicia's former colleague at the Institute Gustav-Roussy, France. The Taiwanese scientists included Dr. Jacqueline Peng-Wang, director of the cancer research division at the National Health Research Institutes, and Dr. Wen-Hsiang Chang, a former postdoctoral researcher in Felicia's laboratory. The conference was insightful and enriching in the coverage of the topics, and there was not a scientist there who did not mention in their scientific lectures about Felicia's outstanding contributions made to their research fields.

A Passion for Life, the documentary on Felicia's life, was scheduled to be screened at the symposium requiem in the afternoon. The film was extremely inspirational. The children and I, my mother, and all of Felicia's and my siblings were at the screening. I was overwhelmed with a multitude of mixed emotions as the screen projected moving images of my life journey with my children. Felicia was beautiful in the documentary, but now I could only see her on the screen. Though she seemed so close, the distance between us was, sadly, an infinity. Tears fell uncontrollably from my eyes. The moving visuals flashed before my eyes and became a blur, and suddenly my mind was a complete blank.

Music was Felicia's passion. So we organized a memorial service with a music tribute to Felicia during the symposium. We invited pianist Hui-Juan Chen to play the Beethoven piano concerto, "Pathetique," one of Felicia's favorites. Our colleagues at the National Health Research Institutes also formed a choir, and they diligently practiced their repertoire during lunch hours. At the memorial service, they sang Felicia's and my favorite song, "Jasmine." Then they sang "Mother," a song full of filial love, expressing the children's loving reminiscence for their mother:

Mother (composed by Gilmour; Chinese lyrics by Yu-Yuan Wang)

Pursuing dreams and fantasies,
I lost my way on Earth.
Coveting flamboyant vanities
Made my heart filled with loneliness.

In my childhood I was innocent and playful,
With no idea of the nature of sin.
Hidden in Mother's bosom, little hands grasping wildly,
Entreating her to sing songs.

In spring, rain fell lightly outside the window
In autumn, the garden was dotted with droplets.
Mother's tears have never dried,
You know who she prays for.

Mother's love makes my heart break,
Heaven above should treat her with grace.
Tired little bird, why not return to the nest?
Don't forget your childhood home.

Kneeling in front of God and burning incense,
She lives eternally among us.

Do not create irrevocable regret,
She is the only one who loves you.

In spring, rain fell lightly outside the window
In autumn, the garden was dotted with droplets.
Mother's tears have never dried,
You know who she prays for.

Upon hearing this song, streams of tears fell from our children's eyes. I had also lost myself. Thinking of Felicia, my soul had scattered and flown away. When they were finally able to stem the flow of their tears, our children, being overcome with gratitude, spoke of how moved they were by everyone's overflowing memories for their mother, and then they spoke of their own feelings for her. They said:

> It is really something special for us to see so many of you here at our mother's memorial. We would also like to thank everyone who has contributed their efforts and thoughts, especially since the three of us are in the States. As you can imagine, it's difficult for us to talk about our feelings about our mother, and there are many aspects about her which cannot be adequately expressed here today.

> Nonetheless, we'd just like to share a few words with you about her from our perspective. We were eulogizing her as our Mom, because it would be much easier to portray her than in a formal speech. As you know, she was very open with her thoughts and feelings, and showed warmth and friendliness, even towards other people. If Mom were here she'd be so happy to see all of you. These get-togethers of all her friends and family, such as the gala dinner at David's wedding, or our parents' anniversary parties, always made her so happy. Our Mom felt such wonderful feelings for all of you and it showed: she'd be talking and smiling, eating and having fun, or dancing and singing. Of course, there'd be one of us kids around snapping photographs. She was also eager to introduce us, her children, to her friends, family, and colleagues. She was so friendly that she loved to look for connections between people, because we believe she cared for many people just like her own family. She was also

honest and sincere with everyone. As you look through the commemorative book, you can see the sheer energy in her eyes and the joy in her smile. She cherished every moment with her family, us, and you.

This past year, we've been through a lot, and have thought much about her. It's hard to comprehend that Mom is no longer here with us, but the feeling of her being here is strong. She is everywhere. The way she touches our lives every day, even when she is not around, reminds us that our bond is not broken. We each remember how we would hug, how she would take our arms when we walked together, how she would call us for a meal or to get ready to go out. We see her in the things around us — the clothes we bought together, and the cutlery and cooking utensils she got us. We can see her smile; we can hear her voice at times — encouraging us to feel good about ourselves, to find the perfect balance in life, not to worry too much and be happy.

Still, it's been over a year and half since we last sat down together for our dinner at a restaurant in Taipei amidst the noisy buzz and busy bustle. Now there is only silence and stillness. And so we have tried over the past one year to visualize that she is happily united with our loved ones who have also passed on — our grandparents and Margie, who lived with us like our family member for fourteen years. We pray that they are all taking care of one another in Heaven as we would care for one another in the family — Mom taught us to love not only members of our family, but also our friends and acquaintances.

She may not be with us in body and flesh, but she is here, here within our hearts, living strong. She left in us the seeds of her spirit, which we try to nurture in ourselves as best as we can. We hope too that her spirit continues on in all of us, which we believe will be our best tribute to her.

I thanked the children for their words about their mother. Their words represented the feelings of our entire family. That day, my mind was like a blank canvas, and I was struggling within to express my thoughts and feelings, but I was filled with immense gratitude and thanked all the scientists and friends who had come from all over the world to attend the conference in honor of Felicia. I also expressed my sincere and utmost gratitude to our colleagues at the National Health Research Institutes and the Institute of Biomedical Sciences.

One year has already passed. Although I live each day in reminiscence of Felicia, I had accepted the fact that she had already left. At the time of her death, our family tomb was still being constructed, so we placed her ashes temporarily at the Long-Quan Cemetery in Hsin-Dian. One year later when the family tomb was completed and the children came home to attend the symposium in memory of their mother, I chose an auspicious day to relocate her ashes to our family tomb in Lin-Kou.

That day, with David holding his mother's urn of ashes, Faith, Albert, Felicia's and my siblings were at the family tomb to put Felicia at her final resting place. I said to Felicia, "This is the Wu family tomb; today I have brought you home. Fallen leaves return to their roots; all living things that wither will return to the earth. The children and I will always think of you. In future this will also be the place where I will be buried; I only hope that we will be together forever, never to be separated again."

It was only after putting Felicia at her final resting place that I finally felt that I had accomplished an unfulfilled wish at last. After one year, I have gradually become accustomed to the reality of Felicia being gone, but I still light a stick of incense every day. The swirling smoke from the incense, I hope, would carry thoughts and stories of my daily life to Felicia. I believe Felicia understands my longing for her.

Felicia's biography later became another outlet for me to release my feelings. I poured my feelings into this book. I told myself, I would never forget, and even a thousand years later I still need not worry the memory would disintegrate by forces of nature. While writing Felicia's biography, I relived the deep and enriching life that Felicia gave me, and for that, I came to appreciate it even more.

I still remember the day of Felicia's funeral. I decorated the mourning hall, where Felicia's body lay, with white organza and fresh flowers. I hoped Buddha would guide Felicia to a pure land without illness, without pain, without worries, one that is filled only with love and happiness. I also hoped that Felicia would be able to let go of the burden of pain and illness that she suffered on earth and ascend in lightness to the highest heavens.

That morning as I saw the fluttering drapes of white organza cascading like snowflakes, I broke down in tears, I was at a loss to face the days ahead without Felicia.

If I say my sorrow has lessened to some extent, I would attribute that to Felicia's encouragement. The second day of the Spring Festival this year, 2001, I drove to the family tomb, taking with me flowers, fruit, and incense to offer my prayers to my father and Felicia. The weather in Taipei was clear and bright on that day. However, as soon as I turned into the mountain roads of Jia-Bao Village in Lin-Kou, the sky turned cloudy, the mountain was shrouded in a mist and the trees on both sides of the road swayed vigorously. I turned on the car lights and thought, it couldn't be that Felicia knew I was coming and had especially laid drapes of white organza on the mountain slopes, as an indication to me that she knew I had come. The car ran into a narrow, muddy lane. As it was impossible to proceed any further, I got out of the car and trod on the muddy road. After only a few steps, I lost my foothold and nearly slipped into the mud swamp. At that very instant, the sky suddenly cleared. I walked to the front of the family tomb and looked. Before my eyes lay a picturesque scenery where the ocean met the azure blue sky in the horizon, and the lush green trees shimmering in the sun like stars. That indeed was a beautiful view which Felicia loved. With Felicia's urn back at the family tomb, she could now rest in peace.

After offering my prayers, I opened the door of the tomb and entered the chamber. I saw Felicia's urn of ashes resting on the soil. I sat down and spoke softly to her, sharing with her my thoughts. But I knew though Felicia and I were separated, she understood the feelings in my heart.

Grass thrive in summer, waves surge in winter, flowers bloom in spring and the moon shines the brightest in autumn, and such is life as we experience sorrow, joy, separation and reunion in our lifetime. I sped in my car as I left the family tomb and returned to Taipei. I said to Felicia, "Rest in peace, Felicia! Time vanishes without a trace, but our beautiful memories are etched in eternity. From now on, I will continue to live happily and work even harder because of you. Up in Heaven, you should be at peace and smile."

Timeline of the Main Events in Felicia's Life

February 27, 1939
Born in Taipei, Taiwan.

1945 – 1951
Attended Peng Lai Elementary School in Taipei City.

1957
Received Taipei First Girls' High School's first gold medal and the "Model Youth Award" conferred by the government of the Republic of China.

1957 – 1961
Guaranteed admission, without sitting for the entrance examination, into the chemistry department at National Taiwan University; also received the President's Scholarship.

1961 – 1963
Pursued a Master's degree program in organic chemistry at the University of Minnesota, U.S.A.

November 10, 1963
Returned to Taiwan and married Cheng-Wen (Ken) Wu.

1963 – 1965
Served as a medical technician and special assistant in the biochemistry department at the United States Naval Medical Research Unit 2 (NAMRU-2) in Taipei.

January 25, 1966
Gave birth to David Wu.

1965 – 1969
Attended and graduated from Case Western Reserve University with a Ph.D. in organic chemistry.

1969 – 1971
Conducted postdoctoral research at Cornell University in the department of biochemistry and molecular cell biology.

January 25, 1971
Gave birth to Faith Wu.

1971 – 1972
Conducted postdoctoral research at Yale University Medical School's pharmacology department.

June 13, 1973
Gave birth to Albert Wu.

1972 – 1979
Served as lecturer in the biophysics department and subsequently, assistant professor in the biochemistry department at the Albert Einstein College of Medicine in New York City. Researched on the function of intrinsic zinc ions and mechanisms of genetic transcription in RNA polymerase.

1979 – 1980
Served as a visiting professor at the Institute Pasteur and the Institute Gustave-Roussy in France.

1980 – 1990
Served as associate professor and subsequently promoted to full professor in the pharmacology department in the School of Medicine at SUNY Stony Brook, conducted research and taught biochemical pharmacology. Researched on the proteins involved in gene regulation, and found that the Xenopus transcription factor, TFIIIA, contains zinc. "Intrinsic zinc" was the basis for the future discovery of "zinc fingers."

September 27, 1982
Felicia's mother Ti-Yen Chen (born February 23, 1911) passed away at the University of Iowa Hospital in Iowa City.

1986
Onset of breast cancer; underwent surgery and chemotherapy.

July 1988 – July 1999
Returned to Taiwan with Ken Wu in order to jointly establish the Institute of Biomedical Sciences at Academia Sinica, and served as Special Medical Chair and the head of the cancer research division. Her main research topics included: the anti-cancer mechanisms of Vitamin K3, the cancer suppression properties of the adeno-associated virus, gene gun techniques, and the action mechanism of anti-metastasis agents.

August 1994
Represented Taiwan in a conference held in China sponsored by the Natural Science Foundation; had the opportunity to meet Chairman Ze-Min Jiang of the People's Republic of China.

September 1994
Breast cancer migrated to the liver; marked the beginning of an agonizing five-year struggle against cancer.

November 7, 1994 – November 11, 1994
The American Association for Cancer Research and the Institute of Biomedical Sciences jointly sponsored and organized a special conference entitled, "Modern Developments in Cancer Therapeutics"; Felicia attended and gave a speech despite her cancer recurrence.

June 1995 – October 1995
Traveled to the United States to undergo high dose chemotherapy and autologous BMT.

May 1995
Gave her first public lecture at the Ministry of Transportation and Communications in Taipei. The topic was "The Fight against Cancer: The Experience of One Who is Both Cancer Researcher and Patient." After this, she began her volunteer work to fight cancer, promoting anti-cancer activities on television stations and at alumni associations, clubs, hospitals, and other public venues, as well as actively encouraging cancer patients to fight the disease bravely.

February 1997 – November 1997
Underwent twelve sessions of Taxol treatment.

April 8, 1998
Received the R.O.C. Oncology Society's "Outstanding Cancer Research Award."

April 1999 – June 1999
Underwent hepatic trans-arterial embolization therapy.

July 19, 1999
Passed away at the NTU Hospital as a result of complications arising from cancer, including septicemia and multiple organ failure. She was sixty years old. Over the course of her life, Felicia published over eighty papers in internationally-known journals; she also had over a hundred and sixty conference abstracts.

www.ingramcontent.com/pod-product-compliance
Lightning Source LLC
Chambersburg PA
CBHW050526300426
44113CB00012B/1976